# Keys to Nursing Success

## THIRD EDITION

Janet R. Katz

Carol Carter

Joyce Bishop

Sarah Lyman Kravits

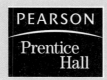

PEARSON

Prentice
Hall

Upper Saddle River, New Jersey
Columbus, Ohio

**Library of Congress Cataloging-in-Publication Data**

Keys to nursing success / Janet R. Katz . . . [et al.]. — 3rd ed.
    p. ; cm.
  Includes bibliographical references and index.
  ISBN-13: 978-0-13-513085-8 (pbk.)
  ISBN-10: 0-13-513085-9 (pbk.)
1. Nursing. 2. Nursing—Study and teaching. 3. Nursing—Vocational
guidance. 4. Test-taking skills. I. Katz, Janet R., 1953-
  [DNLM: 1. Nursing. 2. Career Choice. 3. Education, Nursing. WY 16
K44 2009]
  RT71.K49 2009
  610.73—dc22                                    2008010118

**Vice President and Executive Publisher:** Jeffery W. Johnston
**Executive Editor:** Sande Johnson
**Development Editor:** Bryce Bell
**Project Manager:** Kerry Rubadue
**Editorial Assistant:** Lynda Cramer
**Production Coordination:** Thistle Hill Publishing Services, LLC
**Design Coordinator:** Diane C. Lorenzo
**Cover Designer:** Jeff Vanik
**Cover Image:** Jupiter Images
**Production Manager:** Susan Hannahs
**Director of Marketing:** Quinn Perkson
**Senior Marketing Manager:** Amy Judd
**Marketing Coordinator:** Brian Mounts

This book was set in Sabon by S4Carlisle Publishing Services. It was printed and bound by Edwards Brothers. The cover was printed by Phoenix Color Corp/Hagerstown.

Pearson Education Ltd. London
Pearson Education Singapore Pte. Ltd.
Pearson Education Canada, Inc.
Pearson Education–Japan

Pearson Education Australia PTY. Limited
Pearson Education North Asia Ltd. Hong Kong
Pearson Educación de Mexico, S.A. de C.V.
Pearson Education Malaysia Pte. Ltd.
Pearson Education Upper Saddle River, New Jersey

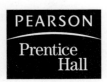

10 9 8 7 6 5 4 3 2 1
ISBN 13: 978-0-13-513085-8
ISBN 10: 0-13-513085-9

This book is your guide to college and nursing. College and nursing are your path to change and a better life. Change is part of daily life. For instance, last year you may have worn flared leg jeans and this year they are straight leg. What was your favorite song last year? Is it the same this year? Can you even imagine what you will be wearing, fashion- and style-wise, in five years? You will have new friends, new ideas, and new kinds of fun. Today, the idea of learning and memorizing every bone, muscle, tendon, and nerve in the human body may not be your idea of fun. But, later, when you take anatomy, it will be. So keep an open mind as you use this book. Change is happening.

In writing this book, I kept you in mind. I think of you as young as 18 years old and as old as 45 or even 55 years old. I think you are women. I think you are men. Some of you are Muslim, Jewish, Christian, Baha'i, Buddhist, and many other religions. Some of you are atheists. I hope that many of you come from ethnic backgrounds that are different from the majority white female nurse. I know you are Mexican American, Latino, African American, American Indian, Alaska Native, Chinese American, Japanese American, and combinations of these. Many of you may be far from home in an environment unlike any you've been in before. You might look around and see few, if any, faces that look like yours. If so, seek out support: Look for student groups or teachers who can help you adjust.

I see nursing students from many countries, too: Vietnam, India, Africa, and even the island of Yap in the Pacific. I know that some of you are learning English as you progress in college and your career. I work with many students from countries around the world and know you have special challenges. I also know you can succeed: I see you graduating with a degree in nursing. I have seen you come to nursing school full of anxiety about succeeding and I have seen you graduate with honors. I also know that you add to our schools and to nursing. As one student from Iran said, "We are role models for the American students." He said, "We show them that even with all the adversity we have had in our lives, and not having English as a first language, we can make it. We inspire them, too."

I know that many of you have little idea of what nursing is all about and probably are wondering what college will be like. Please use this book to help you reach your goals. You deserve the best, and through your progress you will ease suffering and pain in our world. I welcome you to college, to nursing, and to this book!

*Janet R. Katz, PhD, RN*

# Photo Credits

All individual photos for Q & A Blue Sky Questions Down-to-Earth Answers provided by photo subjects.

Michal Heron/PH College, p. 78; Image Source, p. 134; BSIP/Phototake NYC, p. 240; Doug Menuez/Getty Images–Photodisc, p. 300; David Young-Wolff/PhotoEdit Inc., p. 336; EyeWire Collection/Getty Images–Photodisc, p. 364; Digital Vision, p. 394.

Hemera Technologies Inc., pp. 89, 94, 99, 153, 164, 165, 167, 199, 212, 215, 222, 230, 236, 245, 246, 247, 249, 259, 262, 281, 282, 323, 345, 358, 368, 378, 413, 415.

All other chapter-opening and marginal photos in this text from Corbis Images, Digital Graphics, Digital Vision, EyeWire, Hemera Technologies Inc., and PhotoDisc royalty-free sources.

# Brief Contents

# Contents

## Chapter 1

### EXAMINE: RESEARCHING YOUR NURSING EDUCATION: Collecting the Basic Data    2

## Chapter 2

### INVESTIGATE: DISCOVERING NURSING: Exploring Your Options    46

# Chapter 6

# Chapter 7

## Chapter 11

## Chapter 12

# Chapter 13

**NOTE:** *Every effort has been made to provide accurate and current Internet information in this book. However, the Internet and information posted on it are constantly changing, so it is inevitable that some of the Internet addresses listed in this textbook will change.*

# Preface

In writing the third edition of *Keys to Nursing Success* we asked this question: How can students get the most out of college and use what they learn to achieve their goals in an ever-changing world? We found an important answer in the concept of successful intelligence, developed by psychologist Robert Sternberg.[1]

## New to the third edition of *Keys to Nursing Success*

### Building on successful intelligence

Successful people, says Sternberg, are more than their IQ score. Focus on the two most important parts of Sternberg's message and you can change your approach to education in a way that will maximize your learning and *life success.*

**One:** *Successful intelligence gives you tools to achieve important goals.* Successful intelligence goes beyond doing well on tests (analytical thinking). Only by combining that analytical skill with the ability to come up with innovative ideas (creative thinking) and the ability to put ideas and plans to work (practical thinking) will you get where you want to go.

**Two:** *Intelligence can grow.* The intelligence you have when you are born does not stay the same for the rest of your life. You can build and develop your intelligence in the same way that you can build and develop physical strength or flexibility.

Every chapter of *Keys to Nursing Success* helps you to build successful intelligence. How?

- *Chapter coverage:* The theme is covered in detail in the thinking chapter (Chapter 5) and continued throughout the book. Successful intelligence concepts are referenced throughout chapters of the text.
- *In-text exercises:* Three exercises within the chapter text—*Get Analytical! Get Creative!,* and *Get Practical!* develop each skill in the context of the chapter material and your personal needs.
- *Synthesis exercise:* At the end of each chapter, the *Putting It All Together* exercise gives you an opportunity to combine all three skills and apply them toward a meaningful task.

## This book connects you with the ideas and experiences of others

- *Chapter-opening Q & A* highlights questions posed by actual students as they begin college. Each question is answered by another person who offers ideas and advice.
- *Descriptions of real students' experiences,* often accompanied by quotes from the students, have been woven into the text in areas where they enhance the topic being discussed.
- *A focus on cultural competence,* in Chapter 10, shows the value of going beyond tolerance to actively adapt to and learn from people different from you. References to cultural competence and diversity are also woven throughout every chapter, showing how diversity is part of many aspects of school, the workplace, and personal life. In this edition there is renewed effort to emphasize the importance of being culturally aware and sensitive in nursing. Part of cultural competency is increasing the diversity of nursing and that includes recruiting more men.
- *Personal Triumph* stories, real-life accounts of how people have overcome difficult circumstances in the pursuit of education and

fulfillment, appear near the end of every third chapter. These inspiring stories motivate you to step up your personal efforts to succeed.

- *Chapter summaries* introduce a word or phrase from a language other than English and suggest how you might apply the concept to your own life.

- A *continuing focus on multiple intelligences* highlights individual diversity and confirms that each individual has a unique way of learning, no one way being better than another. Chapter 3 introduces and explains this concept, and subsequent chapters include grids with strategies for applying various learning styles to the chapter content.

### This book provides strategies and resources that help you do your work

With successful intelligence as the foundation of this edition and cultural competence as an underlying theme, *Keys to Nursing Success* presents these learning tools and materials that will help you succeed in college and beyond:

**A college primer:** Because there's so much to know right off the bat, the section *Quick Start to College* appears in Chapter 1. *Quick Start* helps you get a feel for the structure of your college, the people who can help you with academic and life issues, the resources available to you, and expectations from instructors, administrators, and fellow students.

**Skills that prepare you for college, nursing, and life:** The ideas and strategies that help you succeed in college also take you where you want to go in your career and personal life. Three parts of this text help you develop a firm foundation for lifelong learning.

- *Defining yourself and your goals:* Chapter 1 provides an overview of nursing by giving the facts. Chapter 2 and Chapter 3 get you on track with a focus on opportunities in nursing and ways to manage yourself effectively, focusing on values, goal-setting strategies, time-management skills, and handling stress. Chapter 4 helps you identify complementary aspects of your learning style (your Multiple Intelligences and your Personality Spectrum), choose strategies that make them work for you, and begin to think about your major.

- *Developing your learning skills:* Chapter 5 puts your learning into action by exploring the concept of successful intelligence in depth, helping you build analytical, creative, and practical thinking skills and put them together to solve problems, make decisions, and achieve goals. The next few chapters build crucial skills for the classroom and beyond—*Reading and Studying* (Chapter 6), *Listening, Note Taking, and Memory* (Chapter 7), *Test Taking* (Chapter 8), and *Researching and Writing* (Chapter 9).

- *Creating success:* Recognizing that success includes more than academic achievement, Chapter 10 focuses on developing the interpersonal and communication skills you need in a diverse society. Chapter 11 helps you manage the stress and wellness issues that so many college students face, and Chapter 12 covers the money-management and career-planning skills you need in college and beyond. Finally, Chapter 13 helps you think expansively: What is in the future of nursing? What are ethical questions in health care and nursing? What path have you traveled during the semester? What plans do you have for your future?

**Skill-building exercises:** Today's graduates need to be effective thinkers, team players, writers, and strategic planners. The set of exercises at the end of each chapter—*Building Skills for College, Career, and Life Success*—encourages you to develop these valuable skills and to apply thinking processes to any topic or situation:

- *Developing Successful Intelligence: Putting It All Together:* These exercises encourage you to combine your successful intelligence thinking skills and apply them to chapter material.

- *Team Building: Collaborative Solutions:* This exercise gives you a chance to interact, problem solve, and learn in a group setting, building your teamwork and leadership skills in the process.

- *Writing: Discovery Through Journaling:* This journal exercise provides an opportunity to express your thoughts and develop your writing skills.

- *Career Portfolio: Plan for Success:* This exercise helps you gather evidence of your talents, skills, interests, qualifications, and experience. The *Career Portfolio* exercises build on one another to form, at the end of the semester, a portfolio of information and insights that will help you in your quest for the right career and job.

**Particular help with test taking:** At three places in the text, a segment called *Study Break* appears. Each segment features a test-taking topic and helps you develop your test-taking skills throughout the semester in addition to your work on the test-taking chapter.

## This book changes with your needs

As we revise, we are in constant touch with students and instructors who tell us how we can improve. From our work with students, student editors, instructors, and experts all over the country, we have made important changes to better focus this new edition on what you need to succeed now. Here's what's new:

- The textwide theme of successful intelligence is presented—the way to achieve goals and success through analytical, creative, and practical thinking
- A new focus in Chapter 1 on the nursing shortage in the way it is currently being discussed in the nursing literature and among nursing professional organizations. Based on research by nurses, such as Linda Aiken and colleagues at the University of Pennsylvania, the discussion has turned to making the workplace better. It has also turned to the faculty shortage. It is understood now that many qualified candidates are being turned away from schools because there are not enough faculty to teach them.
- Chapter 2 has new information about roles that are changing in nursing, especially in advanced practice. The doctorate of nursing practice and the clinical nurse leader are examples of this change. In addition, areas of practice within nursing, such as emphasis on bioterrorism and aspects of disaster nursing, are growing.

Three in-chapter exercises in each chapter—one building analytical thinking skill, one building creative thinking skill, and one building practical thinking skill:

- A new first exercise at the end of each chapter—*Developing Successful Intelligence: Putting It All Together*—to encourage the synthesis of successful intelligence thinking skills
- Revision of learning styles material in Chapter 4 to delineate more clearly the two learning styles assessments and enhance their usefulness
- Extensive revision of Chapter 5—the thinking chapter—to focus on successful intelligence and how it makes problem-solving and decision-making happen
- Earlier placement of test-taking material (in Chapter 8) as well as in the *Study Break* segments
- Revision of Chapter 10—the diversity chapter—to focus on cultural competence, along with added cultural references throughout the text
- New student stories included within the text to heighten relevance of the material and the readers' ability to connect to it
- Newly revised end-of-chapter exercises to increase relevance and usefulness and to help students build on what they learn throughout the semester

## This book is just a start—only you can create the life of your dreams

As you work through this course and move forward toward achieving your goals, keep this in mind: Studies have shown that when students believe they have a fixed level of intelligence, they improve less, put less effort into their work, and have a harder time in the face of academic challenges. However, students who feel they can become more intelligent over time are more likely to improve, tend to work harder, and handle academic challenges with more success.[2] *Believe that your intelligence can grow*—and use this book to develop it this semester, throughout your college experience, and afterward as you build the future of your dreams.

**Students and instructors:** Many of our best suggestions have come from you. Send your questions, comments, and ideas about *Keys to Nursing Success* to Janet Katz, jkatz@wsu.edu. We look forward to hearing from you, and we are grateful for the opportunity to work with you.

## Notes

1. Successful intelligence concepts from Robert Sternberg, *Successful Intelligence* (New York: Plume, 1997).
2. David Glenn, "Students' Performance on Tests Is Tied to Their Views of Their Innate Intelligence, Researchers Say," *The Chronicle of Higher Education* (June 1, 2004). Available: http://chronicle.com/daily/2004/06/2004060103n.htm.

## Nurse Katz's Top Three Rules for Success

The top three rules for *success* are based on consistent behaviors that lead to gaining a healthy dose of knowledge and skill acquisition while you are in college. These are the top three rules you will need to follow to succeed as a nursing major:

1. Go to class.
2. Learn to study.
3. Take school seriously (study).

# Acknowledgments

This significant revision has been produced through the efforts of an extraordinary team. Many thanks to:

- Robert J. Sternberg, IBM Professor of Psychology and Education at Yale University, for his ground-breaking work on successful intelligence and for his gracious permission to use and adapt that work as a theme for this new edition.

- Our reviewers, whose input is invaluable.

*Sixth-edition reviewers:* Renee Hoeksel, Washington State University, Vancouver; Linda B. Hureston, Chicago State University; Linda S. Johanson, Lenoir-Rhyne College; Laura McQueen, North Carolina A&T State University; Deb Stanford, The University of North Carolina, Greensboro.

*Fifth-edition reviewers:* Peg Adams, Northern Kentucky University; Veronica Allen, Texas Southern University; Angela A. Anderson, Texas Southern University; Robert Anderson, The College of New Jersey; Joyce Annette Deaton, Jackson State Community College; Ray Emett, Salt Lake Community College; Jacqueline Fleming, Texas Southern University; Ralph Gallo, Texas Southern University; Jennifer Guyer-Wood, Minnesota State University; Laura Kauffmann, Indian River Community College; Quentin Kidd, Christopher Newport University; Patsy Krech, University of Memphis; Curtis Peters, Indiana University Southeast; Margaret Quinn, University of Memphis; Corliss A. Rabb, Texas Southern University; Rebecca Samberg, Housatonic Community College; Karyn L. Schulz, Community College of Baltimore County–Dundalk; Jill R. Strand, University of Minnesota–Duluth; Toni M. Stroud, Texas Southern University; Cheri Tillman, Valdosta State University

*Reviewers from previous editions:* Fred Amador, Phoenix College; Manual Aroz, Arizona State University; Glenda Belote, Florida International University; Todd Benatovich, University of Texas at Arlington; John Bennett Jr., University of Connecticut; Ann Bingham-Newman, California State University–LA; Mary Bixby, University of Missouri–Columbia; Barbara Blandford, Education Enhancement Center at Lawrenceville, NJ; Jerry Bouchie, St. Cloud State University; Mona Casady, SW Missouri State University; Kara Craig, University of Southern Mississippi; Leslie Chilton, Arizona State University; Jim Coleman, Baltimore City Community College; Sara Connolly, Florida State University; Janet Cutshall, Sussex County Community College; Valerie DeAngelis, Miami-Dade Community College; Rita Delude, NH Community Technical College; Marianne Edwards, Georgia College and State University; Judy Elsley, Weber State University in Utah; Skye Gentile, California State University, Hayward; Bob Gibson, University of Nebraska–Omaha; Sue Halter, Delgado Community College; Suzy Hampton, University of Montana; Karen Hardin, Mesa Community College; Patricia Hart, California State University, Fresno; Maureen Hurley, University of Missouri–Kansas City; Karen Iversen, Heald Colleges; Laura Kauffman, Indian River Community College; Kathryn K. Kelly, St. Cloud State University; Nancy Kosmicke, Mesa State College; Frank T. Lyman Jr., University of Maryland; Marvin Marshak, University of Minnesota; Kathy Masters, Arkansas State University; Barnette Miller Moore, Indian River Community College; Rebecca Munro, Gonzaga University; Sue Palmer, Brevard Community College; Bobbie Parker, Alabama State University; Virginia Phares, DeVry of Atlanta; Brenda Prinzavalli, Beloit College; Jacqueline Simon, Education Enhancement Center at Lawrenceville, NJ; Carolyn Smith, University of Southern Indiana; Joan Stottlemyer, Carroll College; Thomas Tyson, SUNY Stony

Brook; Eve Walden, Valencia Community College; Marsha Walden, Valdosta State University; Rose Wassman, DeAnza College; Angela Williams, The Citadel; Don Williams, Grand Valley State University; William Wilson, St. Cloud State University; Michelle G. Wolf, Florida Southern College

• Our student editor, Dylan Lewis, for his wisdom, guidance, and hard work.

• The PRE 100 instructors at Baltimore City Community College, Liberty Campus, for their ideas and support, especially college president Dr. Jim Tschechtelin and coordinator Stan D. Brown.

• Those who generously contributed personal stories, exhibiting courage in being open and honest about their life experiences:

Beverly Andre, Triton College; Stephen Beck, Learn-to-Learn Company; Joyce Bishop, Golden West College; Carol Carter, LifeBound Inc.; Peter Changsak, Sheldon-Jackson College; Rosalia Chavez, University of Arizona; Carol Comlish, University of Alabama; Darrin Estepp, Ohio State University; Rachel Faison, Bard College; Jacqueline Fleming, Texas Southern University; Ramona Z. Locke, Vice President Senior Financial Consultant, Merrill Lynch Private Client Group; Parisa Malekzadeh, University of Arizona; Joe A. Martin Jr., University of West Florida; Gustavo Minaya, Community College of Baltimore County, Essex Campus; Raymond Montolvo Jr., University of Southern California; Afsaneh Nahavandi, Arizona State University West; Nisar Nikzad, Community College of Denver; Julia Nolan, University of California, Davis; Michael Nolan, Oregon State University; Morgan Paar, Academy of Art College; Morgan Packard, Tulane University; Shyama Parikh, DePaul University; Joe Pullen, University of Detroit; Lisa Rabinowitz, Bloomfield College; Randy Ust, University of Mary; Tracy Ust, St. Cloud University; Dr. Benjamin Victorica, University of Florida; Tonjua Williams, St. Petersburg College

• Jessica Ovitz, Cynthia Nordberg, Dr. Frank T. Lyman, and Dan Laukitis for their invaluable advice and assistance.

• Michael Jackson for his writing samples and advice.

• Our terrific editor Sande Johnson, who through her leadership was able to put together a team of people whose combined efforts took this edition to a new level. Special thanks to developmental editor, Bryce Bell, for his comprehensive vision, hard work, and insightful ideas, and to editorial assistant Lynda Cramer for all her efforts and attention to detail.

• The following reviewers of and contributors to the instructor's manual, for their insight:

Todd Benatovich, University of Texas at Arlington; Amy Bierman, student, Old Dominion University; Jennifer Cohen; Jodi Levine, Temple University; Geri MacKenzie, Southern Methodist University; Gene Mueller, Henderson State University; Tina Pitt, Heald College; Dan Rice, Iowa State University; Michael and Frances Trevisan, Washington State University; Karen Valencia, South Texas Community College; Eve Walden, Valencia Community College; Don Williams, Grand Valley State University; William Wilson, St. Cloud State University; Nona Wood, North Dakota State University

• Our production team for their patience, flexibility, and attention to detail, especially Pam Bennett, Kerry Rubadue, Angela Urquhart and Renata Butera at Thistle Hill, and typesetters at S4 Carlisle Publishing Services.

• Our marketing gurus, especially Amy Judd, our marketing manager; Quinn Perkson, director of marketing; and our student success sales directors Brian Mounts, Marketing Coordinator; and Student Success Sales Directors Connie James, Patty Ford, Deb Wilson, Matt Christopherson, and Lynda Sax.

• Publisher Jeff Johnston, President of Education, Nancy Forsyth, and President Tim Bozik, for their leadership and their interest in and commitment to the Student Success list.

• The Prentice Hall representatives and management team, who help us bring our mission to instructors all over the country.

• Our families and friends, who have encouraged us and put up with our commitments.

- We extend a very special thanks to Judy Block, whose research, writing, and editing work was essential and invaluable.

Finally, for their ideas, opinions, and stories, we would like to thank all of the students and professors with whom we work. Joyce, in particular, would like to thank the thousands of students who have allowed her, as their professor, the privilege of sharing part of their journey through college. We appreciate that, through reading this book, you give us the opportunity to learn and discover with you—in your classroom, in your home, on the bus, and wherever else learning takes place.

# About the Authors

**Janet R. Katz** has practiced nursing in cardiac rehabilitation as well as acute and critical cardiac care. She earned her PhD in educational leadership and now teaches community health as assistant professor for Washington State University's Intercollegiate College of Nursing. Janet is the author of several articles on nursing. Her research focuses on the area of recruiting and retaining Native American students into nursing and on community-based participatory research that is culturally competent, such as on health promotion for Native American teenagers. She is active in advancing the profession of nursing and its mission of disease prevention, health promotion, and health care advocacy for individuals, families, and communities, both locally and globally. She lives in Spokane, Washington.

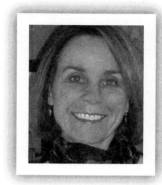

**Carol Carter** is founder of LifeBound, a career coaching company that offers individual coaching sessions and seminars for high school students, college students, and career seekers. She has written *Majoring in the Rest of Your Life: Career Secrets for College Students* and *Majoring in High School*. She has also co-authored *Keys to Preparing for College, Keys to College Studying, The Career Tool Kit, Keys to Career Success, Keys to Study Skills, Keys to Thinking and Learning,* and *Keys to Success*. She has taught welfare-to-work classes, team-taught in the La Familia Scholars Program at the Community College of Denver, and conducted numerous workshops for students and faculty around the country. Carol is a national college and career expert and interviewed regularly in print, on the radio, and for television news programs. In addition to working with students of all ages, Carol thrives on foreign travel and culture; she is fortunate enough to have been a guest in more than 40 foreign countries. Please visit her website and write her at www.lifebound.com.

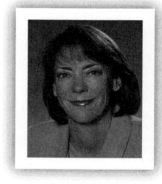

**Joyce Bishop** holds a PhD in psychology and has taught for more than 20 years, receiving a number of honors, including Teacher of the Year for 1995 and 2000. For five years she has been voted "favorite teacher" by the student body and Honor Society at Golden West College, Huntington Beach, California, where she has taught since 1987 and is a tenured professor. She worked with a federal grant to establish Learning Communities and Workplace Learning in her district, and she has developed workshops and trained faculty in cooperative learning, active learning, multiple intelligences, workplace relevancy, learning styles, authentic assessment, team building, and the development of learning communities. Joyce is currently teaching online and multimedia classes, and she trains other faculty to teach online in her district and region of 21 colleges. She coauthored *Keys to College Studying, Keys to Success, Keys to Thinking and Learning,* and *Keys to Study Skills*. Joyce is the lead academic of the *Keys to Lifelong Learning Telecourse,* distributed by Dallas Telelearning.

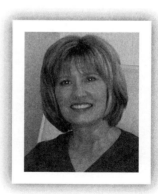

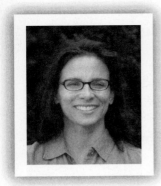

**Sarah Lyman Kravits** comes from a family of educators and has long cultivated an interest in educational development. She coauthored *Keys to College Studying, The Career Tool Kit, Keys to Success, Keys to Thinking and Learning*, and *Keys to Study Skills* and has served as program director for LifeSkills, Inc., a nonprofit organization that aims to further the career and personal development of high school students. In that capacity she helped formulate both curricular and organizational elements of the program, working closely with instructors as well as members of the business community. She has also given faculty workshops in critical thinking. Sarah holds a BA in English and drama from the University of Virginia, where she was a Jefferson Scholar, and an MFA from Catholic University.

# Keys to Nursing Success

## THIRD EDITION

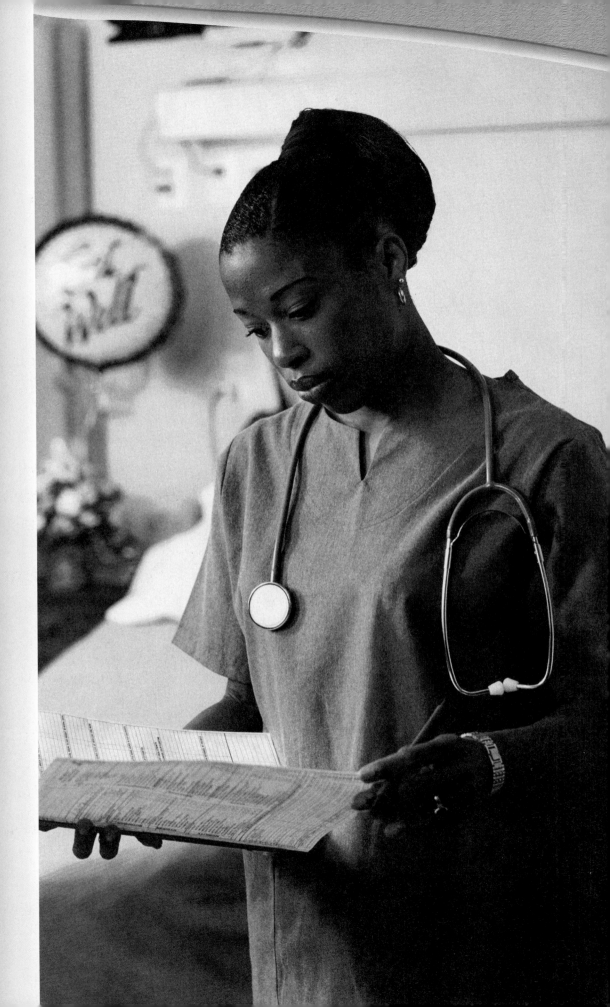

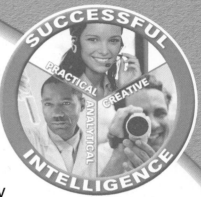

**W**elcome—or welcome back—to an education in nursing. Whether you are just coming out of high school, returning to student life after working for some years, or continuing on a current educational path, you are facing new challenges and changes. Every person has a right to seek the self-improvement, knowledge, and opportunity that an education can provide. By choosing to pursue nursing, you have given yourself a strong vote of confidence and the chance to improve your future. *And nursing needs you: There is a nursing shortage that is expected to grow. A large part of that involves a shortage of diverse nurses. If you are a student of color there are many opportunities for you in nursing. The same holds true for men.*

This book helps you fulfill your potential as a nursing major by giving you keys—ideas, strategies, and skills—that can lead to success in school, on the job, and in life. Chapter 1 gives you an overview of the nursing education world. It starts by looking at today's nursing students—who they are and how they've changed—and at the connection between a nursing education and success. You will also discover in this chapter how various resources can help you deal with problems and how teamwork plays a role in your success. To discover what a nurse is, and will be in the future, see Figure 1.1.

*IN THIS CHAPTER …*

*you will explore answers to the following questions:*

- What are three ways to become an RN? 6
- Who are RNs today, and what challenges do students face? 10
- What is the role of diversity in nursing? 12
- How does an education in nursing promote success? 21
- Why do you need to study a variety of arts and sciences? 26
- What basics should you know as you begin school? 29

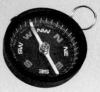

| FIGURE 1.1 | The future vision for nursing |

*"Nursing is the pivotal health care profession, highly valued for its special-ized knowledge, skill and caring in improving the health status of the pub-lic and ensuring safe, effective, quality care.*

*The profession mirrors the diverse population it serves and provides leadership to create positive changes in health policy and delivery systems.*

*Individuals choose nursing as a career, and remain in the profession, because of the opportunities for personal and professional growth, support-ive work environments and compensation commensurate with roles and responsibilities."*

*Source:* American Nurses Association (April 2002). "Nursing's Agenda for the Future: A Call to the Nation." www.ana.org.

## Q&A BLUE SKY QUESTIONS DOWN-TO-EARTH ANSWERS

### What can I do to prepare myself for the future?

I started my nursing education in Tokyo, Japan, which is where I come from. For a short while, I worked in a hospital there, too. Although I liked the work, I realized that, though working one on one with patients can be very satisfying, I wanted to do more. There are many fields of study in the nursing profession, and I wasn't sure what to choose until I took a course in community health. From this class I discovered that I might be able to use my education to affect entire populations of people. One day I hope to help improve community health in a developing country.

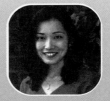

Eiko Kawaide
Senior, Elmira Nursing
College, Elmira, New York

I started learning English a few years ago in order to work someday as a community health nurse in the developing world. Through studying English at an English school, I got a chance to go to the United States by winning a scholarship to Elmira College. I saw this as a great chance for me to both master English and deepen my knowledge of medicine and nursing. I was sure that studying in the United States would help me to achieve my life goals.

In this branch of nursing, I would be able to involve myself in many exciting issues. Maybe I could support public policy to better serve the health care needs of developing countries. One problem that needs addressing is how to plan and implement primary health care effectively. I am also interested in helping child survival in underprivileged countries and communities. I recently read a book about child survival. Just giving medicine or food doesn't help much, unless we focus on the context of poverty and underdevelopment. Many children are suffering from hunger and disease, and they are less resistant to disease because of lack of adequate nutrition. I really want to deal with such kinds of problems and help to decrease infant and under-five mortality rates.

Global programs like WHO's "Health for All by the Year 2000" are very intriguing to me. I also think about the possibilities of improving connections between Japan and developing countries to help more people who are suffering from health problems. I know these are big dreams, but I've heard that nursing care is moving out of the hospitals and into the community—including the international community.

## PRACTICAL ANSWERS

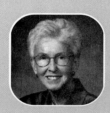

**Margretta Madden Styles**
Dr. Styles was the immediate past president, International Council of Nurses, Geneva, Switzerland, at the time of this interview. She was a nurse scholar and leader. Styles was the recipient of seven honorary doctorates and, according to the American Nurses Association Hall of Fame, "Styles had a global impact on the profession."
Margretta Madden Styles
1930–2005

*You are well on your way. Just continue down the path you have chosen.*

Nurses have always played a very active role in public health, liberally applying their commitment and expertise throughout the world. Public health focuses on health promotion and prevention and involves all members of the community. Therefore, it offers the most for your investment.

Indeed, nursing has been moving out of hospitals for many decades, more so in some countries than in others. In many developing nations, where resources are scant, public health and community nursing has long been the primary mode of health care.

How can you best prepare for the future? There are four keys to developing a career in nursing, as well as other professions. *Education, education, education* is the number-one factor. So you are headed in the right direction.

*Mentors and linkages* are the second and third keys. As an aspiring professional, you will need the support and advice of persons who are successful and well recognized in your field. They will share with you the wisdom of their experiences and guide you toward the achievement of your own goals. Good mentors will also assist you in connecting with individuals, organizations, and other resources essential to the development of your career.

To achieve your goals relating to international public health, pursue linkages through three major sectors:

- *School-to-school linkages.* Inquire at your university about institutional relationships with schools in other nations. Is this a route available to you to connect with nurses in their "sister" schools?
- *Health sector linkages.* Are your governmental health authorities able and willing to introduce you to nurses within your WHO region or with the WHO itself?
- *The world network of nurses associations.* This may be the best linkage of all. In this you are very fortunate. The Japanese Nurses Association (JNA) is the largest in the world, with connections through the International Council of Nurses to counterparts, such as the American Nurses Association, in 120 nations. The JNA is well known for its assistance to and work with other nations. The president of the JNA is a world leader in the profession.

*Focused expertise* is the fourth key to professional success. Define your specialty. What particular expertise do you want to develop and practice throughout your career? Focus! Then through education, mentors, and linkages make yourself one of the most informed, scholarly, and well-recognized authorities within your specialty. Be the best in your field.

# What Are Three Ways to Become an *RN?*

In the late 1800s, Florence Nightingale founded formal nursing education. Nightingale's work in the Crimea War, along with Mary Seacole, a black nurse from Jamaica, greatly affected views of health care and nursing. After making many reforms in how injured and sick British soldiers were treated, Nightingale set out to make major reforms in hospitals and nursing education. At that time, there were no formal training courses for nurses. So, along with reforms in the military system, Nightingale changed hospitals, was one of the first to keep biostatistics, instituted mandatory hand washing, and developed the first training of professional nurses. In the United States, the first nursing school associated with a university was opened in 1909 at the University of Minnesota. However, most nursing education was based in hospitals, rather than universities, until the end of World War II.

Today, there are three ways to become a registered nurse (RN): (1) by earning a bachelor's degree in nursing (BSN), (2) by earning an associate's degree in nursing (ADN), or (3) by obtaining a diploma. Becoming an RN means you attend a nursing program that makes you eligible to sit for the national licensing exam, or NCLEX-RN. It is passing that exam that makes you an RN—legally. In other words, you must have a license to work as an RN. Completing a nursing program makes you eligible to sit for the NCLEX-RN (see www.ncsbn.org for more on this exam in your state).

What are the advantages and disadvantages of each type of degree? This is a question that nurses have been debating since the formation of the ADN programs shortly after World War II. The advent of the community college system combined with a nursing shortage helped the ADN programs to come about. Following is a description of the three ways to become an RN.

## BSN

Many professional organizations argue that nurses are better prepared to deal with the complexities of health care and to work in a variety of roles if they have a BSN. It takes at least four years to obtain this degree. Some places, such as the Veterans' Administration, require that RNs have a BSN. Here is how the American Association of Colleges of Nursing (AACN) association argues the point:

> The BSN nurse is the only basic nursing graduate prepared to practice in all health care settings—critical care, ambulatory care, public health, and mental health—and thus has the greatest employment flexibility of any entry-level RN.
>
> The BSN curriculum includes a broad spectrum of scientific, critical-thinking, humanistic, communication, and leadership skills, including specific courses on community health nursing not typically included in diploma or associate-degree tracks. These abilities are essential for today's professional nurse who must be a skilled provider, designer, manager, and coordinator of care. Nurses must

make quick, sometimes life-and-death decisions; understand a patient's treatment, symptoms, and danger signs; supervise other nursing personnel; coordinate care with other health providers; master advanced technology; guide patients through the maze of health resources in a community; and teach patients how to comply with treatment and adopt a healthy lifestyle.[1]

Furthermore, research in 2003 from Linda Aiken, PhD, RN, of the University of Pennsylvania School of Nursing, showed that in hospitals with higher rates of BSN nurses, rather than ADN nurses, surgical patients had fewer deaths.[2] AACN also encourages programs that support two-year, or associate-degree nurses, in going back to school to earn a bachelor's degree in nursing. AACN notes the following:[3]

- Formal articulation agreements between ADN and BSN programs is making nursing education easier. Articulation helps avoid repeating course work.
  - Thirty-two states have broad articulation agreements.
  - Eight states mandate credit transfer between ADN and BSN programs.
  - Eighteen states are developing or improving their agreements.
- In 2004, according to the Bureau of Labor Statistics, there were 600 RN-to-BSN programs in the United States.[4]
  - In 2004, there were 165 accelerated BSN programs. Accelerated BSN programs also are for those who have a bachelor's or higher degree in another field. Programs last 12 to 18 months and provide the fastest route to a BSN for individuals who already hold a degree.[5]
  - In 2004, there were 137 RN-to-MSN programs. Accelerated master's degree programs combine one year of an accelerated BSN program with two years of graduate study.[6]

## ADN

The ADN degree takes two to three years. One advantage of community college programs is that they are often more easily accessible than university programs. An outstanding cardiac nurse, Judy Meyers, said, "If it wasn't for community college I may never have become a nurse." Judy lived in a small town in Idaho that was too far away from a university, but it did have a community college. Eventually Judy moved and earned her BSN and then a master's degree in nursing. Today she is a professor of nursing with a PhD. Many excellent nurses have ADN degrees. Here is how the National Organization of Associate Degree Nurses (NOADN) argues the value of the degree:

Associate degree nursing (ADN) education provides a dynamic pathway for entry into registered nurse (RN) practice. It offers accessible, affordable, quality instruction to a diverse population. Initiated as a research project in response to societal needs, ADN education is continually evolving to reflect local community needs and current health care trends. ADN graduates are prepared to function in multiple health care settings, including community practice sites.

Graduates of ADN programs possess a core of nursing knowledge common to all nursing education routes. They have continuously demonstrated their competency for safe practice through NCLEX-RN pass rates. These nurses provide a stable workforce within the community. The majority of ADN graduates are adult learners who are already established as an integral part of the community in which they live. They exhibit a commitment to lifelong learning through continuing education offerings, certification credentialing, and continued formal education.[7]

## Diploma

There are not as many diploma programs as there used to be, but they do exist. Diploma nurses focus on clinical skills in their training and for this reason graduate from their programs ready to go to work as an RN. The disadvantage is that nurses with diplomas have a difficult time advancing without a college degree. Diploma programs take two to three years to complete.

## Additional Paths to Nursing Degrees

Other paths for obtaining nursing degrees are available as programs designed for those who already have their ADN and wish to obtain a BSN or MSN, and for those who have a bachelor's degree in a non-nursing area.

### RN to BSN

RN-to-BSN programs exist within most departments, schools, or colleges of nursing. Some are offered completely online, others via a video system, and many on campus. Basic college requirements must be met, but programs may transfer most of your credits from the ADN program you attended.

### Accelerated Programs

If you already have a bachelor's degree in another area, you can earn a BSN or an MSN. These programs are called accelerated, bridge, or fast-track options, and they incorporate previous education with nursing education. There is an increasing drive to offer programs via the Internet. Here is information from the AACN about accelerated programs:[8]

#### Program Basics

- Accelerated BSN programs offer the quickest route to become an registered nurse (RN) for adults who have already completed a bachelor's or graduate degree in a non-nursing discipline.
  - Fast-track baccalaureate programs take between 11 and 18 months to complete, including prerequisites.
  - Fast-track master's degree programs generally take about 3 years to complete.

#### Fast-Track Nursing Education

- Admission standards for accelerated programs are high with programs typically requiring a minimum of a 3.0 grade point average (GPA) and a thorough prescreening process. Students enrolled in accelerated programs are encouraged *not* to work given the rigor associated with completing degree requirements.

- Accelerated baccalaureate and master's programs in nursing are appropriately geared to individuals who have already proven their ability to succeed at a senior college or university. Having already completed a bachelor's degree, many second-degree students are attracted to the fast-track master's program as the natural next step in their higher education.

- Graduates of accelerated programs are prized by nurse employers who value the many layers of skill and education these graduates bring to the workplace. Employers report that these graduates are more mature, possess strong clinical skills, and are quick studies on the job.

- AACN's 2005 survey found that 7,829 students were enrolled in accelerated baccalaureate programs, up from 6,090 in 2004 and 4,794 students in 2003. The number of program graduates has also increased with 3,769 graduates in 2005 as compared to 2,422 and 1,352 graduates in 2004 and 2003, respectively. In accelerated master's degree nursing programs, 3,200 students were enrolled and 674 students graduated in 2005. By comparison, in 2004, there were 2,666 students enrolled and 542 graduates from these programs.

# Data on Enrollment in All Nursing Programs

Students are enrolled in all three types of programs. The latest statistics from the National League of Nursing show the following:[9]

In 2005, 53% of nursing students enrolled in ADN, 43% in BSN, and 4% in diploma programs.

Full-time versus Part-Time Students: In the 2004–2005 school year, 88.3% of BSN students were enrolled full time and 11.7% part time. For ADN students, 54.2% were enrolled full time and 45.8% part time.

Applicants: In 2005, close to 350,000 students applied to nursing schools. Of those 67% were considered qualified and 38% were accepted, 12% were placed on waiting lists, 17% were rejected, and 33% of total applicants were not considered qualified.

Retention: After the first year of school, 72% of BSN students and 64% of ADN students remained in school.

Ethnicity of Students: From 2002 to 2005, the enrollment of minority nursing students decreased by 2%, indicating the critical need to recruit and retain students of color into nursing.

Percentage of students enrolled in colleges and in nursing schools by ethnicity:

| African American | | Hispanic | | Asian | | American Indian | |
|---|---|---|---|---|---|---|---|
| College | Nursing | College | Nursing | College | Nursing | College | Nursing |
| 12.3 | 12.6 | 10.5 | 5.3 | 6.0 | 5.6 | 1.0 | 0.9 |

Age of students: In 2005, 72% of BSN students were under 25 years old, whereas in the ADN program 28.5% were under 25 years old.

Tuition and required fees: In the 2004–2005 school year, full-time nursing students in a public college or university BSN program paid close to $5,000 per year. In a private school, they paid under $20,000.

Full-time ADN students in public programs paid around $2,500 per year.

## Who Are RNs Today, and What Challenges Do Students Face?

To get an idea of who is going into nursing, review these facts from the AACN:[10]

- Nurses comprise the largest single component of hospital staff, are the primary providers of hospital patient care, and deliver most of the nation's long-term care.

- Although often working collaboratively, nursing does not "assist" medicine or other fields. Nursing operates independent of, not auxiliary to, medicine and other disciplines. Nurses' roles range from direct patient care to case management, establishing nursing practice standards, developing quality assurance procedures, and directing complex nursing care systems.

- With more than four times as many RNs in the United States as physicians, nursing delivers an extended array of health care services, including primary and preventive care by advanced, independent nurse practitioners in such clinical areas as pediatrics, family health, women's health, and gerontological care. Nursing's scope also includes care by certified nurse-midwives and nurse-anesthetists, as well as care in cardiac, oncology, neonatal, neurological, and obstetric/gynecological nursing and other advanced clinical specialties.

The National Survey of Registered Nurses is one of the most important sources for statistical data on RNs. The survey is published every four years. Following are interesting statistics about nursing:[11]

- There are 2.9 million RNs in the United States.

- The average salary for a full-time RN was $57,784. The average for a nurse working in a hospital in 2007 was $60,970 (Bureau of Labor Statistics, http://www.bls.gov/oes, May 17, 2007).

- Degrees held by RNs:

  | BSN | 34.2% |
  |---|---|
  | ADN | 33.7% |
  | Diploma | 17.5% |
  | Master's or doctoral degree | 13% |

- Employment setting and percentage of RNs working in them:

| | |
|---|---|
| Hospitals | 56.2% |
| Community or public health | 15% |
| Ambulatory health | 11.5% |
| Nursing education | 2.6% |
| Nursing homes/Extended care facilities | 6.3% |
| Other, including occupational health, insurance claims/benefits, long-term care, and prison or jail | 8.5% |

- Type of position and annual average earnings (MSN is a master's in nursing):[12]

| Nursing Position | ADN | BSN | MSN | Doctorate |
|---|---|---|---|---|
| Administrator or assistant | $60,442 | $68,696 | $92,831 | $97,275 |
| Nurse practitioner | — | — | $71,265 | — |
| Staff nurse | $51,477 | $54,003 | $59,436 | — |

- Distribution of RNs employed in hospitals by dominant function:[13]

| | |
|---|---|
| Direct patient care | 59.1% |
| Critical care | 16.2% |
| Emergency Department | 7.8% |
| Administration | 5.2% |
| Teaching | 2.6% |
| Consultation | 1.5% |
| Research | 0.8% |
| Patient coordinator | 5.7% |
| Other | 1% |

## Student Life: Facts and Challenges

- Nursing students comprise more than half of all students in the health professions.
- More women enrolled in college than men earn associate, bachelor's, and master's degrees. In addition, the number of women receiving all types of degrees (not just nursing) has increased at a faster rate than for men. Between 2002 and 2003, 58% of bachelor's degrees were awarded to women.[14]
- In 2002–2003, 67% of degrees were earned by non-Hispanic white students; 22% went to Hispanic, African American, Native American/Pacific Islanders, and Asian American students.[15]
- Between 1994–1995 and 2004–2005, prices at public colleges rose by 30%, and those at private colleges increased by 26%, after adjustment for inflation.[16]

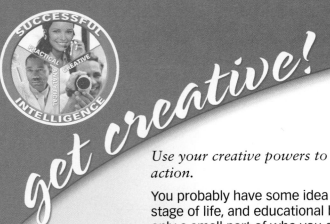

## See Yourself at Your Best

*Use your creative powers to improve your opinion of yourself and inspire action.*

You probably have some idea of where you fit into the student body—your age, stage of life, and educational background. However, your "student status" is only a small part of who you are.

Imagine that students gained entry into college by writing personal ads and posting them on the admissions website. Write a personal ad that you feel would give you the best possible chance to get in. In it, talk about

- What makes you unique and anything but "average."
- What is special about you that will make the college a better place.
- How your college education will bring you personal and professional success.

The decision to take advantage of a nursing education is in your hands. You are responsible for seeking out opportunities and weaving school into the fabric of your life. You may face some of these challenges:

- Handling the responsibilities and stress of parenting children alone, without a spouse
- Returning to school as an older student and feeling out of your element
- Learning to adjust to the cultural and communication differences in the diverse student population
- Having a physical disability that presents challenges
- Having a learning disability such as dyslexia or attention-deficit/hyperactivity disorder
- Balancing a school schedule with part-time or even full-time work
- Handling the financial commitment college requires

Your school can help you work through these and other problems if you actively seek out solutions and help from available support systems around you.

## What is the Role of *Diversity* in Nursing?

As seen in Figure 1.2, from the most recent U.S. National Sample Survey of Registered Nurses, 81.8% of nurses were white. Yet U.S. census data show that the total U.S. population in 2004 was 67.9% white. To meet the

## FIGURE 1.2

Comparison of 1996 and 2000 national sample survey of percentage of registered nurses in the U.S. population

| Ethnic/Racial Group | 2000 RN | 2000 U.S. | 2004 RN | 2004 U.S. |
|---|---|---|---|---|
| African American | 4.9 | 12.1 | 4.6 | 12.2 |
| Hispanic | 2.0 | 12.5 | 1.8 | 13.7 |
| Asian/Pacific Islander | 3.7 | 3.7 | 3.3 | 4.1 |
| Native American/Alaska Native | 0.5 | 0.7 | 0.4 | 0.7 |
| White (non-Hispanic) | 86.6 | 69.1 | 88.4 | 67.9 |

Adapted from *The National Sample Survey of Registered Nurses,* 2000 and 2004.

challenges of increasing diversity in the United States, nursing needs to recruit men and women of color into the profession.[17] It is more encouraging to look at the latest enrollment data for nursing schools. In BSN and ADN programs 71% to 72% of students are white non-Hispanic, 12% to 13% are black, 5% to 6% are Asian, 4% to 6% are Hispanic, and 1% are American Indian.[18]

## Why Isn't Nursing More Diversified?

Historically, African Americans, American Indians, and Latinos have suffered from more illness and death from diseases than non-Hispanic whites in the United States. Differences in the health of groups of people are called *health disparities*. Receiving poorer quality health care is one reason many organizations have called for changes to eliminate health disparities. One suggestion by the Institute of Medicine is to increase the diversity of health care providers.[19]

Diversity as defined by the AACN includes race and ethnicity, class, gender, age, religion, sexual orientation, and disabilities.[20] Beverly L. Malone, past president and only the second African American president of the American Nursing Association, views the United States as a country of many being led by the one, and she identifies "the one" as those who are primarily of European descent. Malone notes that nursing is an institution that has maintained the dominance of one group over the other but, at the same time, as a majority female profession, nurses are especially aware of the "harsh realities of oppression and victimization by others."[21] Because of this, Malone reasons, nurses may be partially excused. However, she considers that given its professional philosophy mandating quality care for all people, nursing should be particularly sensitive to others.

The Sullivan Report, called *Missing Persons: Minorities in Health Professions*, also makes note of the history of racism in the United States leading to health care systems and health care professions education programs that favored whites. This history is seen in the numbers that show 25% of the U.S. population is African American, American Indian, and Hispanic, but only 9% of nurses, 6% of doctors, and 5% of dentists come from these groups. The Sullivan Report has these encouraging words about increasing the diversity of all health professions:[22]

> From the streets of Harlem to the barrios of East Los Angeles, the Commission saw shining examples of young students and professionals who can lead to this new era. Many share a dream of returning to their communities as physicians, dentists, and nurses to provide care for friends, neighbors, and relatives. They face huge financial obstacles, but new financing mechanisms can put a health professions education within their reach. Further reducing the debt burden will broaden access to a health professions education.
>
> "I had incredible support that allowed me to pursue my dreams and fight to get my education," testified Claribel Sanchez, a University of California, Berkeley, student born and raised in East Los Angeles, a neighborhood that has seen more than its share of crime and violence. "Even if I'm here on loans, I'm not letting money become an issue. It's the only way I can get through and I'm not going to give up."
>
> With change, new role models will provide hope to medically underserved communities which currently see health care as a luxury, not a reality. New ways for providing quality care to those who now receive little will be discovered.
>
> Tracy Brewington, a nursing student at Howard University, told the Commission: "I'm looking forward to going back home to Philadelphia, to the inner city, where I will have the opportunity to give back to my community. I feel like even if just one person could do something to try to eliminate these health disparities, it could be me. I'm here to make a difference."

## Why Does Nursing Need Diversity?

The Institute of Medicine says that "disparities in the health care delivered to racial and ethnic minorities are real."[23] Studies from The Center for Health Professions indicate that increasing the diversity of health care providers can remove cultural barriers, which, in turn, can lead to a population's improved health status.[24] The Institute of Medicine calls for a systematic and sustained effort to enroll and graduate ethnic minority students prepared for health sciences careers, such as nursing.[25] Likewise, in the PEW Health Professions Commission report, U.S. senator George Mitchell is quoted as saying, "Ours is a nation of minorities. This is not just about race, and it's not about quotas. This is about a national need for health care providers who are best qualified to meet the needs of their patients and society."[26] The Institute of Medicine and the PEW Commission unequivocally call for a solution to the harmful deficit in minority health care professionals. The American Nurses Association also actively supports a health care environment in which registered nurses reflect the diversity of the U.S. population.[27] Effective recruitment and retention strategies are needed to increase men and nurses of color in the profession.[28] Role models, mentors, financial aid, study skills assistance, and a welcoming environment are all ways to increase recruitment and retention of students.

## Men in Nursing

Nursing is predominantly a female profession, but that is changing. In 2004, 5.4% of RNs were men.[29] In 2005, 12% of students in nursing schools were men. A considerable increase was made in the 1990s but has since leveled off.[30] Surveys of college men suggest they would be more likely to choose nursing if they had more information. Men enter nursing for the same reasons women do: They want to help people, they are interested in science, they want a secure career with a decent salary, and they want a career with a great deal of opportunity.

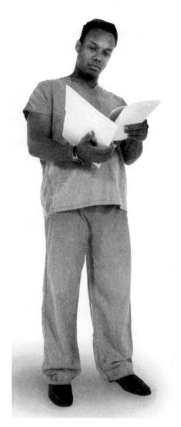

Men tend to be drawn to areas in nursing that are more technical such as emergency departments, intensive care units, anesthesia, and flight nursing. Many men in nursing also become managers and administrators. However, there are men who become oncology nurses (working with cancer patients), pediatrics nurses, and work in labor and delivery. Some men have even trained to be nurse-midwives.

Attitudes toward men in nursing are changing slowly. On one hand, patients often mistake the man who is a nurse for the doctor. Coworkers may have biases about men in nursing. These biases may be seen in asking men to help with lifting and moving patients, assuming men don't know much about labor and delivery, or babies. On the other hand, the men are perceived as ready for leadership roles, male physicians may treat male nurses with more respect, and they make more money. One study in 2002 showed that men in nursing made 12% more than women.[31]

Encouraging men to enter nursing needs to be a priority for nursing. Ways to achieve this include changing perceptions that men cannot be in a caring profession, showing images of nurses that include men, working in high schools to encourage young men to choose nursing, and changing the idea that the word *nurse* means a woman.

One group working to support and promote men in nursing is the American Assembly for Men in Nursing (www.aamn.org). The purpose of this organization is "to provide a framework for nurses, as a group, to meet, to discuss and influence factors which affect men as nurses."

The historical perspective in Figure 1.3 is adapted from the University of Iowa College of Nursing.[32]

Why don't more men go into nursing? Some say it is because of the persistent stereotype that nurses are female and that nursing is women's work. But that was not always the case. As you have just read, historically, nursing has been the realm of men. Read what men in nursing are saying and some of their suggestions to help men get into a great profession.

## African American Nurses

In *Black Women in White*, it was noted that the racism at the end of the 19th century made it nearly impossible for black women to obtain nursing degrees.[33] Yet, since their arrival in the Americas, black women provided health care to both blacks and whites.[34] The training of black nurses was first implemented by hospital schools in the North that imposed racial quotas. The New England Hospital for Women and Children in Boston was where the first black professional nurse, Mary Eliza Mahoney, received her diploma in 1879. At that time the school admitted one black and one Jewish student each year.[35] The philanthropists John D. Rockefeller and his

**FIGURE 1.3**   A brief history of men in nursing

**500 BC**
- In Ayur-Veda, the books from ancient India that discuss the prevention and cure of disease, the "Nurses" mentioned are always male.

- In the New Testament, the Good Samaritan paid the male innkeeper to provide care for an injured man. This story turned particular attention toward the sick poor, and by so doing also affected nursing, medicine, and charity.

**AD**
- The first five centuries of the Christian era (1–500) witnessed the rise of a religious and social movement that enabled the systematic development of organized nursing.

**300**
- Men risked their lives to provide nursing care in every plague that swept Europe. The Parabolani was initiated in 300 A.D. during the Black Plague epidemic.

- When Western Europe succumbed to Barbarism (500–1000 A.D.) the care of sick men was assigned to monks.

**500**
- The order of Benedictines, established in the sixth century by St. Benedict of Nursia, decreed nursing the sick would be a chief function and duty of community life. 500 A.D.

**1000**
- Military nursing orders known as Knights Hospitalers surfaced in the 1100s. They nursed the sick and defended the Holy Land during the Crusades.

- The Order of the Santo Spirito or Holy Ghost, established in 1070, was identified with the development of general hospitals within city walls.

- An order of men established in 1095, the Antonines (Hospital Brothers of St. Anthony), devoted themselves to sufferers of "St. Anthony's Fire," probably the ergotism which caused hallucinations.

**1200**
- St. Dominic also founded orders to take nursing out among the people (Dominican order founded 1206).

- St. Francis of Assisi (1182–1226) established three religious nursing orders including the Gray Friars, distinguished by grey robes with a rope girdle. This order chose to identify itself with the care of lepers and contributed to a public health movement (Franciscan order founded 1211).

- St. Louis IX was another saint whose endeavors with lepers were well known. Louis personally tended to the sick and devoted his life to humane treatment for all individuals (inherits throne of France 1226).

- The brotherhood of Misericordia was started in Florence in 1244. Founded primarily as a volunteer ambulance society, they became known as the "Masked Brotherhood." This name arose from the members' belief that their contributions would gain spiritual reward only if they prevented themselves from being recognized by others.

**1300**
- The Alexian Brothers were organized in the 1300s to provide nursing care for the victims of bubonic plague in the Netherlands.

**1500**
- The Brothers of Mercy, (also known as the Brothers of St. John of God or the order of the Fatabene-Fratelli), was founded in Spain in 1538 by John Ciudad. They were mendicants who devoted themselves to nursing, hospital work, the distribution of medicines, the tender care of the mentally ill and abandoned children, and the visitation of the sick at home.

- In the sixteenth century St. Camillus founded the Nursing Order of Ministers of the Sick who pledged themselves to the work of nursing doing hospital work and caring for those stricken with the plague in Rome in 1590.

**1860**
- Large numbers of men and women volunteered as nurses during the American Civil War. Walt Whitman served as a volunteer Civil War nurse in Washington, D.C. He described his experiences in a collection of poems.

**1898**
- In 1886 the School for Male Nurses was established in connection with the New York City Training School for Nurses on Blackwell's (Welfare) Island; In 1888 the Mills College of Nursing was established in Bellevue Hospital in New York, the first nursing college for men.

**1928**
- The Congregation of the Alexian Brothers established two schools for men nurses in their hospitals in Chicago (1898) and St. Louis (1928) which provided all types of care for men and boys.

**1940**
- According to the U.S. Census, the number of men in nursing in 1940 was approximately 2% of the total number of graduate and student nurses.

- Although the U.S. government badly needed nurses during WWII, they refused to allow males to receive equal opportunity in the Military. Although female nurses received full commission rank in U.S. military service in 1947, the first men were not commissioned as nurses until 1955.

**1960**
- Philip E. Day became the first male to be elected president of a state nurses' association in 1960.

**1966**
- A congressional bill authorizing appointment of male nurses to the regular forces of the Air Force, Army, and Navy Nurse Corps was signed by President Lyndon Johnson in 1966. Men constituted 22% of the Army's total nursing population.

**1974**
- Male nurses face the sex stereotyping and cultural pressures that define nursing as a woman's profession.

- The American Assembly for Men in Nursing was established in 1974.

*Source:* University of Iowa College of Nursing. "Men in Nursing."

# NURSING PROFILES
## MEN IN CLINICAL NURSING[36]

**David Hughes, RN**
**Software Architect**
**University of Washington School of Nursing**
**Seattle, Washington**

How I became a nurse and the paths I have taken during my career is a question I often ponder. I have had an extremely rewarding experience; something I will always be thankful for. I did not enter nursing as the result of a conscious decision to become a nurse. I started college with the intent of getting a degree in biology and pre-med then entering a MD/PhD program so that I could conduct biomedical research.

I was an undergrad at the University of New Mexico in Albuquerque, NM. I was in the biology program and assisting the research efforts of the department chair. I spent a summer in Mexico studying the zonation of tapeworms in the spiral gut of stingrays; believe it or not it was exciting work. I also volunteered at the medical school as a lab tech in a cardiology research lab. I became even more interested in research and medicine during these experiences and enjoyed working with gifted individuals and intriguing tools. Over time I transitioned into the lab manager position and thought my career path was set. I was going to become a researcher with a medical/clinical background. I would think nothing of spending days and nights in the lab conducting research, developing my computer skills, working with flow cytometers, measuring intracellular calcium using immunofluoresence and confocal laser microscopes. . . it was captivating! I felt good about contributing to the body of knowledge that healthcare providers used in treating patients.

wife, Laura Spelman Rockefeller, established the first black nurses' training program in 1881 at the Atlanta Baptist Female Seminary, commonly referred to as Spelman College.[37]

Efforts by the black community to train black nurses faced financial problems and discrimination. In 1868, the Harlem Dispensary was founded to care for the area's poor. In 1887, it became the Harlem Hospital, and in 1910, when Harlem went from a majority white to majority black neighborhood, concerns were raised by whites about white women caring for black men. In 1923, the Harlem Hospital School of Nursing was established to educate black women nurses who could care for the black patients. Yet administrators and physicians were still white. Black female students and staff were mistreated. It was not until 1945 that Alida Cooley Daily became the first black director of the Harlem school.[38]

In the 1920s, there were approximately 3,000 black nurses.[39] Petra Pinn, one of these nurses, graduated from the Tuskegee Institute training school in 1906 and became the head nurse of the Hale Infirmary in Montgomery, Alabama. By the 1920s, she was superintendent and manager of the Benevolent Society Hospital in Greenville, South Carolina. Nursing provided Pinn "a route to personal prestige and administrative autonomy, and a means to serve her people."[40] Although white nurses did not recognize black nurses as colleagues, within black communities, they were respected and admired and "next to the teacher, they were the highest ideal of black womanhood."[41]

By the mid-1930s, 25 years after the first baccalaureate program was established for white students, only one black college, Florida A & M in Tallahassee, offered a bachelor's degree in nursing. Black nurses worked together for change. For example, the National Association of Colored Graduate Nurses (NACGN), founded in 1908, fought for and won the right for black nurses to serve in the army and the navy in World War II.

Black nurses were excluded from state exams needed for licensing as registered nurses. Ludie C. Andrews, who graduated from Spelman College in 1906, spent 10 years working to allow black nurses the right to take the Georgia State Board licensing exam. Previous to her victory in 1920, the state of Georgia issued licenses to black nurses based on different standards and procedures than for white nurses. Black nurses were also denied membership in the American Nurses Association (ANA).[42] Two black nurses were instrumental in changing the ANA, Geneva Estelle Massey Riddle Osborne and Mabel Keaton Staupers. Riddle Osborne was the first black nurse in the United States to earn a master's degree and the first black instructor at New York University and at the Harlem Hospital School of Nursing. She also served as the president of the NACGN from 1934 to 1939. Stauper, born in 1890 in Barbados, West Indies, and raised in New York City, had led efforts to integrate the Army Nurse Corp during World War II.[43]

In 1939, Riddle was invited to speak at the ANA meeting in New Orleans about the status of black nurses, but due to Jim Crow laws, was unable to enter the St. Charles hotel, where the meeting took place.[44] The ANA's intolerance was noted as incongruent when those who "desire to insure basic and human rights of all people have not been able to impress hotel managers and other less enlightened individuals with the importance of this principle."[45] Integration of the ANA finally occurred in 1948, and Estelle Massey Riddle Osborne was elected to the board of directors. In 1951, the NACGN was dissolved because Staupers felt that black nurses, now integrated into the ANA, held the leadership positions they needed.[46]

Large societal changes in addition to work within black communities enabled black nurses to make policy changes that have resulted in "the advance of all minorities within nursing."[47] But racism and marginalization of minority nurses continues today.[48]

The National Black Nurses Association (NBNA) was formed in 1971 with their first leader, Dr. Lauranne Sams, former dean and professor of nursing, School of Nursing, Tuskegee University, Tuskegee, Alabama, carrying on the work of advancing professional black nursing.[49]

The NBNA is active today and has several professional publications. The organization has approximately 150,000 African American nurse members from around the world, including the United States, eastern Caribbean, and Africa. The "NBNA mission is to provide a forum for collective action by African American nurses to "investigate, define and determine what the health care needs of African Americans are and to implement change to make available to African Americans and other minorities health care commensurate with that of the larger society."[50]

## Asian and Pacific Islander Nurses

People who identify as Asian American and Pacific Islander are counted together for the U.S. census, but they represent a great variety of countries, cultures, and experiences.[51] Many from these groups have been in the

United States longer than white immigrant groups, such as Germans or Irish.[52] Asian and Pacific Islander nurses comprise 3.3% of all RNs. Even though Asian and Pacific Islanders rank high socioeconomically in the United States, they are not well represented in leadership roles in nursing and in educational systems.[53]

Asians and Pacific Islanders suffer health disparities with higher rates of lung cancers, heart disease, hepatitis B, and tuberculosis. To alleviate health disparities, nurses who are culturally competent and who represent all groups in the United States are needed. The need for nurses who can provide culturally competent care is increasing significantly.[54] Even though the Registered Nurses Sample Survey (2001) showed that the 3.3% of nurses who are Asian/Pacific Islander is close to the percentage in the U.S. population, 4.1%, these numbers do not reflect the real need. Data is not necessarily accurate because people from many subgroups are combined into one large ethnic group.[55]

The professional association, Asian American/Pacific Islander Nurses Association (AAPINA), began in 1991.[56] The goals of AAPINA include identifying and supporting the health care of Asian Pacific Islanders (API) internationally, taking action on issues such as registration and policies affecting the health of APIs, working with others in health care, and identifying and supporting professional nursing issues of concern to API nurses.

## Hispanic and Latino Nurses

The Hispanic population is the fastest growing ethnic minority group in the United States, and Hispanics represent many countries, including Mexico, Puerto Rico, Cuba, and the countries in Central and South America. The number of Hispanics in the United States is increasing, but Hispanics suffer many health disparities.[57] Much more cultural diversity is needed within nursing to help improve Hispanic and minority health. Furthermore, the highest educational degree most Hispanic nurses obtain is the associate's degree, and like other nurses of color, this education means that Hispanic nurses may be less likely to be in leadership positions. There have been few Hispanic directors, or deans, in the history of nursing schools in the United States.[58]

Historically and culturally, barriers to attaining leadership roles outside the home may be attributed to Hispanic culture that encourages men to work outside the home and women to work as housewives.[59] Gender roles may also explain why more Hispanic women than men go into nursing.[60] To increase the number of Hispanic nurses, recruitment and retention problems must be addressed from a Hispanic perspective.[61] Education may be presented not only as a personal benefit to the individual student but as a family benefit.[62]

The National Association of Hispanic Nurses (NAHN) was started in 1975 by Laura Murillo Rohde, RN, PhD, ND, FAAN. It includes chapters in the District of Columbia and Puerto Rico. NAHN began as a committee formed at an American Nurses Association conference as the Spanish-Speaking/Spanish Surnamed Nurses' Caucus. One year later, it was renamed the National Association of Spanish-Speaking/Spanish-Surnamed Nurses. Finally, in 1979, it was renamed the National Association of Hispanic Nurses.[63]

MISSION

Promoting Hispanic nurses to improve the health of our communities.

PHILOSOPHY

NAHN strives to serve the nursing and healthcare delivery needs of the Hispanic community and the professional needs of Hispanic nurses. NAHN is designed and committed to work toward improvement of the quality of health and nursing care for Hispanic consumers and toward providing equal access to educational, professional, and economic opportunities for Hispanic nurses. (Available from http://thehispanicnurses.org)

## Native American and Alaska Native Nurses

The first school of nursing for Native American students was located on the Navajo reservation in northeastern Arizona at Ganado.[64] The school was started in the fall of 1930 and closed in 1952.[65] The school has since reopened and now offers a bachelor's degree in nursing with the support of the University of Northern Arizona. Ganado is one of a few schools of nursing located on a reservation; the others are the Salish Kootenai College in Montana and Sisserton Wapheton College and Oglala Lakota College, both located in South Dakota.[66]

Lillian Tom-Orme, a Navajo, past president of the Native Alaska Native American Indian Nurses Association (NANAINA), is a policy analyst and professor at the University of Utah. Responding to changes in health care systems and to the health needs of Native Americans, Tom-Orme noted that nursing could help restore the balance and harmony that is important to Indian nations by having Indian nurses provide care for Indian communities.[67] Tom-Orme proposed that Indian nurses partner with other nurses and health care professional while retaining the values of caring, spirituality, and "the core of all that we do as American Indian nurses."[68]

Increasing the number of Native American nurses is not just a matter of increasing educational opportunities but includes the need to increase understanding of the challenges Native American nurses face. Native American nurses often value and practice traditional holistic nursing.[69] Integrating traditional values with the culture of nursing is needed.[70]

Role models have been identified by Native American nurses as fundamental in their decisions to become nurses.[71] One Navajo nurse educated at Georgetown University in Washington, D.C., said that her reason for becoming a nurse was her grandmother and the hospice nurse who cared for her grandmother when she had cancer.[72] Another nurse from the Fond du Lac reservation said she was encouraged by her mother, who was a nurse's aide, to become an RN.[73] The first Hopi nurse told interviewers that she became a nurse, despite barriers such as her fear of evil spirits, catching illnesses, and learning white man's ways, because of a nurse in her local clinic who served as her role model.[74]

There is a long tradition of Native American women becoming medical practitioners.[75] In the early 19th century, graduation lists from black colleges show that Native American women attended the colleges and became nurses. An Omaha Indian woman, Susan La Fesche, was one of the first Native Americans to receive formal training as a physician and became a leader for her tribe in legislative actions to promote health and to recognize tribal land rights.[76]

Susie Walking Bear Yellowtail, a Crow Indian woman, is considered one of the first Native American nurses. Yellowtail graduated from a nursing program in Massachusetts in 1921, but she eventually returned to her Montana reservation to promote health and become a national leader in Indian health policy.

The National American Indian Native Alaskan Nurses Association (NANAINA) was started after the American Indian Nurses Association and later, the American Indian Alaska Native Nurses Association. The organization holds annual conferences, publishes a newsletter, and provides scholarships to members.

The goals of NANAINA from their website http://www.nanainanurses.org/index.html include:

Continuing to support Alaska Native and American Indian students, nurses and allied health professionals through the development of leadership skills and continuing education.

Continuing to advocate for the improvement of health care provided to American Indian and Alaska Native consumers.

Working at increasing culturally competent health care provided to Alaska Native and American Indian consumers.

### International Students

Many students come to the United States to study nursing, and many RNs come to work. In 2004, 3.5% of U.S. RNs were from countries other than the United States. Nurses from the Philippines (50.2% of foreign-educated RNs) and Canada (20.2%) make up the majority of foreign-born nurses. RNs also come from the United Kingdom (8.4%), Nigeria (2.3%), Ireland (1.5%), India (1.3%), Hong Kong (1.2%), Jamaica (1.1%), Israel (1.0%), and South Korea (1.0%). Twelve percent of RNs are from 47 other countries. The majority of foreign-born RNs have a BSN degree.[77]

If you are an international student considering nursing, go to the All Nursing website U.S. Nursing Schools for International Students: http://www.allnursingschools.com/faqs/international.php. Here you will find questions and answer useful to your admissions process.

### *Journey*

"A journey of a thousand miles must begin with a single step."

LAO-TZU

# How Does an Education in Nursing Promote *Success?*

Nurses make up the majority of the nation's health care workers, with 2.9 million registered nurses. Yet misinformation from news stories, television, and other media continues to confuse the public with inaccurate images of

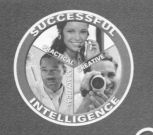

get practical!

# Face Your Fears

*Use practical skills to conquer a fear of yours that stems from the experience of starting college.*

First, describe your fear—and be specific.

Now, list three small activities that get you closer to working through that fear. If you don't want to start a project because you fear failure, for example, you can begin by reading a book on the subject, brainstorming what you already know about it, or making up a project schedule.

1. _____

2. _____

3. _____

Commit yourself to one step that you will take within the next two days. State it here. Include the time and date you will begin and how much time you will spend.

What reward will you give yourself for taking this step?

Did taking this step help ease your fear? If so, describe how.

Affirm that you have taken that first step and are on the way to success by signing your name here and writing the date.

Name _____ Date _____

nurses. As you plan an education in nursing, consider the following facts about nurses from the AACN:[78]

- The U.S. Bureau of Labor Statistics projects that employment for registered nurses will grow faster than the average for all occupations through 2014.

- Though often working collaboratively, nursing does not "assist" medicine or other fields.

- Nursing operates independent of, not auxiliary to, medicine and other disciplines. Nurses work under their own license, independent of other health professions, yet they work closely with doctors and others.

- There are more than four times as many RNs in the United States as physicians.

- Nursing delivers all health care services, including primary and preventive care by advanced, independent nurse practitioners (NPs), in such clinical areas as pediatrics, family health, women's health, and gerontological care.

- Most health care services involve some form of care by nurses. Although approximately 56.2% of all employed RNs work in hospitals, many are employed in a wide range of other settings, including private practices, public health agencies, primary care clinics, home health care, outpatient surgical centers, health maintenance organizations, nursing school–operated nursing centers, insurance and managed care companies, nursing homes, schools, mental health agencies, hospices, the military, and industry. Other nurses work in careers such as college educators or as researchers.

- Nurses can be certified nurse-midwives (CNMs) and nurse-anesthetists (CRNAs), as well as certified in cardiac, oncology, neonatal, neurological, or obstetric/gynecological nursing, and other advanced practice clinical specialties.

## Shortage of Nurses

An aging population, (i.e., the baby boomers) is living longer. This means there is a demand for nurses with knowledge of gerontology (taking care of elders), long-term care, and taking care of people with chronic illnesses. Demand has intensified for more BSN nurses with skills in critical thinking, case management, and health promotion skills across a variety of inpatient and outpatient settings. There is also a need for nurses to be culturally competent.

Pointing out the emergence of a disastrous nursing shortage, the AACN projects the following statistics:[79]

- Some 1.2 million new nurses will be needed by 2014.
- Currently, there are 118,000 vacancies, a vacancy rate of 8.5%.
- An estimated 55% of nurses working now plan to retire by 2020.

A 2006 Fact Sheet from the AACN on the nursing shortage states many reasons for the nursing shortage, including a greater demand for nurses than the supply and the aging workforce.[80]

- Supply of new nurses has decreased even though applications were up 9.5%.
- Supply of nurses is adversely impacted by faculty shortages in nursing schools, making it difficult to increase the number of students nationwide.
- A decrease in the number of new nurses means the average age of a nurse is increasing. An aging workforce means more nurses will be retiring soon, increasing the shortage. In other words, there are not enough new nurses coming into the profession to replace, much less increase, the ones who will be leaving. The average age for a nurse in 2004 (the latest statistics) was 46.8 years old. That is up from the average age in 2000 of 45.2 years.

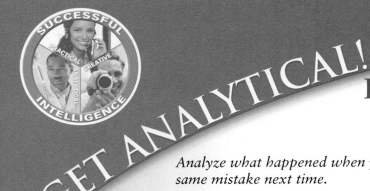

# Learn from a Mistake

*Analyze what happened when you made a mistake in order to avoid the same mistake next time.*

Describe an academic situation—you didn't study enough for a test, you didn't complete an assignment on time, you didn't listen carefully enough to a lecture and missed important information—where you made a mistake. What happened?

What were the consequences of the mistake?

What, if anything, did you learn from your mistake that you will use in similar situations?

This shortage increases stress on nurses there are fewer nurses to take care of patients. Linda Aiken has studied the affect of the shortage on nurses. She and her colleagues found that nurses reported more job dissatisfaction and emotional exhaustion when they were responsible for more patients than they can safely care for. She concluded that "failure to retain nurses contributes to avoidable patient deaths."[81]

## Salaries in Nursing

An education in nursing prepares you for a career that is rewarding in many ways, including financially.

Consider the latest (May 2005) salary data from the Bureau of Labor Statistics.[82] The average annual wage of workers in the most common health care occupations were in these ranges:

$25,380 for pharmacy technicians

$36,210 for licensed practical nurses (LPNs)

$56,880 for RNs

$88,650 for pharmacists

$140,370 for family and general practitioners

$45,950 for dieticians and nutritionists

$22,200 for nurses' aides

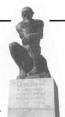

## *Understanding*

"Understanding is joyous."

CARL SAGAN

# Can *Graduate* School Help?

The health system's increasing demand for front-line primary care providers and the accelerating trends toward prevention and cost efficiency are driving the nation's need for nurse practitioners, certified nurse-midwives, and other registered nurses with advanced practice skills.

## Advanced Practice Nursing

Here are a few facts about advanced practice nurses (those with master's or doctorate degrees in a clinical specialty):

- Nurse practitioners and midwives earn an average of $75,905 per year. Clinical nurse specialists earned $75,294 per year in 2000.[83]

- For the highest paying specialty area, nurse anesthetists, the average salary (according to salary.com) was $164,172.[84] Approximately 46% of the nation's 36,000 nurse anesthetists and student nurse anesthetists are men, compared with about 8% in the nursing profession as a whole. In 2001, the CRNA professional association's most recent figure, the average salary was $113,000.[85]

- Mounting studies show that the quality of care by NPs and midwives is equal to, and at times better than, comparable services by physicians.[86]

See Figure 1.4 for a percentage breakdown of advanced nurses by roles.

---

**FIGURE 1.4**    More education is likely to mean more income

Median annual income of persons with income 25 years old and over, by gender and highest level of education, 2000.

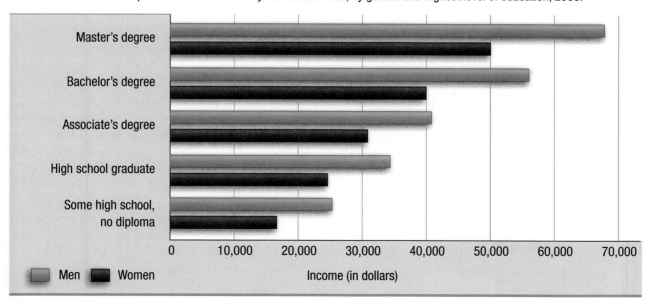

Source: U.S. Department of Commerce, Bureau of the Census, *Current Population Reports,* Series P-60, "Money Income of Households, Families, and Persons in the United States," 2002.

# Why Do You Need to Study a *Variety* of Arts and Sciences for Nursing?

You probably already know the reasons why a good science background is important: to keep up with rapid advances that affect daily life. With newspaper headlines announcing "Scientists urge more prudent use of antibiotics" and magazine articles discussing robotics, DNA, and the "geometry lesson of the marching ants," it takes only basic observation to see that life is rapidly changing owing to advances in science and technology. If you are 18 years old and just beginning college, think back 10 years. What kind of computer did you have? What kind of treatments were available for HIV? If you are older and returning to school, the contrast is much more vivid. Do you remember a time when you didn't own a DVD or a cell phone? Did you always have e-mail? Do you remember a time when no one talked about greenhouse gases or global warming? And almost everyone can remember a time when complex genetic engineering, cloning, or stem cell research were not occurring.

Examples of how technology and science affect our lives abound, and it is for this reason that a knowledge of science and math is needed. You need this knowledge even if you do not pursue a nursing career; you need it to be an active citizen and a responsible family member. For instance, you must be able to understand the implications, both ethical and practical, of genetic testing and therapy; of spread of viruses; and of disappearing wetlands, rain forests, and other natural habitats. Can you understand the research presented in the articles you read? Can you discern reality from sensationalism? If you read about a new study on exercise, engines, or equilibrium, can you put it to use?

All of us are called on to make political, social, and personal decisions regarding everything from health care to finances, from international foreign aid to environmental protection, and from genetically engineered tomatoes to gene therapy for a host of diseases. The decision to major in nursing is a good one and one that will be useful to you in many ways. Science and math knowledge and skills teach you critical thinking, creativity, teamwork, and all-around good work **habits**; each one is essential to any kind of career you pursue.

Studying the humanities and arts gives you the needed knowledge to think in different ways and to understand new perspectives. For instance, think about studying art. Learning about the evolution of painting from romantic realism to impressionism can help you understand how social changes affect human thinking and actions. If this seems far removed from nursing, consider health practices. In the past, people relied completely on physicians to tell them what to do. With today's technology and increased access to information, people are assuming responsibility for their health. It is common now for people to work with their care providers to come to solutions rather than accept what someone else tells them. Technological and social changes affect human behavior, and the health care system is evolving to meet these needs. People want more preventive care and disease prevention, which is exactly what nurses provide. Nursing is the study of human beings and their response to health and illness. That response is based on many things, such as culture, social learning, politics, and history.

**HABIT**
A preference for a particular action that you do a certain way, and often on a regular basis or at certain times.

The more you learn in college the better prepared you'll be to work with all kinds of people.

A major purpose of going to college is to broaden your worldview by taking time to study subjects not specifically related to a major or career goal. The purpose of this book is to help you learn to succeed in nursing, whether you remain in nursing your entire life or decide in your senior year to become an art major. And if this is the case, your science background will help you with painting (chemistry), sculpting (physics and geometry), ceramics (chemistry and physics), and designing jewelry (metallurgy, physics, and anatomy). Remember, your goals may change as you go through college, but what you learn in the physical and life sciences, math, and humanities will help no matter what you decide.

## How Education, Not Just Nursing Education, Promotes Life Success

If your work in college only helped you succeed in the classroom, the benefit of your learning wouldn't last beyond graduation day. However, learning is a tool for life, and a college education is designed to serve you far beyond the classroom. Here are a few important "life success goals" that college can help you achieve:

*Life Success Goal: Increased Employability and Earning Potential.* Getting a degree greatly increases your chances of finding and keeping a high-level, well-paying job. College graduates earn, on average, around $20,000 more per year than those with a high school diploma (see Figure 1.5). Furthermore, the unemployment rate for college graduates is less than half that of high school graduates (see Figure 1.6).

**FIGURE 1.5**    More education is likely to mean more consistent employment

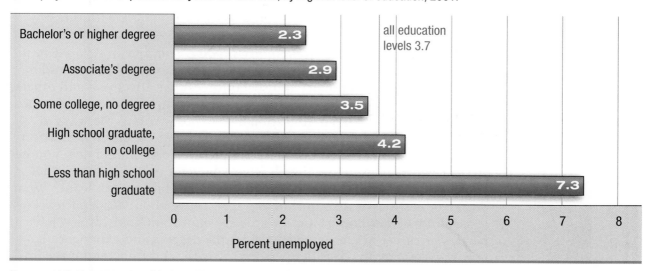

Unemployment rates of persons 25 years old and over, by highest level of education, 2001.

*Source:* U.S. Department of Labor, Bureau of Labor Statistics, Office of Employment and Unemployment Statistics, unpublished tabulations of annual averages from the Current Population Survey, 2002.

FIGURE 1.6

## Registered nurses prepared for advanced practices, March 2004

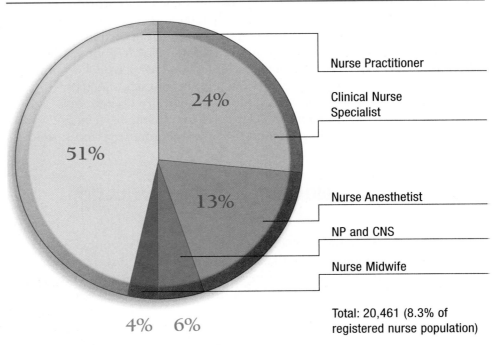

Nurse Practitioner

Clinical Nurse Specialist

Nurse Anesthetist

NP and CNS

Nurse Midwife

Total: 20,461 (8.3% of registered nurse population)

*Source:* National Sample Survey, 2004.

*Life Success Goal: Preparation for Career Success.* Your course work will give you the knowledge and hands-on skills you need to achieve your career goals. It will also expose you to a variety of careers related to your major, many of which you may not have even heard of. Completing college will open career doors that are closed to those without a degree.

*Life Success Goal: Smart Personal Health Choices.* The more educated you are, the more likely you are to take care of your physical and mental health. A college education prepares you with health-related information that you will use over your lifetime, helping you to practice wellness through positive actions and to avoid practices with the potential to harm.

*Life Success Goal: Active Community Involvement and an Appreciation of Different Cultures.* Going to college prepares you to understand complex political, economic, and social forces that affect you and others This understanding is the basis for good citizenship and encourages community involvement. Your education also exposes you to the ways in which people and cultures are different and how these differences affect world affairs. Thinking about these big-picture goals should help you begin to brainstorm, in more detail, what you want out of college. What courses do you want to take? What kind of schedule do you want? What degree or certificate are you shooting for? Think about academic excellence and whether honors and awards are important goals. If you have a particular career in mind, then consider the degrees and experience it may require. Finally, consider personal growth, and think about the importance of developing friendships with people who will motivate and inspire you.

In Chinese writing, this character has two meanings: one is "chaos"; the other is "opportunity." The character communicates the belief that every challenging, chaotic, demanding situation in life also presents an opportunity. By responding to challenges in a positive and active way, you can discover the opportunity that lies within the chaos.

Let this concept reassure you as you begin college. You may feel that you are going through a time of chaos and change. Remember that no matter how difficult the obstacles, you have the ability to persevere. You can create opportunities for yourself to learn, grow, and improve.

# Quick Start to College Resources

## What Basics Should You Know as You Begin School?

One of the first steps in creating your own success is learning what your college expects of you—and what you have a right to expect in return as a consumer of higher education.

### WHAT YOUR COLLEGE *EXPECTS* OF YOU

If you are clear on what it means to be a college student before classes start, you will minimize surprises that may be obstacles later on. What is expected of you may be different from anything you encountered in high school or in other educational settings.

Specific expectations involve understanding curriculum and graduation requirements, registering for classes, pursuing academic excellence, following school procedures, getting involved in extracurricular activities, and mastering the college's computer system. Do your best to understand all these areas and, if you need it, ask for help—from instructors, administrators, advisers, mentors, experienced classmates, and family members.

Additional/resources to assist you include your college catalog and student handbook. Your *college catalog* contains a wealth of information. It may give general school policies such as admissions requirements, the registration process, and withdrawal procedures. It may list the departments to show the range of subjects you may study. It may outline instructional programs, detailing core requirements as well as requirements for various majors, degrees, and certificates. It may also list administrative personnel as well as faculty and staff for each department. The college catalog is an important resource in planning your academic career. When you have a question, consult the catalog first before you spend time and energy looking elsewhere.

Your *student handbook* describes important policies such as how to add or drop a class, what the grading system means, campus rules, drug and alcohol policies, what kinds of records your school keeps, and safety tips. Keep your student handbook where you can find it easily, in your study area at home or someplace safe at school. The information it provides can save you a lot of trouble when you need to find out about a resource or service. For example, if you call for locations and hours before you visit a particular office, you'll avoid the frustration of dropping by when the office is closed.

Your student handbook also looks beyond specific courses to the big picture, helping you to navigate student life. In it you will find some or all of the following, and maybe even more: information on available housing (for on-campus residents) and on parking and driving (for commuters); overviews of the support offices for students, such as academic advising, counseling, career planning and placement, student health, disabled student services, child care, financial aid, and individual centers for academic subject areas such as writing or math; descriptions of special-interest clubs; and details about library and computer services. It may also list hours, locations, phone numbers, and addresses for all offices, clubs, and organizations.

### EXPLORING YOUR CURRICULUM AND GRADUATION REQUIREMENTS

Use your college catalog and website to explore your course requirements, and then complete the following:

- What are your course requirements for graduation?
- What are the requirements to major in a department that interests you? List, on a separate page if necessary, the courses in the order they must be taken.
- What grade point average must you maintain to remain in good standing at your college and to major in your area of interest?

Identify two study-related activities you will start in the next month to help ensure that you will achieve that GPA.

GPA:

1. _____
2. _____

## UNDERSTAND CURRICULUM AND GRADUATION REQUIREMENTS

Every college has degree requirements stated in the catalog and website. Among the requirements you may encounter are:

- Number of credits needed to graduate, including credits in major and minor fields
- Curriculum requirements, including specific course requirements
- Departmental major requirements, including the cumulative average needed for acceptance as a major in the department

Among the degrees granted by two-year and four-year colleges are bachelor of arts, bachelor of science, associate of arts, associate of science, and associate of applied science.

## CHOOSE AND REGISTER FOR CLASSES

Your course selections define what you will learn and who will teach you. Course registration can be both exciting and challenging, especially the first time. Scan the college catalog and website and consider these factors as you make your selections:

- Core/general requirements for graduation
- Your major or minor or courses in departments you are considering
- Electives that sound interesting, even if they are out of your field

In most schools, you can choose to attend a class without earning academic credit by *auditing* the class. The main reason students choose to audit is to explore different areas without worrying about a grade, although tuition charges are generally the same.

Once you decide on courses, but before you register, create a schedule that shows daily class times. If the first class meets at 8 A.M., ask yourself if you will be at your best at that early hour. Create one or more backup schedules in case courses or sections you want fill up before you register. Show your ideas to your adviser for comments and approval.

Actual course registration varies from school to school. Registration may take place through your school's computer network, via an automated phone system, or in the school gym or student union. When you register, you may be asked to pay tuition and other fees. If you receive financial aid, make sure that checks from all aid sources have arrived at the college before registration.

## PURSUE ACADEMIC EXCELLENCE

Pursuing academic excellence means doing your very best in every course. You can accomplish this through a series of small but important steps that lead you to success:

- Read all assigned text material ahead of time.
- Attend every class with a positive attitude.
- Arrive on time.
- Complete assignments on schedule.
- Listen attentively, take notes, and participate in discussions.
- Study for exams.
- Seek help if you need it.

When you receive grades, remember that they reflect your work, not your self-worth. A D or an F does not diminish you as a person but rather tells you that your efforts or products are below what the instructor expects. Similarly, an A does not inflate your value as a person but recognizes the high quality of your academic performance.

Most schools use grading systems with numerical grades or equivalent letter grades (see Figure 1.7). Generally, the highest course grade is an A, or 4.0, and the lowest is an F, or 0.0. In every course, you earn a certain number of college credits, called semester hours. For example, Accounting 101 may be worth three hours, and Physical Education may be worth one hour. These numbers generally refer to the number of hours the

| FIGURE 1.7 | Letter grades and equivalent numerical grades per semester hour |

| Letter Grade | A | A− | B+ | B | B− | C+ | C | C− | D+ | D | F |
|---|---|---|---|---|---|---|---|---|---|---|---|
| Numerical Grade | 4.0 | 3.7 | 3.3 | 3.0 | 2.7 | 2.3 | 2.0 | 1.7 | 1.3 | 1.0 | 0.0 |

## FIGURE 1.8  How to calculate your GPA

| COURSE | SEMESTER HOURS | GRADE | GRADE POINTS |
|---|---|---|---|
| Chemistry 1 | 4 | C | 4 credits × 2 points = 8 |
| Freshman Writing | 3 | B+ | 3 credits × 3.3 points = 9.9 |
| Spanish I | 3 | B− | 3 credits × 2.7 points = 8.1 |
| Introduction to Statistics | 3 | C+ | 3 credits × 2.3 points = 6.9 |
| Social Justice | 2 | A− | 2 credits × 3.7 points = 7.4 |
| Total semester hours: 15 Total grade points for semester: 40.3 | | | |

GPA for semester (total grade points divided by semester hours): 40.3 divided by 15 = 2.68
Letter equivalent grade: C+/B−

course meets per week. When you multiply each numerical course grade by the number of hours the course is worth, take the average of all these numbers, and divide by the total number of semester hours you are taking, you obtain your grade point average, or GPA.

Learn the minimum GPA needed to remain in good standing and to be accepted and continue in your major. At some schools, for example, courses with grades below 2.0 may not be counted toward your major requirement. Figure 1.8 shows you how to calculate your GPA.

Inherent in the pursuit of academic excellence is honest, ethical behavior. Your school's academic integrity policy defines the behavioral standards that are expected of you in your studies and in your relationships with faculty, administrators, and fellow students.

### FOLLOW SCHOOL PROCEDURES

Your college has rules and regulations, found in the college handbook and on the website, for all students to follow. Among the most common procedures are:

*Adding or Dropping a Class.* This should be done within the first few days of the semester if you find that a course is not right for you or there are better choices. Late-semester unexcused withdrawals (almost any withdrawal after a predetermined date) receive a failing grade. However, course withdrawals that are approved for medical problems, a death in the family, or other special circumstances have no impact on your GPA.

*Taking an Incomplete.* If you can't finish your work due to circumstances beyond your control—an illness or injury, for example—many colleges allow you to take a grade of Incomplete. The school will require approval from your instructor and your commitment to make up the work later.

*Transferring Schools or Moving from a Two-Year to a Four-Year College.* If you want a change, check out the degree requirements of the new college and complete an application. If you are a student at a community college and intend to transfer to a four-year school, be sure to take the courses required for admission to that school. In addition, be sure all your courses are transferable, which means they will be counted toward your degree at the four-year school. At most community colleges, advisers are available to help students through this process.

*Taking a Leave of Absence.* There are many reasons students take a leave of absence for a semester or a year and then return. You may want time away from academics to think through your long-term goals, or you may be needed for a family emergency. If you are in good standing at your college, leave is generally granted. However, students with academic or disciplinary problems who take a leave may have to reapply for admission afterward.

### GET INVOLVED

Extracurricular activities give you a chance to meet people who share your interests and to develop teamwork and leadership skills. These activities also give you the chance to develop skills that may be important in your career. In addition, being connected to friends and a supportive network of people is one of the main reasons people stay in school.

Some freshmen take on so many activities that they become overwhelmed. Pace yourself the first year. You can always add more activities later. As you seek the right balance, consider this: Studies have shown that students who join organizations tend to persist in their educational goals more than those who don't branch out.[87]

## MASTER YOUR COLLEGE'S COMPUTER SYSTEM

A large part of the communication and work that you do in college involves the computer. Here are just some examples:

- Registering for classes
- Accessing a course syllabus and required-readings list
- E-mailing instructors for assignment clarification; receiving e-mail responses
- Tapping into library databases and the Internet for research
- Completing assignments and writing papers
- Submitting papers via e-mail to instructors
- Creating spreadsheets for math and science
- E-mailing classmates to schedule group/team meetings
- Receiving schoolwide announcements via the college computer network
- Taking interactive quizzes

In most colleges, it is no longer possible to manage without a computer—your own, one borrowed from school, or one available in computer labs. Most dorm rooms are now wired for computers, which gives students access to the campus network. Here are some suggestions for using your computer effectively:

- **Get trained.** Start by getting help to connect to your college network. Then, take training classes to master word processing, data and spreadsheets, and the Internet. If you encounter technical problems, talk to technicians in the computer lab.
- **Use computers to find information.** If you have specific questions about your school, check the college website. You may find the information or the e-mail address of a contact person.
- **Be a safe and cautious user because computers sometimes fail.** To safeguard

your work, create regular backups by saving your work periodically onto the hard drive, CD, or flash drive. In addition, use an antivirus program.

- **Use computers for appropriate tasks.** During study time, try to stay away from Internet surfing and computer games. Set time limits at other times to keep your academic focus.
- **Protect yourself from trouble.** Avoid revealing personal information, including financial data, to strangers you meet on the Internet.

### A WORD ABOUT E-MAIL

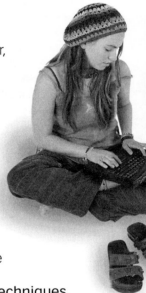

You may be required to communicate with your instructor, submit assignments, and even take exams via e-mail. Following are suggestions for improving your communication:

- **Use your college's E-mail system.** Register for an e-mail account at your school as soon as possible. You'll need this connection to receive schoolwide e-mails and possibly to access the college library.
- **Use effective writing techniques.** To make the best impression—especially when writing to an instructor—take the time to find the right words. Organize your thoughts and use correct spelling, punctuation, and grammar. To make your e-mails easy to read, get to the point in the first paragraph, use short paragraphs, use headings to divide long e-mails into digestible sections, and use lists. Always proofread before hitting "send."
- **Be Careful of Miscommunication.** Try to be diplomatic and pleasant, and think before you respond to upsetting messages. If you write back too quickly, you may be sorry later.
- **Rein in Social E-Mailing.** Prioritize your e-mailing. Respond to the most important and time-sensitive messages first. Save personal e-mail for when you have downtime.

No matter what school or extracurricular activity you are involved in, you will find people who are eager to help you succeed.

## Connecting with People and Support Services

Instructors, administrators, advisers, and a range of support staff are available to help you. This overview will help you identify and connect to the people and services around you. As you read, keep in mind that the names of offices and personnel titles may vary, and remember that some colleges do not offer every resource.

### TEACHING AND LEARNING TAKE CENTER STAGE

The primary mission of most colleges and universities is teaching—communicating to students the knowledge and thinking skills they need to succeed in school and beyond. Responding as an active, engaged learner is your role and responsibility as a student.

In every course, you'll meet one—or sometimes several—instructors. Although the term *instructor* is used in this text, teachers have official titles that show their rank within your college. Instructors with the highest status are full professors. Moving down from there are associate professors, assistant professors, lecturers, instructors, and assistant instructors, more commonly known as teaching assistants or TAs. Adjuncts may teach several courses but are not official staff members.

### ADMINISTRATORS PROVIDE SUPPORT

The administrative staff enables your college—and the student body—to function. Large universities may be divided into schools with separate administrative structures and staffs—for example, a School of Business or a School of Social Work. Each school normally has its own dean, and each department within the school has a chairperson, an instructor who heads the department.

One of the most important administrative offices for students is the Office of the Dean of Student Affairs, which, in many colleges, is the center for student services. Staff members there can answer your questions or direct you to others who can help.

### ADMINISTRATIVE OFFICES DEALING WITH TUITION ISSUES AND REGISTRATION

Among the first administrative offices you will encounter are those involved with tuition payments, financial aid, and registration.

- The *bursar's office* (also called the office of finance, the accounting office, and cashiering services) issues bills for tuition and room and board and collects payments from students and financial aid sources.

- The *financial aid office* helps students apply for financial aid and understand the eligibility requirements of different federal, state, and private programs.

- The *registrar's office* handles course registration, sends grades at the end of the semester, and compiles your official transcript, which is a comprehensive record of your courses and grades. Graduate schools require a copy of your offical transcript before considering you for admission, as do many employers before considering you for a job.

### STUDENT-CENTERED SERVICES

A host of services helps students succeed in college and deal with problems that arise. Here are some you may find useful:

Center for Human Rights
Multicultural Affairs Office
Office of Equity and Diversity

Many schools have offices staffed by specialists who can help you. For instance, if you suspect discrimination or any type of harassment is occurring, seek out the staff in these offices. Such offices are also responsibile for recruitment and retention of diverse students and increasing cultural opportunities and awareness on the campus and in communities. They help assure that different people have a voice in school decision making.

*Academic Enhancement Centers, Including Reading, Writing, Math, and Study-Skills Centers.* These centers offer consultations and tutoring to help students improve skills at all levels.

*Learning Centers and Writing Labs.* Staffed for all students, these centers can be especially useful for students who are learning English. Use their services to help you!

*Academic Computer Center.* Most schools have computer facilities that are open every day, usually staffed by technicians who can assist with computer-related problems. Many facilities also offer training workshops.

*Student Housing or Commuter Affairs Office.* Residential colleges provide on-campus housing for undergraduate students, with many schools requiring lower classmen to live on campus. The housing office handles room and roommate placement, establishes behavioral standards, and deals with special needs (for example, an allergic student's need for a room air conditioner) and problems. Schools with commuting students may have transportation and parking programs.

*Health Services.* Health services generally include sick care, prescriptions for common medicines, routine diagnostic tests, vaccinations, and first aid. All clinics are affiliated with nearby hospitals for emergency care. In addition, psychological counseling is sometimes offered through health services, or you may find it at a separate facility or via the college website. Although services are available, you have to seek them out. Many colleges require proof of health insurance at the time of registration.

*Career Services.* This office helps students find part-time and full-time jobs, as well as summer jobs and internships. Career offices have reference files on careers and employers. They also help students learn to write résumés and cover letters and search job sites on the Internet. Career offices often invite employers to interview students on campus and hold career fairs to introduce companies and organizations. Summer internships and jobs are snapped up quickly, so check the office early and often to improve your chances.

*Services for Students with Disabilities.* Colleges must provide students with disabilities full access to facilities and programs. For students with documented disabilities, federal law requires that assistance be provided in the form of appropriate accommodations and aids. These range from interpreters for the hearing impaired to ramps for students in wheelchairs. If you have a disability, visit this office to learn what is offered. Remember, also, that this office is your advocate if you encounter problems. For specifics on learning disabilities, see Chapter 1.3.

*Veterans' Affairs.* The Office of Veterans' Affairs provides veterans with various services, including academic and personal counseling and current benefit status, which may affect tuition waivers.

Affording college isn't easy, but certain financial-aid resources can help ease the burden. Every school has a system in place to help you understand and apply for financial-aid opportunities. The following overview will help you explore them.

### STUDENT ORGANIZATIONS

Many colleges and universities have student organizations where you can meet and get support from students with similar interests. For example:

Multicultural Student Center
American Indian Students
Asian American Students
Latino Students
International Students
Math Club
Choir
Student Government

Foreign Language Clubs
Intramural Sports Clubs

Please make use of these groups. Many students have benefited from meeting people, finding mentors and tutors, and just getting connected with other students. You need support!

### LEARN ABOUT NURSING STUDENT ORGANIZATIONS

Depending on your school, there will be nursing student organization chapters on or off campus. The National Student Nurses Association (NSNA) may be contacted to find your local chapter. But the simplest method for locating student nurse organizations is to contact your school's nursing adviser. The adviser will know of, or help you contact, other students involved in your local group. These groups will support you in finding and getting into a nursing program of your choice; provide information on all phases of being a student nurse; and, finally, be a great resource for finding jobs after you graduate. They also provide opportunities for experiences in leadership within your school.

NSNA is a membership organization representing 45,000 students in 50 states, the District of Columbia, Guam, Puerto Rico, and the U.S. Virgin Islands.

### NSNA Mission Statement

- Bring together and mentor students preparing for initial licensure as registered nurses, as well as those enrolled in baccalaureate completion programs;
- Convey the standards and ethics of the nursing profession;
- Promote development of the skills that students will need as responsible and accountable members of the nursing profession;
- Advocate for high-quality, evidence-based, affordable, and accessible health care;
- Advocate for and contribute to advances in nursing education;
- Develop nursing students who are prepared to lead the profession in the future[88] (www.nsna.org)

### Understanding and Applying for *Financial Aid*

Financing your education—alone or with the help of your family—involves gathering financial knowledge and making financial decisions. Visit your school's financial aid office in person or on the Internet, research the available options and decide what works best, and then apply early. The types of aid available are student loans, grants, and scholarships.

## FIGURE 1.9    Get the details on federal student loan programs

| LOAN | DESCRIPTION |
|------|-------------|
| Perkins | Low, fixed rate of interest. Available to those with exceptional financial need (determined by a government formula). Issued by schools from their allotment of federal funds. Grace period of up to nine months after graduation before repayment, in monthly installments, must begin. |
| Stafford | Available to students enrolled at least half-time. Exceptional need not required, although students who prove need can qualify for a subsidized Stafford loan (the government pays interest until repayment begins). Two types of Staffords: the direct loan comes from federal funds, and the FFEL (Federal Family Education Loan) comes from a bank or credit union. Repayment begins six months after you graduate, leave school, or drop below half-time enrollment. |
| PLUS | Available to students enrolled at least half-time and claimed as dependents by their parents. Parents must undergo a credit check to be eligible, or may be sponsored through a relative or friend who passes the check. Loan comes from government or a bank or credit union. Sponsor must begin repayment 60 days after receiving the last loan payment. |

*Student Loans.* As the recipient of a student loan, you are responsible for paying back the amount you borrow, plus interest, according to a predetermined payment schedule. The amount you borrow is known as the *loan principal,* and *interest* is the fee that you pay for the privilege of using money that belongs to someone else. Loan payments usually begin after graduation, after a grace period of between six months and a year, and generally last no more than 10 years.

The federal government administers or oversees most student loans. To receive aid from any federal program, you must be a citizen or eligible noncitizen and be enrolled in a program that meets government requirements. Individual states may differ in their aid programs, so check with the financial aid office for details. Figure 1.9 describes the main student loan programs to which you can apply.

*Grants and Scholarships.* Unlike student loans, neither grants nor scholarships require repayment. Grants, funded by federal, state, or local governments as well as private organizations, are awarded to students who show financial need. Figure 1.10 describes federal grant programs. In contrast, scholarships are given for various abilities and talents. They may reward academic achievement, exceptional abilities in sports or the arts, citizenship, or leadership. Scholarships are sponsored by federal agencies and private organizations.

*Researching Financial Aid.* Start digging at your financial aid office and visit your library, bookstore, and the Internet. Guides to funding sources catalog thousands of opportunities.

Additional information about federal grants and loans is available in the current version (updated yearly) of *The Student Guide to Financial Aid*. This publication can be found at your school's financial aid office, or you can request it by mail or phone (1-800-433-3243). The publication is also available online at www.ed.gov/prog_info/SFA/StudentGuide/.

You can find the Free Application for Federal Student Aid (FAFSA) form at your library, at the Federal Student Aid Information Center, through your college's financial aid office or website, or via the U.S. Department of Education's website at www.ed.gov/finaid.html.

If you are receiving aid from your college, follow all the rules and regulations, including meeting application deadlines and remaining in academic good standing. In most cases, you will have to reapply for aid every year. Even if you did not receive a grant or scholarship as a freshman, you may be eligible as a sophomore, junior, or senior. These opportunities often are based on grades and campus leadership, and they may be given by individual college departments.

### Learn More About the Financial Aid Process

You'll find detailed information about the financial aid application process in your college catalog, on the college website, and in federal publications and

| Term/Semester | FAFSA Filing Date |
|---------------|-------------------|
| Fall 200_ | |
| Spring 200_ | |
| Summer 200_ | |

## FIGURE 1.10 Get the details on federal grant programs

| GRANT | DESCRIPTION |
|---|---|
| Pell | Need-based; the government evaluates your reported financial information and determines eligibility from that "score" (called an expected family contribution, or EFC). Available to undergraduates who have earned no other degrees. Amount varies according to education cost and EFC. Adding other aid sources is allowed. |
| Federal Supplemental Educational Opportunity (FSEOG) | Need-based; administered by the financial aid administrator at participating schools. Each participating school receives a limited amount of federal funds for FSEOGs and sets its own application deadlines. |
| Work-study | Need-based; encourages community service work or work related to your course of study. Pays by the hour, at least the federal minimum wage. Jobs may be on campus (usually for your school) or off (often with a nonprofit organization or a public agency). |

websites mentioned in Quick Start. Use these resources to complete the following:

- List the deadlines to submit FAFSA applications during the next year:
- Endowed scholarships may be available through your college. Find out about two scholarships for which you are eligible and describe them here:
  1.
  2.
- Make a commitment to take three actions in the coming year to apply for these scholarships. Describe these actions in the space below.
  1.
  2.
  3.

### USE SUCCESSFUL INTELLIGENCE TO ACHIEVE YOUR GOALS

In Sternberg's view, intelligence is not a fixed quantity; people have the capacity to increase intelligence as they learn and grow. Successful intelligence better predicts life success than any IQ test because it focuses on actions—what you *do* to achieve your goals—instead of just on recall and analysis.

Everyone knows people who fit the conventional definition of "smart." They score well on tests and get good grades. In contrast, other students have a hard time making the grade but are seen as "offbeat," "creative," or "street smart."

Successful intelligence has three parts or abilities: *Analytical* thinking, *creative* thinking, and *practical* thinking.

- **Analytical thinking**—commonly known as

critical thinking—involves analyzing and evaluating information, often to work through a problem or decision. Analytical thinking is largely responsible for school success and is recognized and measured through traditional testing methods.

- **Creative thinking** involves generating new and different ideas and approaches to problems, and, often, viewing the world in ways that disregard convention.
- **Practical thinking** means putting what you've learned into action to solve a problem or make a decision. Practical thinking enables you to accomplish goals despite real-world obstacles.

Here are two examples that illustrate how this works.

*Successful Intelligence in a Study Group—Reaching for the Goal of Helping Each Other Learn*

- **Analyze** the concepts you must learn, including how they relate to what you already know.
- **Create** humorous memory games to help you remember key concepts.
- **Think practically** about who in the group does what best, and assign tasks according to what you discover.

*Successful Intelligence in Considering an Academic Path—Reaching for the Goal of Declaring a Major*

- **Analyze** what you do well, what you like to do. Then analyze the course offerings in your college catalog until you come up with one or more that seem to match up with your strengths.

- **Create** a dream career, then work backward to come up with majors that might support it. For example, if you want to be a science writer, considering majoring in biology and minoring in journalism.
- **Think practically** about your major by talking with students and instructors in the department, looking at course requirements, and interviewing professionals in the fields that interest you.

### Successful Intelligence in Reaching for the Goal of Becoming a Nurse

- **Analyze** your strengths and weaknesses in your college courses. Then analyze the support systems in your college that can help with your weaker course(s) by looking in the catalog, online, or speaking to an adviser or professor. You could start your analysis by going to see someone in academic services. Then, based on your analysis of which option of support works best for you, say a chemistry tutor, proceed to get the help you need.
- **Create** a plan for getting the grade-point average you know you need to get into nursing school. Then create the motivation for your plan by talking to nurses in the nursing school advising office or to other nurses you know. This will help you recreate your motivation to get into nursing school.
- **Think practically** about getting into nursing school by talking with students and instructors in the nursing school or college, reviewing course requirements for admission, and interviewing nurses in practice areas, such as community health or the Emergency Department, that interest you.

Finally, think about what Florence Nightingale said in the 1800s: "Nursing is an art: and if it is to be made an art, it requires an exclusive deviton as hard a preparation, as any painter's or sculptor's work; for what is the having to do with dead canvas or dead marble, compared with having to do with the living body, the temple of God's spirit? It is one of the Fine Arts: I had almost said, the finest of Fine Arts."

You are beginning the journey of your college education and lifelong learning. The work you do in this course will help you achieve your goals in your studies and in your personal life and career. Yale University professor Robert J. Sternberg, the originator of the concept of *successful intelligence,* said that those who achieve success "find their path and then pursue it, realizing that there will be obstacles along the way and that surmounting these obstacles is part of their challenge."[89]

### QUICK START TO COLLEGE RESOURCES

#### Suggested Readings

Chany, Kalman A. *Paying for College Without Going Broke*. New York: Princeton Review, 2004.

Gottesman, Greg, Daniel Baer, et al. *College Survival: A Crash Course for Students by Students*, 5th ed. New York: Macmillan, 1999.

Greene, Howard R., and Matthew Greene. *Ten Principles for Paying for College*. New York: St. Martin's Press, 2004.

Light, Richard J. *Making the Most of College: Students Speak Their Minds*. Cambridge, MA: Harvard University Press, 2001.

Rozakis, Laurie. *The Complete Idiot's Guide to College Survival*. New York: Alpha Books, 2001.

#### Internet Resources

Prentice Hall Student Success Supersite (information about student life, student-to-student bulletin boards, personal stories, opinion polls, and more): **www. prenhall.com/success**.

## Nourish

"Nourish yourself with love of truth, goodness, righteousness, with reverence and admiration for wisdom, beauty, order, wherever such attributes are made manifest."

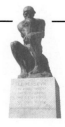

FLORENCE NIGHTINGALE, 1852

## Create Your Future

## DEVELOPING SUCCESSFUL INTELLIGENCE
### *Putting It All Together*

**Evaluating Internet sites.** You will be using the Internet frequently at school and in nursing. This exercise is intended to introduce you to one of the many excellent nursing sites as well as sites that can help you evaluate Internet resources.

**Step 1.** Get together with a group of students and go to your library or computer lab.

**Step 2.** Once on the Internet go to a nursing site. To find one, do a search, say on Google.com, or use a link provided by your school's nursing department or library.

**Step 3.** Bookmark your nursing site, or open a second window, and go to one of these evaluation sites:

    http://www.lib.purdue.edu/ugrl/staff/sharkey/interneteval/

    http://library.albany.edu/usered/eval/eresources.html

    http://nursing.wsu.edu/library/libhelp.asp

**Step 4.** Using the basic criteria for evaluating a site, go back to the nursing site you found and apply them.

**Step 5.** What can you say about the validity and usefulness of your site based on the evaluation criteria?

**Step 6.** What can you do if any of the sites you visited are no longer functioning? How can you find a new site?

## TEAM BUILDING
### *Collaborative Solutions*

**Skills Analysis, or "I'll never forget the time . . ."**
One method for discovering what skills and important interests you have is to tell a story from your life. Start thinking of a time you did something that was fascinating, significant, or in

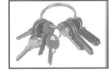

any way particularly memorable. It doesn't have to be anything that seems connected to nursing. Begin with the statement: "I'll never forget the time I . . ." and fill in the rest. You can tell another person your story. After you have told your stories, ask yourself the following questions:

- What was so important to you about this event?
- What underlying feelings and thoughts were associated with it?
- What skills, such as observation, reaction, communication, caution, or humor, did you use?

Write down the answers to these questions, and explore ways they might be connected to a health care field of study such as nursing.

# WRITING

## *Discovery Through Journaling*

*To record your thoughts, use a separate journal or the lined page at the end of the chapter.*

**Reflection.** Writing a journal requires a high level of reflection that goes way beyond a "Dear diary" approach. Reflection is an essential element of nursing and critical thinking. The ability to observe yourself and your thoughts and feelings is a valuable step toward learning to observe the world around you. Observation is one of the most important skills in nursing. Thinking about your thoughts, feelings, and the events that occur each day will assist you in developing an observant mind as well as sharpen your imagination and creativity. All of this will help you to understand and work in nursing.

Start the journal process by writing a detailed description of your environment. You can go into the backyard, into the kitchen, or onto your front porch. Take as long as you need to do this exercise. Minimum: 10 minutes of continuous writing; maximum: several days, or weeks, if that helps you get all the details as precise as possible. (If you need help, consider the following question as a starting point: What do you see, smell, hear, feel?)

# CAREER PORTFOLIO

## *Plan for Success*

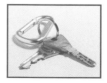

**Career Analysis, or "My three top careers would be . . ."** This exercise can help loosen up your brain and get your thoughts going (often referred to as brainstorming).

1. Begin by making a list of all your favorite ideas for work.
   a. Where do you see yourself working?
   b. Who do you see yourself working with?
   c. What kind of work are you doing?
2. List what you would consider to be your top three jobs incorporating all of the things you said in number 1.

3. Write the name of one person you can think of in a nursing career. If you can't think of anyone, write down someone you think could help you find such a person, for instance, a mentor, a parent, a reference librarian, or a teacher.

_____

_____

_____

4. Find out how to contact this person using either a phone book or an Internet search. Many people in nursing work for universities, so you can often find a way to contact them through the school's website. If the person you have chosen is well known, use a search engine.

_____

_____

_____

5. Call or e-mail the person, and set up an appointment to meet in person (or via e-mail, if that is more convenient for him or her).

6. Ask the person the following questions and add some of your own:
   - What is the most interesting part of your work? The least interesting?
   - If I wanted to pursue this area, what advice would you give?
   - What skills should I be working on in school?
   - How can I get more information?

# *Journal*

Name_____ Date _____

## Definition of Nursing

*Nursing is the protection, promotion, and optimization of health and abilities, prevention of illness and injury, alleviation of suffering through the diagnosis and treatment of human response, and advocacy in the care of individuals, families, communities, and populations.*

American Nurses Association definition of nursing (www.ana.org)

_____

_____

_____

_____

_____

_____

_____

_____

_____

_____

_____

_____

_____

_____

_____

_____

_____

_____

_____

## Suggested Readings

Evers, Frederick T., James Cameron Rush, and Iris Berdow. *The Bases of Competence: Skills for Lifelong Learning and Employability*. San Francisco, CA: Jossey-Bass, 1998.

Jeffers, Susan. *Feel the Fear . . . And Beyond: Mastering the Techniques for Doing It Anyway*. New York: Ballentine, 1998.

Katz, Janet. *A Career in Nursing: Is It Right for Me?* St. Louis: Elsevier, 2007.

Lombardo, Alison. *Navigating Your Freshman Year*. New York: Natavi Guides, 2003.

Simon, Linda. *New Beginnings: A Guide for Adult Learners and Returning Students*, 2nd ed. Upper Saddle River, NJ: Prentice Hall.

Sternberg, Robert. *Successful Intelligence: How Practical and Creative Intelligence Determine Success in Life*. New York: Plume, 1997.

Tyler, Suzette. *Been There, Should've Done That II: More Tips for Making the Most of College*. Lansing, MI: Front Porch Press, 2001.

Weinberg, Carol. *The Complete Handbook for College Women: Making the Most of Your College Experience*. New York: New York University Press, 1994.

## Internet Resources

Student Center: **www.studentcenter.org**

Student.Com—College Life Online: **http://www.student.com**

Prentice Hall Student Success Supersite—Student Union: **http://www.prenhall.com/success/StudentUn/index.html**

Success Stories: **http://www.prenhall.com/success/Stories/index.html**

## Endnotes

[1] American Association of Colleges of Nursing. "Your Nursing Career: A Look at the Facts." Retrieved February 1, 2007, from: http://ww.aacn.nche.edu/education/Career.htm.

[2] Linda H. Aiken, Sean P. Clarke, Robyn B. Cheung, Douglas M. Sloane, and Jeffrey H. Silber, "Educational Levels of Hospital Nurses and Surgical Patient Mortality," *Journal of the American Medical Association* 29 (2003): 1617–23.

[3] American Association of Colleges of Nursing, "Fact Sheet 2006: Articulation Agreements Between Nursing Education Programs." Retrieved February 1, 2007, from: http://www.aacn.nche.edu/Media/FactSheets/AA.htm.

[4] *Bureau of Labor Statistics Occupational Outlook Handbook 2006–2007*. Retrieved February 2, 2007, from: http://www.bls.gov/oco/ocos083.htm#training.

[5] Ibid.

[6] Ibid.

[7] National Organization of Associate Degrees in Nursing. "NOADN Position Statement on Associate Degree Nursing." (2006). Retrieved January 25, 2007, from: http://www.noadn.org/all.php?l=positions.

[8] American Association of Colleges of Nursing, "Fact Sheet: Accelerated Baccalaureate and Master's Degrees in Nursing." Retrieved February 2, 2007 from: http://www.aacn.nche.edu/Media/FactSheets/AcceleratedProg.htm.

[9] National League for Nursing, *Nursing Data Review Academic Year 2004–2005: Baccalaureate, Associate Degree, and Diploma Programs*" (New York: National League for Nursing 2006).

[10] American Association of Colleges of Nursing. "Your Nursing Career: A Look at the Facts." Retrieved February 2, 2007, from: www.aacn.nche.edu/education/nurse_ed/career.htm.

[11] U.S. Department of Health Resources and Services Administration. *The Registered Nurse Population, March 2004: Preliminary Findings:*

*The 2004 National Sample Survey of Registered Nurses* Washington, DC: U.S. Government Printing Office, 2004). Retrieved January 25, 2007, from: http://bhpr.hrsa.gov/healthworkforce/reports/rnpopulation/preliminaryfindings.htm.

[12] U.S. Department of Health Resources and Services Administration. *The Registered Nurse Population, March 2004 National Sample Survey of Registered Nurses.* (Washington, DC: U.S. Government Printing Office, 2004.

[13] Ibid.

[14] U.S. Department of Education, National Center for Education Statistics, *Postsecondary Institutions in the United States: Fall 2003 and Degrees and Other Awards Conferred: 2002–03* (NCES 2005-154) (2005). Retrieved February 1, 2007, from: http://nces.ed.gov/fastfacts/display.asp?id=72.

[15] Ibid.

[16] Ibid.

[17] National League for Nursing, *Nursing Data Review Academic Year 2004–2005: Baccalaureate, Associate Degree, and Diploma Programs* (New York: National League for Nursing, 2006).

[18] Ibid.

[19] Institute of Medicine, "Unequal Treatment: Confronting Racial and Ethnic Disparities in Health Care" (2002). Retrieved January 31, 2007 from: http://www.iom.edu/?id=16740.

[20] R. Warda, "Why Isn't Nursing More Diversified?" In *Current Issues in Nursing* (6th ed.), ed. J. M. Dochterman and H. K. Grace (St. Louis: Mosby, 2001), 483–92.

[21] B. Malone, "Why Isn't Nursing More Diversified?" In *Current Issues in Nursing* (5th ed.), ed. J. C. McCloskey and H. K. Grace (St. Louis: Mosby, 1997), 574–79.

[22] The Sullivan Commission, "Missing Persons: Minorities in Health Professions," in *A Report of the Sullivan Commission of Diversity in the HealthCare Workforce*, 11 (2004). Retrieved January 20, 2007, from: www.aacn.nche.edu/Media/pdf/SullivanReport.pdf

[23] Institute of Medicine, "Unequal Treatment: Confronting Racial and Ethnic Disparities in Health Care" (2002). Retrieved January 31, 2007, from: http://www.iom.edu/?id=16740.

[24] C. Dower, G. Berkowitz, K. Grumbach, and C. Wong. *Action to Health: A Critical Appraisal of the Literature Regarding the Impact of Affirmative Action.* (San Francisco: UCSF Center for the Health Professions and UCSF Institute of Health Policy Studies, 1999).

[25] Institute of Medicine, *Balancing the Scales of Opportunity in Health Care: Ensuring Racial and Ethnic Diversity in the Health Professions.* (San Francisco: Institute of Medicine and National Academy Press, 1994).

[26] M. Stewart and M. Slattery, "Population Diversity Requires More Minority Registered Nurses." Press Release, American Nurses Association (April 16, 1999). Retrieved June 10, 2001, from: www.ana.org/pressrel/1999/pr0416.htm.

[27] Rossman, "Bridging Differences: Montana Nurse Develops Program to Boost Number of Native American Nurses," *American Nurse* 34, no. 1 (2002): 20–21.

[28] H. Bessent, "Closing the Gap: Generating Opportunities for Minority Nurses in American Health Care," in *Strategies for Recruitment, Retention, and Graduation of Minority Nurses in Colleges of Nursing,* ed. H. Bessent, 3–18 (Washington, DC: American Nurses Association, 1997).

[29] U.S. Department of Health Resources and Services Administration. *The Registered Nurse Population, March 2004: Preliminary Findings: The 2004 National Sample Survey of Registered Nurses* (Washington, DC: U.S. Government Printing Office, 2004). Retrieved January 25, 2007, from: http://bhpr.hrsa.gov/healthworkforce/reports/rnpopulation/preliminaryfindings.htm.

[30] National League for Nursing, *Nursing Data Review Academic Year 2004–2005: Baccalaureate, Associate Degree, and Diploma Programs* (New York: National League for Nursing, 2006).

[31] K. L. Chitty, *Professional Nursing: Concepts and Challenges* (St. Louis: Elsevier, 2005).

[32] University of Washington, "Men in Nursing," in *History of Men in Nursing.* Retrieved January 25, 2007, from: http://www.son.washington.edu/students/min/default.asp.

[33] D. C. Hine, *Black Women in White: Racial Conflict and Cooperation in the Nursing Profession, 1890–1950* (Bloomington: Indiana University Press, 1989).

[34] Ibid.

[35] Ibid.

[36] University of Washington School of Nursing, "Men in Nursing. Nursing Profiles." Retrieved January 25, 2007, from: http://www.son.washington.edu/students/min/profiles.asp.

37Ibid.

38Ibid.

39Ibid, 62.

40Ibid, 62.

41Ibid.

42Ibid.

43Ibid.

44Ibid., 131.

45Ibid.

46M. K. Staupers, *No Time for Prejudice* (New York: Macmillian, 1961).

47D. C. Hine, *Black Women in White: Racial Conflict and Cooperation in the Nursing Profession, 1890–1950* (Bloomington: Indiana University Press, 1989).

48Ibid.

49National Black Nurses Association. Retrieved May 5, 2007, from: http://www.nbna.org.

50Ibid.

51A. Kuramoto and K. B. Louis, "Asian/Pacific Islander American Nurses Workforce: Issues and Challenges for the 21st Century," *Journal of Cultural Diversity* 3, no. 4 (1996): 112–115.

52E. B. Merrill, "Culturally Diverse Students Enrolled in Nursing: Barriers Influencing Success," *Journal of Cultural Diversity* 5, no. 2 (1998): 58–67.

53J. Inouye, "Bridging Cultures: Asians and Pacific Islanders and Nursing," in *Current Issues in Nursing* (6th ed.), ed. J. M. Dochterman and H. K. Grace (St. Louis: Mosby, 2001), 520–28.

54A. Kuramoto and K. B. Louis, "Asian/Pacific Islander American Nurses Workforce: Issues and Challenges for the 21st Century," *Journal of Cultural Diversity* 3, no. 4 (1996): 112–15.

55Ibid.

56American/Pacific Islander Nurses Association. Retrieved May 9, 2007, from: http://www.aapina.org/.

57S. Torres and H. M. Castillo, "Bridging Cultures: Hispanics/Latinos and Nursing," in *Current Issues in Nursing*, (6th ed.), ed. J. M. Dochterman, and H. K. Grace (St. Louis: Mosby, 2001), 529–35.

58Ibid.

59Ibid.

60P. I. Buerhaus and D. Auerbach, "Slow Growth in the United States of the Number of Minorities in the RN Workforce," *Image: The Journal of Nursing Scholarship* 31, no. 2 (1999): 179–83.

61A. M. Villarruel, M. Canales, and S. Torres, "Bridges and Barriers: Educational Mobility of Hispanic Nurses," *Journal of Nursing Education* 40, no. 6 (2001): 245–51.

62S. Torres and H. M. Castillo, "Bridging Cultures: Hispanics/Latinos and Nursing," in *Current Issues in Nursing* (6th ed.), ed. J. M. Dochterman and H. K. Grace (St. Louis: Mosby, 2001), 529–35.

63The National Association of Hispanic Nurses. Retrieved May 9, 2007, from: http://thehispanicnurses.org/.

64P. A. Kalisch and B. J. Kalisch, *The Advance of American Nursing*, 3rd ed. (Philadelphia: J. B. Lippincott, 1995).

65Ibid.

66Ibid.

67L. Tom-Orme, "Waters Running Deep, "*Reflections* 24, no. 2 (1998): 20–23.

68Ibid.

69M. A. Plumbo, "Living in Two Different Worlds or Living in the World Differently," *Journal of Holistic Nursing* 13, no. 2 (1995): 155–73.

70R. Struthers, "The Lived Experience of Ojibwa and Cree Women Healers," *Journal of Holistic Nursing* 18, no. 3 (2000): 261–79.

71J. Katz, "'If I Could Do It They Could Do It': A Collective Case Study of Plateau Tribes' Nurses," *Journal of American Indian Education* 44, no. 2 (2005): 36–51.

72B. Keltner, "American Indian, Alaska Native Nurses Blaze Trail of Culturally Competent Care," *The American Nurse* 31, no. 3 (1999): 16.

73Ibid.

74G. Bonnaha, "70+ and Going Strong: A Hopi Pioneer in Nursing," *Geriatric Nursing* 6, no. 6 (1985): 363–64.

75V. S. Mathes, "Native American Women in Medicine and the Military," *Journal of the West* 21, no. 2 (1982): 41–48.

76Ibid.

77U.S. Department of Health Resources and Services Administration, *The Registered Nurse Population, March 2004: Preliminary Findings: The 2004 National Sample Survey of Registered Nurses* (Washington, DC: U.S. Government Printing Office, 2004). Retrieved January 25, 2007, from: http://bhpr.hrsa.gov/

healthworkforce/reports/rnpopulation/preliminaryfindings.htm.

[78]American Association of Colleges of Nursing, "Your Nursing Career: A Look at the Facts." Retrieved February 2, 2007, from: www.aacn.nche.edu/education/nurse_ed/career.htm.

[79]American Association of Colleges of Nursing Fact Sheet (updated September 2006). Retrieved February 5, 2007, from: http://www.aacn.nche.edu/Media/FactSheets/NursingShortage.htm.

[80]Ibid.

[81]Ibid.

[82]Bureau of Labor Statistics, "May 2005 National Occupational Employment and Wage Estimates United States." Retrieved February 7, 2007, from: http://www.bls.gov/oes/current/oes_nat.htm.

[83]Salary.com (2007). "Salary Estimates." Retrieved February 5, 2007, from: http://swz.salary.com/salarywizard/layoutscripts/swzl_newsearchexp.asp.

[84]CRNA Salaries. (2006). Retrieved January 25, 2007, from: http://www.crnajobs.com/crna-careers/main.aspx.

[85]American Association of Nurse Anesthetists. "Nurse Anesthetists at a Glance." CRNA Certified Registered Nurse Anesthetist. Retrieved November 25, 2006, from http://www.aana.com/becomingcrna.

[86]Massachusetts Nurses Association. "Journal of the American Medical Association Study Shows Nurse Practitioners Provide Quality Care on Par with Physicians: Adds to Body of Research Demonstrating NPs Effectiveness." Retrieved September 13, 2007, from: www.massnurses.org/news/2000/000001/jamanp.htm.

[87]W. A. Alexander, *Preventing Students from Dropping Out* (San Francisco: Jossey-Bass, 1976).

[88]National Student Nursing Association, Media Fact Sheet, "Mission Statement." Retrieved February 3, 2007, from: http://www.nsna.org/press/fact_sheet.asp.

[89]R. J. Sternberg, *Successful Intelligence: How Practical and Creative Intelligence Determine Success in Life* (New York: Plume, 1997), 19.

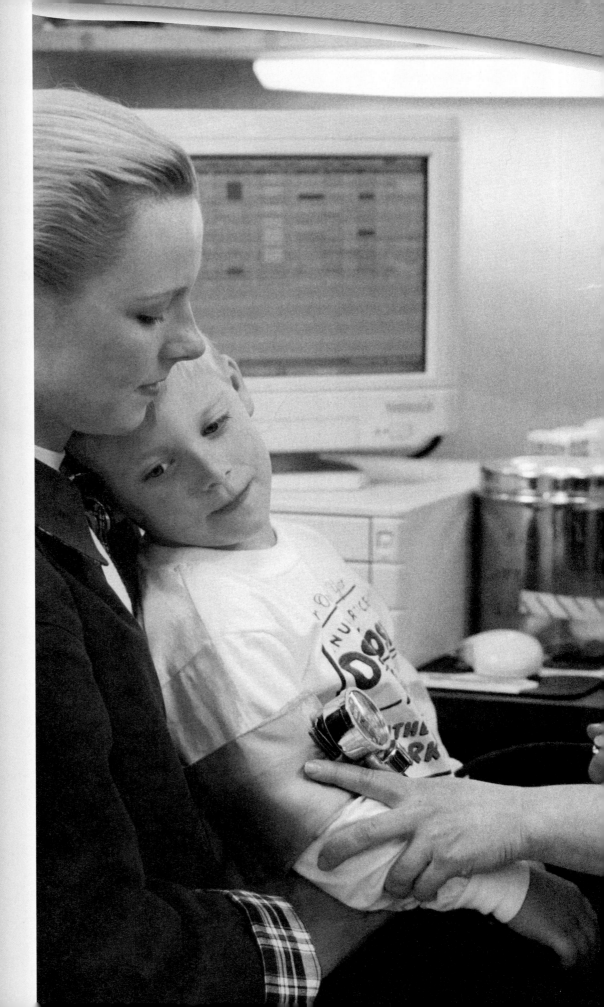

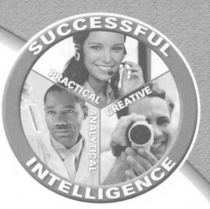

C

ountless opportunities
are available in the profession
of nursing. In this chapter you will
learn what skills you already possess and
what skills you need to develop to succeed
in completing a nursing education. Specific
specialty areas within nursing are explored to
see if one captures your interest. Remember,
consider your values as well as your professional goals as you read this
chapter. Many nurses integrate their values into their work, making a
career in nursing meaningful beyond finding and maintaining a job.
Mariah A. Taylor, RN, MSN, CPNP, and founder of the North Portland
Nurse Practitioner Community Health Clinic in Oregon, put it like this
and it holds true today:

> I base my life on a single principle—love for
> humanity. My love and service stretches to
> include all segments of humanity—all col-
> ors, all creeds, all shapes and sizes, but es-
> pecially humanity's children. I treat all chil-
> dren, from birth to 21 years, with the
> highest quality of care, compassion, and re-
> spect possible. I truly believe health care is
> a right, and not a privilege, especially for
> the underprivileged.[1]

*IN THIS CHAPTER ...*

*you will explore answers to the following questions:*

- Do you realize the opportunities? 49
- What skills do you already have to succeed in nursing? 53
- What skills do you need to develop to succeed in nursing? 55
- What are some of the career options in nursing? 57
- How do health care trends affect nursing? 67
- What can you expect once you are enrolled in school? 69

# Q & A BLUE SKY QUESTIONS DOWN-TO-EARTH ANSWERS

## Given my education, what are my options in psychiatric nursing?

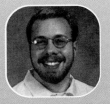

**Mark McIntyre**
Senior, Jacksonville State University, Jacksonville, Alabama

Nursing school has exposed me to many wonderful opportunities to explore my interests. I recently completed an internship for a senior adult day program, and I've also worked for a local mental health clinic. From these experiences, as well as my classes, I've discovered that I love psychiatric nursing. I found out that I prefer to work with people who suffer from pathological disorders rather than behavioral problems. I also liked the senior population because they are very appreciative, and you can see that they benefit so much from the attention and therapy they receive.

Even though I have a strong sense of what I like to do, I'm not sure what direction to take next. Throughout my clinicals, I've felt a little unsure about the setting I want to work in. The work environments in the smaller, local clinics don't appeal to me because most of their patients seem to exhibit conduct and substance-related disorders *rather* than clinical illnesses such as schizophrenia, which is my main interest. I've also heard that there's a high degree of burnout among staff. I don't think I want to work in hospitals, either, but I wonder if that will hinder my nursing career.

Presently I'm working part time as a pharmacy technician for a mental health clinic, and I'm enjoying it. Many people tell me that the field of pharmaceutical sales is wide open and is hiring BSNs right out of college, but I fear that such a position may take me away from patient contact. Because I'm a senior and will be graduating soon, I'm hoping to find my niche. Given my education, what are my options in psychiatric nursing?

## PRACTICAL ANSWERS

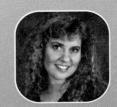

**Laurel Brink**
Graduate student, Gonzaga University, Spokane, Washington

### To determine what you want to be, it is important to know who you want to become.

In her book *From Novice to Expert (1984),* Patricia Benner describes the transitions nurses make from one level of knowledge and competency to another. She says that the gift of being a novice is that it offers a tremendous opportunity for growth and professional development. The challenge is to discover, often by trial and error, strategies that develop the dimensions of psychiatric nursing needed for expertise. It is vital to read professional journals, attend seminars, and join and volunteer in professional psychiatric nursing and mental health organizations to network and form mentor relationships. These relationships can provide invaluable input about this multifaceted field.

In setting realistic goals as a new graduate, I recommend working for at least one year as a community mental health nurse. This can be instrumental in understanding the system all the way from payer sources to direct client services, referral resources, and creating partnerships and connections. Every mental illness has physiological and behavioral components. Schizophrenic clients may have substance abuse problems as well. Hospital experience is difficult to replace. It is in this setting that the schizophrenic client resides when decompensation occurs. In either inpatient or outpatient settings, the psychiatric nurse is the best therapeutic tool for modeling healthy behavior. It is also important to check with your State Nurse Practice Act to see what standards and parameters for practice a bachelor of science registered nurse degree allows.

With breadth of knowledge and experience, psychiatric nurses can serve as client advocates in a special way. Social activism on behalf of this vulnerable, high-risk population is a truly important societal need. Nurses grounded in holistic health, the integration of body, mind, and spirit, can expand and evolve models of psychiatric care. Graduate school preparation will further increase your capacity to develop knowledge, expertise, and credibility that can be translated into action. The importance of education and training throughout one's professional career cannot be stressed enough.

Competence in nursing develops over time. The key to prevention of burnout is setting limits and maintaining principles of self-care. And remember, when you feel overwhelmed and discouraged, staying grounded in your purpose and passion for becoming a nurse will help you endure these growth-producing times. To determine what you want to be, it is important to know who you want to become. Writing a personal mission statement will help you reflect on and define your deepest values, talents, and sense of mission needed to guide your professional development. To stimulate thinking along these lines, I highly recommend Barbara M. Dossey's book *Florence Nightingale: Mystic, Visionary, Healer,* Springhouse Corp. (2000), Springhouse, PA. Our challenge is to continue to grow and take initiative to stimulate positive change in our own lives, as well as work with integrity in the health care institutions we serve. The proud history of nursing provides strength for the journey.

# Do You Realize the *Opportunities?*

If you are choosing nursing as a career, be it as a first or second career, you need to be aware of the intense drive by nursing organizations and health care specialists to increase recruitment of younger people, minorities, and men into nursing. Although part of this is motivated by the critical need to increase diversity in nursing, another reason is the nursing shortage.

The U.S. Department of Health and Human Services (DHHS) reported a shortage of 168,000 nurses nationwide in 2003.[2] By 2015, all 50 states will experience the shortage. The shortage of nurses is rapidly increasing, and by 2020, it is estimated that it will reach 1 million nurses with only 64% of the nurses needed.[3] Areas of shortage vary by state, but in hospitals the worst vacancy rates are seen in critical care units (14.6%) and medical-surgical care (14.1%).[4] The American Hospital Association stated nursing shortages are contributing to emergency department overcrowding and the need to close beds. Geriatrics and community and public health are also areas that are in need of nurses.[5] According to the current DHHS information, the shortage is a problem of both supply and demand.[6]

## The Supply Problem: Not Enough Nurses

There are a number of reasons for the nursing shortage:

- **Enrollment in nursing schools is not growing fast enough.**[7] There has been a 9.6% increase in enrollments, but it is not enough to meet the need for more nurses. A big part of the problem is a shortage of faculty in the schools to teach nurses. Without enough faculty, qualified students are being turned away in record numbers.

- **Aging of the RN workforce.** Without new and younger RNs coming into the workforce, the overall population of nurses are getting older. A third of older nurses today expect to leave nursing—mainly to retire—in the next three years.[8]

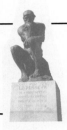

## Attention

*"Tell me to what you pay attention and I will tell you who you are."*

JOSÉ ORTEGA Y GASSETT

The American Association of Colleges of Nursing (AACN) adds the following to the list of supply problems:

- **Job burnout and dissatisfaction.** Nurses are leaving the profession as a result of working conditions that lead to burnout and job dissatisfaction. The AACN reports on a study by Linda Aiken in the October 2002 issue of the *Journal of the American Medical Association* that "nurses reported greater job dissatisfaction and emotional exhaustion when they were responsible for more patients than they can safely care for." Researcher Aiken concluded that "failure to retain nurses contributes to avoidable patient deaths."[9]

- **The shortage is affecting patient access to health care.**[10] Patients are more prone to complications and other problems when there are not enough nurses. Numerous reports and studies have linked nursing care with patient safety and good outcomes. Without nurses, patients and health care suffer.

## The Demand Problem: More Nurses Needed

- **Hospital acuity is increasing.** More nurses are needed in hospitals because the patients are sicker (the patients are more acutely ill). This is referred to as increasing hospital acuity. People do not stay in the hospital as long as they used to, and technology is increasing the capabilities of intensive care units and procedures. More nurses are needed to care for these patients, especially nurses with specialized skills.

The DHHS gave the following as the "driving forces and trends" increasing the demand for more nurses in 2002, and they hold true today:[11]

- **Population growth and aging.** "Recent projections show the nation's population will grow 18% between 2000 and 2020, resulting in an additional 50 million people who will require health care." Baby boomers are expected to increase the numbers of older people, and life expectancy is increasing as well. All in all, there will be more older people who need nursing care.

- **Trends in health care financing.** Although many people remain uninsured, the majority are still able to pay for expensive health care. Technological advances in health care, along with an increase in the disposable income per person in the United States, mean there will be a higher demand for these services by people who can pay for them out of pocket.

# Explore Your Interests

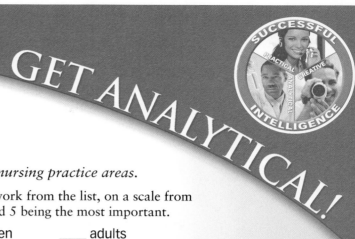

*Evaluate your interests and connect them to nursing practice areas.*

Rate each of the types of populations you could work from the list, on a scale from 1 to 5, with 1 being the least important to you and 5 being the most important.

____ newborns     ____ adolescents     ____ men     ____ adults

____ infants     ____ pediatrics     ____ elders

____ children     ____ families     ____ geriatric

____ maternity     ____ women     ____ hospice

*Rate each of the types of settings you could work in with on the list on a scale from 1 to 5, with 1 being the least important to you and 5 being the most important.*

## Hospital

- Acute care ____
- Critical care ____
- Emergency department ____
- Psychiatric ____

## Ambulatory Care

- Primary care clinics ____
- Family health clinics ____
- Private practices ____
- Other specialty clinics ____
- Outpatient surgical centers ____

## Community, Public Health, and Home Health Nursing

- Community centers ____
- People's homes ____
- City, county, or state health departments ____

## Extended-Stay Facility

- Nursing home ____
- Rehabilitation center ____

*Combine and write your top three choices here:*

1. _____
2. _____
3. _____

*Describe why you are interested in these populations and areas of practice.*

_____

_____

# Curing the Nursing Shortage: Recommendations

The General Accounting Office suggested as early as 2001 that "efforts undertaken to improve the workplace environment may both reduce the likelihood of nurses leaving the field and encourage more young people to enter the nursing profession."[12] This solution is consistent with the problem of nurses leaving the profession because of burnout and dissatisfaction.

Peter Buerhaus and others suggest the following as strategies to help the shortage:[13]

- Improve, or "fix," the problems in the workplace that lead to burnout and job dissatisfaction. Improvements can be made to improve the workplace climate.

- Measure and demonstrate the ways that nurses contribute to quality patient care. Nursing has been undervalued in its role in ensuring quality care. As noted earlier, studies are beginning to show how a lack of nurses can contribute to complications and even death.

- Recruit and retain nurses. Hospitals and health care organizations have to work hard to continuous recruit and retain nurses. This includes long-term methods to make the workplace satisfying and to reduce burnout.

- Increase the capacity to educate nurses. More faculty are needed to meet the demand for more nurses.

- Improve the image of nursing. Through campaigns to educate people about what nurses do and how they contribute to health care, more students will pursue the profession. Career opportunities and the shortage must be highlighted.

- Increase the diversity of nursing through recruiting men and people of different cultures and ethnicities. Nursing is serving an increasingly diverse society. To meet the needs of that society, nursing itself must step up by working hard to improve the diversity of the profession.

The AACN's recommendations focus on unity among nursing organizations. The AACN suggests that leaders from national nursing organizations work together to "ensure safe, quality nursing care for consumers and a sufficient supply of registered nurses to deliver that care."[14] AACN also supports legislative efforts to pass bills such as the Nurse Reinvestment Act, designed to provide financial support to students and potential nursing faculty. Improving nursing's image is also vital to increasing the numbers of nurses.

A shortage of BSN prepared nurses can also affect the quality of patient care. In a study published in the September 24, 2003, issue of the *Journal of the American Medical Association (JAMA),* Linda Aiken and her colleagues at the University of Pennsylvania found that patients cared for by nurses with higher levels of education had better outcomes; specifically, they had a better chance of surviving. "In hospitals, a 10 percent increase in the proportion of nurses holding BSN degrees decreased the risk of patient death and failure to rescue by 5 percent."[15]

The nurse researchers also found that when the nurses did not have too many patients to care for, patient survival improved. And it showed that when there were enough nurses to take care of the patients, the nurses themselves experienced less burnout and job dissatisfaction. Adequate staffing would lead to fewer nurses leaving the profession, which, in turn, would improve the shortage.

## Cultural Diversity

"Knowledge of cultural diversity is vital at all levels of nursing practice."

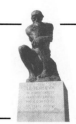

AMERICAN NURSES ASSOCIATION POSITION STATEMENT ON ETHICS AND HUMAN RIGHTS

Nursing offers many career options, which is a plus in terms of employment opportunity, scholarships and grants to attend school, and encouragement from nursing organizations. At the same time, as a professional nurse, you will be faced with many challenges and difficulties in trying to meet the needs of society. But take heart: Opportunities abound, options are abundant, and a life of meaningful work is within your grasp.

# What *Skills* Do You *Already Have* to Succeed in Nursing?

## Science and Humanities

If you love science and are good at it, you have it made. If you love science and are fair at it, you also have it made, although perhaps you will need to work harder. If you love science but have a hard time with it, or if it's been so long since you took a science class that you don't remember much about it anymore, don't give up. Two things will help you succeed: determination and a tutor. Determination is your job and a tutor is your school's. Free tutoring is available because almost all graduate students work in this role as part of their education and training.

Nancy Hoffman, who had been a nursing adviser at Washington State University, confided that when she decided to return to school as a science major after raising her two children, the thought of taking chemistry terrified her. All Nancy could think of was how much she had hated high school chemistry. When she returned to school, the first class she took was biology. Her grade was a C. She said, "I thanked God every day for that C."

Nancy knew that if she was to continue in school with any success, she would have to find a way to get through chemistry. She explained, "Chemistry was like traveling to a foreign land where the people spoke a foreign language. I couldn't understand any of it." So she went to her school's learning center and found a tutor who was a graduate student in chemistry. For the first two months of the semester, Nancy met with him after every class to review the material. Her final grade in organic chemistry? An A.

### How to Find a Tutor

This book will help you become a better student, which will go a long way toward ensuring your success as a nursing major, but part of succeeding is knowing when to ask for help. Tutors are an excellent source of help with any class. Contact your school's Academic Office or adult education center, or ask your adviser, teaching assistant, or instructor to help you find one. The people at your school want to help you succeed in college, and they will likely bend over backward to assist you. It's possible they are sitting in their offices right now, waiting for you to come see them.

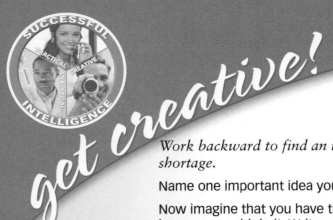

# Map Out a Nursing Shortage Solution

*Work backward to find an interesting solution, all your own, to the nursing shortage.*

Name one important idea you have.

Now imagine that you have the ability to implement that solution. Describe how you would do it. Write your answer here, in a paragraph, as though you were telling someone about the specific steps you would take.

You just created a potential solution! As you begin college and nursing, let your creative mind help you find solutions to problems.

Now Nancy knew how to review on her own, or with other students, and she received A's in all her science classes. She advises all students to visit their school's learning center to find out who, or what, can help them. As Nancy explained, "Don't let embarrassment keep you from asking for help."

## Interest in Health Care and People

Another thing you have going for you is that you want to do something that involves working with other people, or you want to contribute in some way to the health and well-being of someone somewhere. A background in the liberal arts will help you achieve this. Whatever you read in literature courses, view or hear in art courses, and read and write about in sociology and psychology will help you be a better nursing student. All these areas help you understand human nature in all its various forms. Your ability to talk with others is enhanced by your knowledge of different subjects, and talking with others is a key to success in nursing. Communication is one of the most important skills to develop as you go on your way.

An interest in doing something that helps people is a very good start toward a career in nursing. It is also likely that unless you have already worked in a health care setting with nurses or have family members who are nurses and who talk about their work, you do not have a realistic image of what nurses do. If your source about nurses is television or movies, you definitely have a confused image of nursing. Television shows have few positive images of nurses, failing to take into consideration the complexity and responsibility involved in being a nurse.

In one survey, 3,253 college students, with an average age of 25, and over half who were nonwhite females, gave several reasons for wanting to become a nurse.[16] These included that nursing is an interesting career, has a good income, and has good job security. In a second survey from North Dakota, 568 high school students (average age 16.6 years and mostly white) were surveyed about health care and nursing careers. Most students said they planned to attend a four-year college, 38% planned to pursue a career in health care, and of those, 38% planned to become nurses. The students wanting to be nurses gave as their reasons that nurses make a difference in people's lives and the availability of jobs. The majority of all students surveyed agreed that nursing is important and that nurses care for people in times of need.[17]

# What *Skills* Do You Need to *Develop* to Succeed in Nursing?

To determine what skills you need to develop to be successful in nursing, consider a survey of thousands of oncology (cancer) nurses. The nurses were asked to give three words that they thought most accurately describe a good oncology nurse. The top five were *caring, compassion, knowledge, dedication,* and *professionalism.*[18] Add to these *advocacy, creativity, mathematics, observation,* and *critical thinking,* and you have a list of essential nursing attributes.

## Caring

What does caring mean to you? *Caring* is a term that is so strongly associated with nursing, it is usually the first thing people think about being a nurse. Care is the heart and soul of nursing. Caring means taking the time for actively listening; advocating for those in need; valuing and respecting all individuals; being able to examine your own biases and reflect on your thoughts and actions; and such things as making pain relief a priority and the healing process an act of body, mind, and spirit.

## Compassion

Compassion is the ability to be considerate, humane, merciful, and kind. Being considerate of another's needs despite your own beliefs, acting with respect and concern for another's well-being, and being able to assist others toward a full development of their potential in any given circumstance is what compassion is all about.

## Knowledge

Understanding theories used in nursing, including scientific theories, those related to health behaviors, and especially nursing theories and diagnoses, is essential. Knowledge includes the ability to put theory and research into practice using the types of critical thinking and inquiry skills as discussed in Chapter 2.5.

## Dedication

Commitment with diligence is essential in nursing practice. Sticking with a project, despite initial or repeated problems, is especially important in research, in your studies, and in nursing practice. Attention to detail and careful analysis and execution of procedures can be developed in science classes and, later, in nursing school.

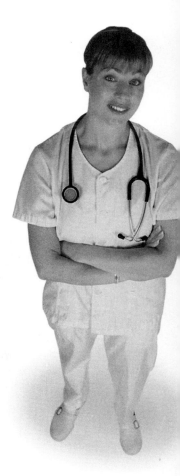

# Professionalism

Professional behavior is developed through belonging to, supporting, and participating in nursing organizations. These organizations, such as the American Nurses Association, work on many levels to promote nursing practice, health and welfare of the public, and health policy through social and political action. Professional actions include respect for others at all times and acting with integrity and for the best of your clients and fellow nursing colleagues.

# Advocacy

To advocate for yourself, another individual, or a community means that you use your expertise as an RN to protect human rights. RNs may do this by helping others make informed decisions or by acting as a mediator between a client and a doctor, family members, or even the legal system. To advocate is to inform and support a person, provide desired information, and present information in a way that can be understood. It also means understanding that someone may not want information. Advocacy means that an individual's or group's needs are your main concern. It requires you to be assertive, convey concern, understand different communication styles, and practice good working relationships.

# Creativity

Many discoveries and solutions to problems come from creativity or from a mind that can see things just a little bit differently from others. Having a broad education and experience in literature, philosophy, and politics will help you develop the ability to view problems in fresh new ways. Each field of study has its ways of viewing and understanding the world. The more of these you learn, the more flexible and adaptable you will be in your ability and skills as a nursing student and as a nurse.

# Mathematics

You've no doubt heard people freely admit that they have a problem with math, or a "math block." Have you ever heard anyone freely admit that they can't read? Admission of this problem is perceived as shameful, yet saying the same of math is acceptable. What does this say about our view of math skills? The ability to use math is essential in nursing. Most nursing schools require you to take a math test of medication calculations before you can proceed in your course work. You will also need to take a course in statistics to learn about nursing research. Math skills are not optional in the information age of the twenty-first century.

# Observation

Observation is a skill that many nurses will tell you is their greatest asset as a nurse. The ability to study people and nature, see patterns, and notice things that others may not notice requires astute observational skills. All nursing endeavors demand the ability to see, hear, smell, and touch. Observation skills can be enhanced in many ways, such as by taking a course on how to identify plants and trees. Anatomy, microbiology, even art courses allow you plenty of opportunity to practice observing attributes of things you may not have noticed before. Observation is a skill that is developed over time and one that is crucial to the assessment process—a huge part of being a nurse.

## Critical Thinking

Do you question what others say? What you read? What you see? If so, you have what is called healthy skepticism, and healthy skepticism is important to critical thinking. For instance, suppose you read a newspaper article on the effect of marijuana use on mental illness. Your understanding of the article is that there is a link between past use of marijuana and present-day symptoms of depression. In other words, the article implies that marijuana use is a cause of mental illness. However, if you think critically you may question this cause-and-effect statement. One way you might do this is to ask this question: Are people with mental illness, or who have a predisposition to mental illness, more likely to smoke marijuana in the first place? Can you see how this is different from the hypothesis presented in the article? This is an example of healthy skepticism, which causes you to ask this question: Is this right? And it is an example of critical thinking: What else could cause the problem?

As a nurse you will need to do this kind of thinking. Here is another example: A patient comes into the emergency department. She is an elder who has had frequent falls and increasing instability when walking. She is sent off for many tests to rule out neurological problems and chemical imbalances. You, the RN, are thinking of other causes and asking the question: What else could cause the symptoms? You examine her shoes and find that one has a missing heel and a large hole worn through the bottom. After numerous tests at great cost, you discover, by using your critical thinking, that her shoes have been the source of the problem all along. Critical thinking will save lives, save money, and improve your patients' quality of life.

# What Are Some of the *Career Options* in Nursing?

Nursing is divided into specialty areas based either on the setting of the practice or the population served. Many of these areas overlap. For instance, you may want to be a pediatric nurse, which is one of the nursing specialty areas based on the population served—children. But will the practice setting be in a hospital, in an outpatient clinic, in home health, or in a clinic for homeless children? The areas described next are intended to give you an idea of some of the many options available in nursing.

## Practice Settings

Nearly all health care services involve care by nurses, and approximately 56% percent of that care occurs in hospitals. But the number of RNs working in other settings is increasing as changes in health care systems lean toward shorter hospital stays and more preventive health care.

## Setting in Detail: What Is Hospital Nursing?

Hospital nurses form the largest group of nurses. Many are staff nurses, providing patient care management and bedside or direct nursing care. They also supervise licensed practical nurses, aides, and unlicensed assistive personnel. Hospital nurses usually choose one area such as surgery, maternity, pediatrics, emergency room, intensive care, or treatment of cancer patients, or they may rotate among departments.

| A Sample of Hospital Departments and Units | |
| --- | --- |
| intensive care | air ambulance |
| step-down or acute care | home health |
| outpatient | hospice |
| operating room | research |
| postoperative recovery room | chemical dependency |
| labor and delivery | psychiatric |
| emergency | |

**The roles.** Hospital nurses work as staff nurses on units or in departments. They also work as managers and administrators; as educators for current and new staff; as computer specialists; and in quality management, infection control, and research.

**Educational preparation.** Hospitals hire many new graduates. Depending on the hospital's size, specialty area, and location, your degree will matter. Management and education positions may require a BSN, a master's degree in nursing (MSN) with specialization as a clinical nurse specialist (CNS), or possibly in a developing role as the clinical nurse leader (CNL), or a doctorate in nursing (PhD) or in practice (DNP). Critical care and other specialty units such as the emergency department may require several years of experience in other nursing units.

## Setting in Detail: What Is Ambulatory Care Nursing?

Ambulatory care nursing takes place in clinics or environments where patients come to be evaluated and treated.

**A Sample of Ambulatory Care Settings**

Outpatient departments
Nurse-managed centers
Physician or nurse practitioner group practices/clinics

**The roles.** The definition that best captures the work of ambulatory care nursing is one that defines the role, rather than the setting. The American Academy of Ambulatory Care Nursing provides core values to define the practice. In summary, these values include sharing responsibility of care among patients, families, and members of the health care team; providing education to help patients and families make informed decisions (remember the definition of advocacy mentioned earlier in this chapter); giving continuity of care; and providing care that balances quality, patient needs, cost, and resource use.[19]

**Educational preparation.** Most nurses working in ambulatory care have some experience in nursing and a BSN. The expansion of the role requires increasing coordination and management in the health care network and community. One area that is expanding is telehealth (see later), a new subspecialty in which nursing care is provided using telephones, computers, and videos. New graduates may be hired if they have school experience in ambulatory care settings.

## Setting in Detail: What Is Community and Public Health Nursing?

Community and public health nursing in the United States and other countries around the world has been the backbone of health care for millions of people. Changes in health care are influencing community nursing by increasing the need for nurses who can assess entire populations (rather than just individual clients), determine areas of the greatest need for services, provide cost-effective care in teams, and evaluate future trends and practices that save money and maintain high quality. If that sounds like a big job, it is!

Public health nurses work in government and private agencies and clinics, schools, retirement communities, and other community settings. They focus on populations, individuals, and families to improve the overall health of communities. They also work as partners with communities to plan and implement programs. Public health nurses instruct individuals, families, and other groups in health education, disease prevention, nutrition, and child care. They arrange for immunizations, blood pressure testing, and other health screening. These nurses also work with community leaders, teachers, parents, and physicians in community health education.

The Pan American Health Organization (PAHO)/World Health Organization (WHO) describes public health nursing this way:

> Public health practice is characterized as much by the way the world is viewed as it is by any specific activity. The thinking of a public health worker is primarily focused on groups or populations, rather than individuals. . . . Public health professionals are deeply concerned that individuals receive the primary health care and emergency care they need. But the major focus of attention is on building the systems within which people can be healthy: safe drinking water, safe disposal of waste of all kinds, safe and nutritious food supply, safe workplaces, health education as a part of basic education.[20]

| A Sample of Community and Public Health Settings | |
| --- | --- |
| hospice | occupational health/industry |
| home health/home care | nursing school–operated nursing centers |
| mental health | insurance and managed care companies |
| rural health | schools |
| the military | disaster areas |

**Telehealth.** The New Hampshire Board of Nursing defines telehealth nursing as using the nursing process to provide care for individual patients or defined patient populations over the phone or other electronic communication media. The goal of telephone triage is appropriate patient referral to the appropriate level of care within an appropriate period of time.

Areas of nursing practice in telehealth:

- Telephone triage (which may include symptom assessment, counseling, home treatment advice, referral, and crisis intervention)[21]
- Health information and education
- Disease management
- Interactive two-way video technology (i.e., home care)

**The roles.** To understand the roles, you must think about factors that influence community and public health. They include many social problems and conditions such as illiteracy, unemployment, poverty, homelessness, substance abuse, the return of infectious diseases such as tuberculosis, chronic illnesses, women's health, violence, teen pregnancy, sexually transmitted diseases, human immunodeficiency virus/acquired immunodeficiency syndrome (HIV/AIDS), and well-child care. Community and public health nurses cannot rectify these problems alone, but through their practice they can educate, enact policy reforms, and care for the public from birth to death.

**Educational preparation.** Many community and public health nurses think that education in politics must accompany nursing education. From the list of areas that influence public health, it is easy to see why understanding health policy and politics is necessary. As with ambulatory nursing and other types of nursing, an increase in the health care system's complexity and client needs means a demand for more education. The area of greatest growth in community and public health nursing is likely to be for community nurse specialists and other advanced practice nurses with graduate degree education.

## Populations

Nurses work with all kinds of people in all stages of development and in all areas of the world. The list provided here is categorized by developmental stages, but other population categories could include people at high risk of stroke; people with diabetes, hypertension, or asthma; or those with heart disease. These divide people up based on a health condition. Following are examples of the populations served by nurses:

| | | |
|---|---|---|
| newborns | adolescents | men |
| infants | pediatrics | elders |
| children | families | geriatric |
| maternity | women | hospice |

### Population in Detail: What Is Maternity Nursing?

In maternity nursing you will work with women who are pregnant. If you think about it, this could take place in a number of settings depending on when in the pregnancy you are working with patients or what kinds of problems they are having. For instance, you could work with a pregnant woman in an office setting doing prenatal checks and education. You could work with a pregnant woman in the hospital if she comes in with a problem or to actually deliver the baby. Or, if you are a public health nurse, you might work with a pregnant woman in her home helping her prepare and doing education.

# What Do Nurses Do?

This is a difficult question to answer because the work of nurses covers so many areas. But to summarize, nurses promote health, prevent disease, and help patients cope with illness. They act as advocates and health educators for patients, families, and communities, as well as provide direct patient care by observing, assessing, and recording symptoms, reactions, and progress. RNs work with physicians and advanced practice nurses and manage client care through nursing care plans. The following sections are intended to give you an idea of a *few* areas within nursing, the setting, the roles, and the educational preparation involved.

# Advanced Practice Nursing

### What Are Advanced Registered Nurse Practitioners (ARNPs)?

Advanced practice nursing, as discussed in Chapter 1, is a growing area of nursing. At the advanced level, nurse practitioners (NPs) provide an example. NPs provide basic primary health care. They diagnose and treat common acute illnesses and injuries. NPs can prescribe medications in most states. Other advanced practice nurses include clinical nurse specialists (CNSs), certified registered nurse anesthetists (CRNAs), and certified nurse-midwives (CNMs). New roles in development include the clinical nurse leader (CNL) and the doctorate in nursing practice (DNP). The DNP will likely replace the NP, and the CNL may be added to the CNS role.

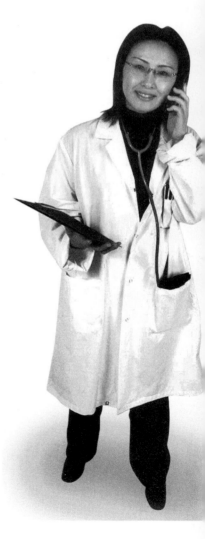

**A Sample of Advanced Practice Settings**
Nurse clinics
Reservation clinics
Physician offices
Community and public health clinics
Hospitals: all units, including emergency and critical care
Schools
Colleges
Industrial settings
Home health agencies

**The roles.** ARNPs often work in a specialty area, such as pediatrics, cardiology, or geriatrics, to name a few. They perform many functions, including primary care interventions, health assessment, risk appraisal, health education and counseling, diagnosis and management of acute minor illnesses and injuries, and management of chronic conditions.

CNSs work with patients and families in addition to acting as consultants for other nursing staff. Many serve in hospitals and on university teaching faculty. CNS roles may include clinical research, teaching, consultation, leadership, and administration. See Figure 2.1 for more information on CNSs as well as on CNMs, CRNAs, and NPs.[22]

FIGURE 2.1 Specialty areas for advanced registered nurse practitioners

| Advanced Practice Nurses | Application of Advanced Knowledge and Skills | Patient Population Served | Practice Settings |
|---|---|---|---|
| Certified Nurse-Midwife | Well-women health care: management of pregnancy, childbirth, antepartum, and postpartum care, health promotion | Childbearing women | Homes, hospitals, birthing centers, ambulatory care |
| Clinical Nurse Practitioner (Specialist) | Management of complex patient health care problems in various clinical specialty areas through direct care, consultation, research, education, and administration | Individuals with physical or psychiatric illness or disability, or maternal or child health problems | Hospitals, ambulatory care, community care, home health, rehabilitation |
| Nurse Anesthetist | Preoperative assessment, administration of anesthesia, recovery | Individuals in all age groups undergoing surgical procedures | Hospitals, operating rooms, ambulatory care, surgical settings |
| Nurse Practitioner | Management of a wide range of health problems through physical examination, diagnosis, treatment, and family/patient education and counseling; primary care and health promotion | Individuals and families, women, infants, children, elderly, adults, and others | Primary care, long-term care, ambulatory and community care, hospitals |

*Source:* Adapted from the American Association of Colleges of Nursing, 2002.

**Nurse practitioners.** About 51% of ARNPs are nursing practitioners.[23] NPs conduct physical exams; diagnose and treat common acute illnesses and injuries; provide immunizations; manage high blood pressure, diabetes, and other chronic problems; order and interpret X-rays and other laboratory tests; and counsel patients on adopting healthy lifestyles and health care options.

In addition to practicing in clinics and hospitals in metropolitan areas, the nation's estimated 141,209 NPs also deliver care in rural sites, inner cities, and other locations not adequately served by physicians, including populations such as children in schools and the elderly.[24] Many NPs work in pediatrics, family health, women's health, and other specialties, and some have private practices. NPs can prescribe medications in all states and the District of Columbia, and many states have given NPs authority to practice independently without physician collaboration or supervision. A growing number of states allow NPs to write prescriptions independently.

**Clinical nurse specialists.** Some 24% of ARNPs are clinical nurse specialists.[25] Clinical nurse specialists (CNSs) provide care in a range of specialty areas, such as cardiac, oncology, neonatal, and obstetric/gynecological nursing, as well as pediatrics, neurological nursing, and psychiatric/mental health. Working in hospitals and other clinical sites, CNSs provide acute care and mental health services, develop quality assurance procedures, and serve as educators and consultants. An estimated 75,521 CNSs are currently in practice nationwide.[26]

**Certified nurse-midwives.** Four percent of ARNPs are nurse-midwives.[27] The nation's approximately 13,643 CNMs provide prenatal and gynecological care to normal healthy women; deliver babies in hospitals, private homes, and birthing centers; and continue with follow-up postpartum care.[28]

**Certified registered nurse anesthetists.** An estimated 13% of ARNPs are nurse anesthetists.[29] More than 32,523 certified registered nurse anesthetists (CRNAs) administer more than 65% of all anesthetics given to patients each year, and they are the sole anesthesia providers in approximately a third of U.S. hospitals, according to the American Association of Nurse Anesthetists (AANA).[30] A total of 49% of CRNAs are men, a proportion much higher than in the rest of the RN population.[31] Working in the oldest of the advanced nursing specialties, CRNAs administer anesthesia for all types of surgery in settings ranging from operating rooms and dental offices to outpatient surgical centers.

## Other Nursing Roles Requiring Graduate Education

These roles include college instructors and professors, case managers, health policy and government workers, nurse entrepreneurs, parish nursing, nursing informatics, researchers, executives, and international leaders. You should be able to see that nursing is not without opportunity for just about any interest you may have. The career field is growing in all directions, and the only limit is your imagination, education, and experience.

**Educational preparation.** ARNPs, or those in any advanced nursing role, have met higher educational and clinical practice requirements beyond the basic nursing education and licensing required of all RNs. At this time this requires an master's degree, which usually takes two to three years to earn. It also includes special licensing and certification examinations, depending on the specialty area. Of nurses working in education, the majority have a master's or doctorate degree. If you think you will want to take on an advanced role, plan on continuing your education for up to four years after you earn your undergraduate degree.

## What Are Some Less Common Nursing Roles?

A number of other jobs are available to nurses, including

- Entrepreneur/consultant
- Medical editor/writer
- Nursing informatics
- Pharmacy/medical sales
- Bioterrorism and disaster response nurse
- Flight nurse
- Forensic nurse
- International nurse
- Military nurse

- Parish nurse
- Research nurse
- Alternative therapy nurse
- Travel nurse

## Less Common Roles in Detail: What Is International Nursing?

The International Council of Nurses (ICN) plays a role in international nursing. The ICN's goals are to influence health, social policy, and professional and socioeconomic standards worldwide, and to empower national nursing associations to act on behalf of nurses and the public.[32]

With globalization, what happens in one place on the globe affects us all. A disease in one country can more easily find its way to another than ever before (see later section, "How Do Health Care Trends Affect Nursing?"). Many schools and colleges of nursing are using international student exchange as a method for educating nursing students about important global issues. If you have an opportunity to do an exchange, take advantage of it. Even an experience within the United States that is different from where you live will be beneficial.

**Resources.** For further information on international nursing opportunities, begin with the following:

**International Council of Nurses:** www.icn.ch/abouticn.htm. This site has links to international health sites, nursing practice guidelines, policy statements, and nursing employment opportunities.

**International Nursing:** http://nursingworld.org/inc/. This site offers links to WHO and PAHO. It offers information on job opportunities and nursing publications.

## Less Common Roles in Detail: What Is Alternative and Complementary Therapy in Nursing?

More than 40% of people in the United States are using therapies such as massage, chiropractics, aromatherapy, hypnosis, acupuncture, herbal medicines, and yoga. This represents only a few of the alternative, or complementary, treatments. These kinds of therapies are consistent with a nursing value of providing holistic care. The treatments are a part of holistic care, but, as with other medicine and therapies, they do not constitute all of it. Alternative therapy is often used adjunctly with more accepted Western medicine, thus the term *complementary*. Nurses act both as providers of therapy and as patient educators. Nurses need to educate patients about the safety and efficacy of alternative therapy as well as the benefits. For more information on alternative therapies and on holistic nursing in all its forms, visit http://ahna.org or search the Internet. Holistic nursing practice is now recognized by the American Nurses Association as a specialty practice.

The Hospice and Palliative Nurses Association provides the following definitions of terms:[33]

Alternative therapies: Complementary and other unconventional therapies used instead of conventional medical and surgical therapies.

Complementary therapies: Used together with conventional medicine.

Integrative therapies: Combine mainstream medical therapies and alternative therapies with scientific evidence of safety and effectiveness.

## Less Common Roles in Detail: What Is Parish Nursing?

Parish nursing is growing in the United States. This type of nursing is similar to community health nursing except that the population of interest is generally a congregation of people involved in one church, temple, or mosque. Since 1997, the ANA has recognized parish nursing as a nursing specialty. Some characteristics are common among parish nurses. They are RNs, are part of the ministry staff, have taken courses in parish nursing, and focus on holistic care that includes health promotion and disease prevention with emphasis on spiritual care.

Following are the "Assumptions Regarding Parish Nursing Practice and the Curriculum" from the International Parish Nurse Resource Center:[34]

- The participant is a registered nurse with a current license or a student in a baccalaureate nursing education.
- Parish nursing is considered a calling in which ministry shapes the practice.
- The practice of parish nursing requires specialized knowledge and skills.
- The practice of parish nursing encourages a partnership model between parish nurses, individuals, families, congregations, and communities across the life span.
- Parish nursing contributes to the health of the faith community.
- Parish nursing values Faith Community Nursing: Scope and Standards of Practice (ANA/HMA, 2005), in the United States; parish nurses in other countries are accountable to their own specific standards of practice.

## Less Common Roles in Detail: What Is Forensic Nursing?

The International Association of Forensic Nurses (IAFN) is the only international professional organization of registered nurses formed exclusively to develop, promote, and disseminate information about the science of forensic nursing. Forensic nursing applies nursing to public and legal processes. It includes health care in

> the scientific investigation and treatment of trauma and/or death of victims and perpetrators of abuse, violence, criminal activity and traumatic accidents. The forensic nurse provides direct services to individual clients, consultation services to nursing, medical and law related agencies, as well as providing expert court testimony in areas dealing with trauma and/or questioned death investigative processes, adequacy of services delivery and specialized diagnoses of specific conditions as related to nursing.[35]

For more information, search the Internet or visit the IAFN's website at www.iafn.org.

## Less Common Roles in Detail: What Is Travel Nursing?

Many nurses consider the opportunity to travel and work a good one. Agencies generally help nurses locate the places they want to go and negotiate the conditions of their work agreements. You must be an RN with recent nursing experience and good references. Length of positions vary but may last from one to three months. Until nursing has interstate licensing, you have to obtain a license for each state in which you work. Many agencies provide housing and, sometimes, may include health benefits and travel reimbursement. There are many agencies and an International Traveling Nurses Association. For more information, search the Internet for "traveling nurses."

## Less Common Roles in Detail: What Is Bioterrorism and Disaster Response Nursing?

Disaster response and relief are not new to nursing. Across the globe, nurses have had to face this problem during times of war and acts of terrorism, and with the terrorist events of 9/11, it is now an even greater concern for nurses in the United States. Hospitals, communities, and health care agencies are working on disaster preparedness in light of spreading fears of anthrax and smallpox. The American Nurses Association is involved with other nursing organizations on this front. Teams are being formed in many communities to respond to disasters.

Public health nursing includes all aspects of disaster nursing. According to the Washington State Nurses Association, the system may not be in such good shape to face future threats:

> Public health is also our first line of defense in responding to bioterrorism and in disaster preparedness. Through decades of neglect and erosion in funding, the ability of our public health nurses and local public health departments to perform core functions has been drastically reduced. It is absolutely critical that we have an adequate and long-term stable funding source for public health.
>
> With the continuing threats of terrorist attacks, natural disasters and pandemic flu, we simply cannot wait. The solution is a dedicated long-term stable and adequate source of funding for our public health infrastructure, one in which the role of public health nurses are fully recognized and utilized.[36]

Following are the types of information nurses are interested in related to bioterrorism:

How to care for patients
How to protect yourself
How to prepare your hospital/community
Developing a national nurses response team

Information on these topics and more can be found through the American Nurses Association website at www.nursingworld.org/news/disaster/.

# How Do Health Care *Trends* Affect Nursing?

Health care trends will affect your work as a nursing student and as a nurse. The curriculum and what you learn should reflect the changes occurring in health care. For instance, one of the drivers for the increase in health costs is technology. Technology is also a tool to make health care better. Technology is advancing quickly, and many useful tests, treatments, and diagnostics are being developed. In school you will learn about technology such as nursing informatics and research. But technology and other trends also raise many questions—ethical, legal, and economic.

In terms of being a nurse, an RN, and a professional, you must think *big*. Thinking about health care trends is thinking big. And thinking big also means knowing how to ask questions. This may be the most important skill you can learn, and it will bring you back to critical thinking. Health care trends will change, and your thinking and questioning will change as well. Will you be ready to work with the new trends? Anticipate them and work proactively? This will take some work, but the *trend* in nursing is critical thinking and taking a leadership role in health care.

The major trends in health care have been written about by most of the major policy and professional nursing organizations. A report from the Institute of Medicine, *The Quality Chasm,* described current thinking about how health care needs to change. Following are examples of how we have to change how we view health care:[37]

1. Current: Care is based on face-to-face visits. New: Care is continuous healing relationships. Patients receive care when needed, including by Internet and telephone.

2. Current: Professional autonomy drives variability in how and what type of care is given. New: Care is customized according to patients' needs and values.

3. Current: Professionals control care. New: The patient is the source of control. Patients get information and opportunity to exercise the degree of control they choose over the decisions that affect them.

4. Current: Information is a record. New: Knowledge is shared freely. Patients have access to their own medical information and to clinical knowledge.

5. Current: Decision making is based on training and experience. New: Decision making is based on evidence. Patients should receive care based on the best available scientific evidence.

6. Current: "Do no harm" is an individual responsibility. New: Safety is a system property. Patients should be safe from injury caused by the care system.

7. Current: Secrecy is necessary. New: Transparency is necessary. The health care system should make information available to patients and their families including information describing the system's performance on safety, evidence-based practice, and patient satisfaction.

8. Current: The system reacts to needs. New: Needs are anticipated. The health care system should anticipate patients' needs rather than simply reacting to events.

9. Current: Cost reduction is sought. New: Waste is continuously decreased. The health care system should not waste resources or patients' time.

10. Current: Preference is given to professional roles over the system. New: Cooperation among clinicians is a priority. Clinicians and institutions should actively collaborate and communicate. (Cooperation is a primary professional obligation, "trumping" traditional roles associated with degree, profession, or gender.)

Reading the IOM list, it is not hard to see why nurses and other health care providers need more education to work with complex systems. Other trends are related to the health care environment. From the National League for Nursing comes a list of the top-10 health care trends:[38]

1. Changing demographics and increasing diversity

2. Technological explosion

3. Globalization

4. Era of the educated consumer, alternative therapies and genomics, and palliative care

5. Shift to population-based care and the increasing complexity of patient care

6. Cost of health care

7. Impact of health policy and regulation

8. Collaborative practice

9. Current nursing shortage

10. Advances in nursing science and research

Many of these trends are directly tied to either the demand for more nurses or the supply shortage of nurses. Changing demographics include the need for more nurses as the population grows older. Changing demographics also mean that in the United States more nurses of color are needed to reflect the changing population. Globalization means that diseases are crossing borders and that interdependence is more important than ever. Increases in HIV/AIDS in other countries affect the United States as we increase humanitarian foreign aid to help others and to protect ourselves. The rise of tuberculosis is another example of how globalization affects the United States. Immigrants may increase the risk of infection, and public health nurses are involved in programs to test and administer treatments. If you look at the top-10 list you can probably think of many other ways nursing is involved with health care trends.

Read the following statement by the Joint Commission on Accreditation of Healthcare Organizations, and then refer back to the list of trends to see how nurses play a key role in affecting these trends:

Nearly every person's health care experience involves the contribution of a registered nurse. Birth and death, and all the various forms of care in between, are attended by the knowledge, support and comforting of nurses. Few professions offer such a special opportunity for meaningful work as nursing. Yet, this country is facing a growing shortage of registered nurses. When there are too few nurses, patient safety is threatened and health care quality is diminished. Indeed, access even to the most critical care may be barred. And, the ability of the health system to respond to a mass casualty event is severely compromised. The impending crisis in nurse staffing has the potential to impact the very health and security of our society if definitive steps are not taken to address its underlying causes.[39]

## How Will *Changes* in Educational Preparation Affect RNs?

For many years attempts have been made to raise the educational requirements for the initial RN license, or entry into practice, to a bachelor's degree and, possibly, to create new job titles. These changes, should they occur, have to be made through state legislation. Changes in licensing requirements will not affect RNs currently licensed with diplomas or associate degrees, who would be "grandfathered" into the new laws.

The Bureau of Labor Statistics (2006–2007) says on this matter, "Individuals considering nursing should carefully weigh the pros and cons of enrolling in a B.S.N. program, since their advancement opportunities are broader. In fact, some career paths are open only to nurses with bachelor's or advanced degrees. A bachelor's degree is generally necessary for administrative positions, and is a prerequisite for admission to graduate nursing programs in research, consulting, teaching, or a clinical specialization."[40]

# What Can You *Expect* Once You Are *Enrolled* in School?

To preview what you can expect once you are accepted and enroll in a school or college of nursing, read what the *Occupational Outlook Handbook* for 2006–2007 says about nursing education:

> Nursing education includes classroom instruction and supervised clinical experience in hospitals and other health facilities. Students take courses in anatomy, physiology, microbiology, chemistry, nutrition, psychology and other behavioral sciences, and nursing. Course work also includes liberal arts classes. Supervised clinical experience is provided in hospital departments, such as pediatrics, psychiatry, maternity, and surgery. A growing number of programs include clinical experience in nursing homes, public health departments, home health agencies, and ambulatory clinics.[41]

Nursing school is not easy. It takes hard work, commitment, and time to attend classes, study, attend clinical fully prepared, and work on projects and exams. Many schools are working to accommodate students who may not be able to attend school full time. Some offer schedules that make it possible to take fewer courses at any one time. This can allow students with families, or who need to work during school, more flexibility. Some courses are offered for students who do not live near the university. For instance, at

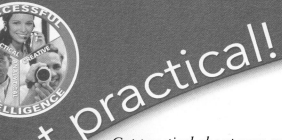
# Discover New Options

*Get practical about new areas in nursing you haven't considered.*

Go to one of the nursing websites listed at the end of this chapter. Explore the sites to find a field of nursing that you had not considered in the past but one that looks potentially interesting.

List three reasons why this area interests you:

1. _____
2. _____
3. _____

After examining these reasons, decide what you could do, or who you could talk to, to learn more about it.

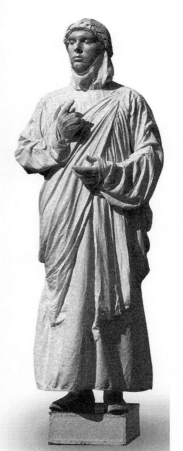

Washington State University the main nursing college is in Spokane, but students take courses from four different sites around the state via live video and the Internet.

If you plan to go to nursing school, you will need to consider the commitment carefully. You will also want to talk to advisers at the schools you are considering to discuss such topics as schedules and accommodations for working students and students with families. Talk to advisers about their admissions criteria so you can plan ahead. Many schools today are turning students away because of a nursing faculty shortage.

Nursing school is a rewarding experience. It will open you to a whole new way of seeing the world. It will prepare you for a lifelong career that is exciting and rewarding. You will be changed forever by attending nursing school; you will make new friends, learn incredible amounts of knowledge, change behaviors, and become a professional. Preparing for this experience is vital. Talk to other nursing students, advisers, and nurses to help you get ready.

# *Docendo Discimus*

This Latin phrase means "we learn by teaching." As a student you may think you are doing all the learning and your instructors all the teaching. But you teach when helping other students in laboratories and in study groups, and you teach your instructors through inquiring questions, thoughtful answers, and describing life experiences. The concept that people learn as they teach emphasizes the cyclical and ongoing nature of education.

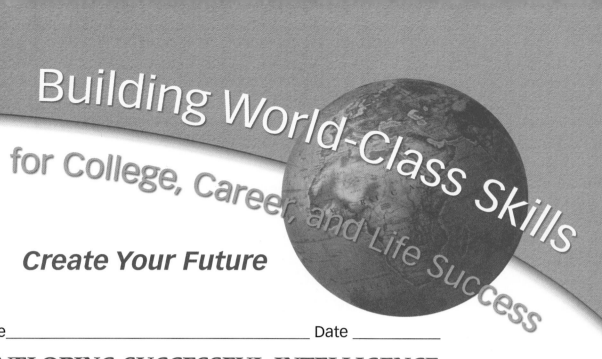

# Building World-Class Skills
## for College, Career, and Life Success

### Create Your Future

Name_____ Date _____

# DEVELOPING SUCCESSFUL INTELLIGENCE
## *Putting It All Together*

### Learning from Others

*Tools to Use*

College catalog

Other students

Instructors and professors

Career center

Student organization members

Faculty websites

Using any or all of these tools, choose one person who works in a nursing practice area of interest to you. Base your decision on the recommendations of others or on information from faculty Web pages. This person may also have research experience. He or she should be available to you, that is, have on-campus office hours. Call the person and request a meeting.

Ask the following questions and add any of your own:

1. What is your educational background?

   _____

2. How did you decide on this area?

   _____

   _____

   _____

3. Was it hard to find work in this area, and how did you go about it?

   _____

   _____

   _____

4. What areas are related to this work?

_____

_____

5. Do you ever have students work with you?

_____

6. Can I contact you later if I have more questions?

_____

# TEAM BUILDING

## *Collaborative Solutions*

**Alertness to Real-World Research in the News**. To be a success in nursing, you must study all aspects of it, including what is in the news. Pay attention to what appears in the popular press (newspapers, magazines, television news) and in scientific journals.

1. For one week, review a local newspaper and the local television news. Keep notes on the health news presented.
2. In class, divide into small groups and discuss your notes, looking for common threads between the newsworthy information and other social or political trends.
3. In small groups, discuss whether there is a great deal of information about nurses or very little. Discuss why.

**Alertness to Nursing Images on TV and in the Movies**.  A new campaign is under way by a Baltimore-based Center for Nursing Advocacy. The center says that medical dramas on television such as Fox's *House* and ABC's *Grey's Anatomy* are misleading in showing nurses as insignificant in patient care. The shows feature physicians and interns doing things that in real life nurses would be responsible for. Shows frequently portray nurses as uneducated or subservient. The shows, if they do portray an intelligent nurse, show that person as leaving nursing to become a doctor instead of highlighting the advancement opportunities in nursing. The American Nurses Association is concerned that misleading television shows will affect young people's decisions to become nurses, worsening the shortage. TV producers justify their actions saying it is for entertainment, not to be realistic.

Nurses on TV or in the movies are fictional characters meant to make simulations of supposed real-life emergencies realistic and, at least, dramatic. The purpose of this exercise is to discover images that are positive and those that are negative. Remember, absence of nurses in situations in which nurses would normally be present is a negative image. It makes nursing work invisible and unimportant, or it implies that others do the work of nurses.

1. Write down your image of a nurse, using as much description of who, what, why, and where as you can think of.

   _____

   _____

   _____

   _____

2. List a movie or television show you have seen that you think shows what nurses do in their practice. Describe the nurse you see in this situation.

   _____

   _____

   _____

   _____

3. Compare answers from questions 1 and 2. How do they differ? How are they the same? What do they tell you about how you see the career of nursing? What would you like to do as a nurse?

   _____

   _____

   _____

# WRITING

## Discovery Through Journaling

*To record your thoughts, use a separate journal or the lined page at the end of the chapter.*

**Observing What You Already Observed**. Return to your first journal entry and read it through. Next, return to the initial observation site and begin observing it again. Record all new observations in your journal. Spend a minimum of 10 minutes of continuous, uninterrupted writing. When you are finished, read what you wrote. Think about how your first and second observations differed and how they were the same. Reflect on this observation process and write your thoughts or feelings about it.

# CAREER PORTFOLIO

## Plan for Success

**Interests, Majors, and Careers**. On a separate sheet, write for 5 to 10 minutes on the following, and then share in small groups: What in your view is the most important thing that influenced you to think about a career in nursing? Write a story about that situation or idea. Be as specific as you can, using sights, smells, feelings, places, times. In the small group, talk about why you think your story was influential in your career decision.

*(continued)*

Prepare to write by listing activities and subjects you like:

1. _____
2. _____
3. _____
4. _____
5. _____
6. _____

Name three practice areas that might relate to your interests and help you achieve your career goals.

1. _____
2. _____
3. _____

For each area, name someone in that area you could contact. Use the Sigma Theta Tau International Nursing Honor Society website, www.nursingsociety.org/career.

1. _____
2. _____
3. _____

## Suggested Readings

Katz, Janet. *A Career in Nursing: Is It Right for Me?* St. Louis: Elsevier, 2007.

## Internet Resources

Discover Nursing by Johnson and Johnson
http://www.discovernursing.com

The National Student Nurses Association
http://www.nsna.org

The American Association for Men in Nursing
http://www.aamn.org

National League for Nursing
http://www.nln.org/Careers/resources.htm

The American Association of Colleges of Nursing
http://www.aacn.nche.edu/Education/nurse_ed/careerresources.htm

Nursing Careers in the Indian Health Service
http://www.his.gov

The Military
http://www.careersinthemilitary.com/index.cfm?fuseaction=main.careerdetail&mc_id=120

Nursing World
http://www.nursingworld.org

Sigma Theta Tau International, Honor Society of Nursing
http://www.nursingsociety.org/

Nursing Voices: The Stories
http://www.hodes.com/industries/healthcare/features/nursingvoices/readstories.asp

Career Voyages
http://www.careervoyages.gov/healthcare-main.cfm

Futures in Nursing
   http://www.FuturesInNursing.org/basics/index.
   shtml

Nursing Spectrum's Student Corner
   http://www.nursingspectrum.com/
   StudentsCorner/CareersInNursing/

Nurse Zone
   http://www.nursezone.com/
   student_nurse_center/default.asp

Nurses for a Healthier Tomorrow
   http://nursesource.org/nursing_careers.html

Choose Nursing
   http://www.choosenursing.com/

The Voice for Global Health
   http://www.globalhealth.org/

Diversity Rx
   http://www.diversityrx.org/HTML/DIVRX.htm

# Endnotes

[1] Mariah A. Taylor, "The Clinic of Last Resort," *Reflections on Nursing Leadership* 25, no. 2, (1999): 24–30.

[2] U.S. Department of Health and Human Services, "What Is Behind HRSA's Projected Supply, Demand, and Shortage of Registered Nurses?" Health Resources and Services Administration, Bureau of Health Professions, National Center for Health Workforce Analysis. (April 2006). Retrieved February 7, 2007, from: http://bhpr. hrsa.gov/healthworkforce/reports/ behindrnprojections/index.htm.

[3] Ibid.

[4] American Association of Colleges of Nursing, "Fact SheetUpdated September 2006 Nursing Shortage." Retrieved February 7, 2007, from: http://www.aacn.nche.edu/Media/FactSheets/ NursingShortage.htm.

[5] Ibid.

[6] U.S. Department of Health and Human Services, "Projected Supply, Demand, and Shortages of Registered Nurses: 2000–2020." Health Resources and Services Administration, Bureau of Health Professions, National Center for Health Workforce Analysis. (July 2002). Retrieved November 21, 2002, from: http://bhpr. hrsa.gov/healthworkforce/rnproject/report.htm.

[7] American Association of Colleges of Nursing, "Fact Sheet Updated September 2006 Nursing Shortage." Retrieved February 7, 2007, from: http://www.aacn.nche.edu/Media/FactSheets/ NursingShortage.htm.

[8] U.S. Department of Health and Human Services, "What Is Behind HRSA's Projected Supply, Demand, and Shortage of Registered Nurses?" Health Resources and Services Administration, Bureau of Health Professions, National Center for Health Workforce Analysis. (April 2006). Retrieved February 7, 2007, from: http://bhpr. hrsa.gov/healthworkforce/reports/ behindrnprojections/index.htm.

[9] American Association of Colleges of Nursing, "Fact Sheet Updated September 2006 Nursing Shortage." Retrieved February 7, 2007, from: http://www.aacn.nche.edu/Media/FactSheets/ NursingShortage.htm.

[10] Ibid.

[11] U.S. Department of Health and Human Services, "Projected Supply, Demand, and Shortages of Registered Nurses: 2000–2020." Health Resources and Services Administration, Bureau of Health Professions, National Center for Health Workforce Analysis. (July 2002). Retrieved November 21, 2002, from: http://bhpr. hrsa.gov/healthworkforce/rnproject/report.htm.

[12] United States General Accounting Office, "Nursing Workforce Emerging Nurse Shortages Due to Multiple Factors." Report to the Chairman, Subcommittee on Health, Committee on Ways and Means, House of Representatives. (July 2001). Retrieved November 30, 2001, from: http://www.gao.gov.

[13] Peter I. Buerhaus, Karen Donelan, Beth T. Ulrich, Linda Norman, Robert and Dittus, "State of the Registered Nurse Workforce in the United States," *Nursing Economics* 24, no. 1 (2006): 6–8.

[14] American Association of Colleges of Nursing, "Fact Sheet Updated September 2006 Nursing Shortage." Retrieved February 7, 2007, from: http://www.aacn.nche.edu/Media/FactSheets/ NursingShortage.htm.

[15] Ibid.

[16] Jean Ann Seago, Joanne Spetz, Dennis Keane, and Kevin Grumbach, "College Students' Perceptions of Nursing: A GEE Approach," *Canadian Journal of Nursing Leadership* 19, no. 2 (2006): 56–74.

[17]Bridget L. Hanson, Patricia L. Moulton, Rebecca Rudel, and Karyn M. Plumm, "North Dakota Nursing Needs: High School Student Survey" (June 2006). Retrieved February 6, 2007, from: http://72.14.253.104/search?q=cache:fNN9h6yVV94J:www.med.und.nodak.edu/depts/rural/rhw/pdf/highschoolstudent_survey.pdf+student+surveys+and+nursing&hl=en&ct=clnk&cd=10&gl=us&client=firefox.

[18]L. U. Krebs, J. Myers, G. Decker, J. Kinzler, P. Asfahani, and J. Jackson, "The Oncology Nursing Image: Lifting the Mist," *Oncology Nursing Forum* 23, no. 8 (1996): 1297–1304.

[19]American Association of Ambulatory Care Nursing, "2004–2009 Strategic Plan." Retrieved February 6, 2007, from: http://www.aaacn.org/cgi-bin/WebObjects/AAACNMain.woa/1/wa/viewSection?wosid=kblh58WyFkpi2zd5WlQ5yzqiqTJ&s_id=1073743905&ss_id=536873398&tName=aboutAAACNStrategicPlan.

[20]Pan American Health Organization and World Health Organization, "Public Health Nursing and Essential Public Health Functions: A Basis for Practice in the Twenty-First Century." Organization and Management of Health Systems and Services (HSO), Division of Health Systems and Services Development (HSP). (November 2001). Retrieved November 30, 2002, from: www.paho.org/search/DbS_Return.asp.

[21]The New Hampshire Board of Nursing, "Telehealth Nursing" (2006). Retrieved February 6, 2007, from: http://www.nh.gov/nursing/practice/TelehealthNursing.htm.

[22]American Association of Colleges of Nursing. "Hallmarks of the Professional Nursing Practice Environment." Washington, DC, p. 4 (January 2002). Retrieved November 8, 2002, from: www.aacn.nche.edu/publications/position/hallmarks.htm.

[23]U.S. Department of Health Resources and Services Administration, *The Registered Nurse Population, March 2004: Preliminary Findings: The 2004 National Sample Survey of Registered Nurses* (Washington, DC: U.S. Government Printing Office, 2004). Retrieved January 25, 2007, from: http://bhpr.hrsa.gov/healthworkforce/reports/rnpopulation/preliminaryfindings.htm.

[24]Ibid.

[25]Ibid.

[26]Ibid.

[27]Ibid.

[28]Ibid.

[29]Ibid.

[30]American Association of Nurse Anesthetists. "Becoming a Nurse Anesthetist." Retrieved February 7, 2007, from: http://www.aana.com/BecomingCRNA.aspx?ucNavMenu_TSMenuTargetID=8&ucNavMenu_TSMenuTargetType=4&ucNavMenu_TSMenuID=6&id=108.

[31]Ibid.

[32]International Council of Nursing. "About ICN: ICN Mission." Retrieved December 22, 2002, from: www.icn.ch/abouticn.htm.

[33]Hospice and Palliative Nurses Association, "HPNA Position Statement Complementary Therapies." Retrieved January 31, 2007, from: http://www.hpna.org/DisplayPage.aspx?Title=Quality%20Resources.

[34]International Parish Nurse Resource Center, "Assumptions Regarding Parish Nursing Practice and the Curriculum." Retrieved February 6, 2007, from: http://ipnrc.parishnurses.org/InformationEducators.phtml?header=intlinfoeducate.gif#Curriculum.

[35]International Association of Forensic Nurses, "About IAFN." Retrieved December 1, 2002, from: www.forensicnurse.org/about/default.html.

[36]Washington State Nurses Association, "About Public Health Nursing." Retrieved February 6, 2007, from: http://www.wsna.org/publichealth/.

[37]Donald M. Berwick, "A User's Manual for the IOM's 'Quality Chasm,'" *Report Health Affairs* 21, no. 3. Retrieved February 7, 2007, from: content.healthaffairs.org/cgi/reprint/21/3/80.pdf.

[38]B. R. Heller, M. T. Oros, and J. Durney-Crowley, "The Future of Nursing Education: Ten Trends to Watch." Retrieved February 7, 2007, from: http://www.nln.org/nlnjournal/infotrends.htm.

[39]The Joint Commission on Accreditation of Healthcare Organizations, "Nursing Shortage Poses Serious Health Care Risk: Joint Commission Expert Panel Offers Solutions to National Health Care Crisis at the Crossroads: Strategies for Addressing the Evolving Nursing Crisis." Retrieved February 6, 2007, from: http://jcsearch.jcaho.org/cgibin/MsmFind.exe?RE SMASK=MssResEN.msk&CFGNAME=MssFind EN.cfg&AND_ON=N&QUERY=health%20care %20at%20the%20crossroads.

[40]Bureau of Labor Statistics, *Occupational Outlook Handbook, 2006–07 Edition. Registered Nurses.* Retrieved February 7, 2007, from: http://www. bls.gov/oco/ocos083.htm#training.

[41]Ibid.

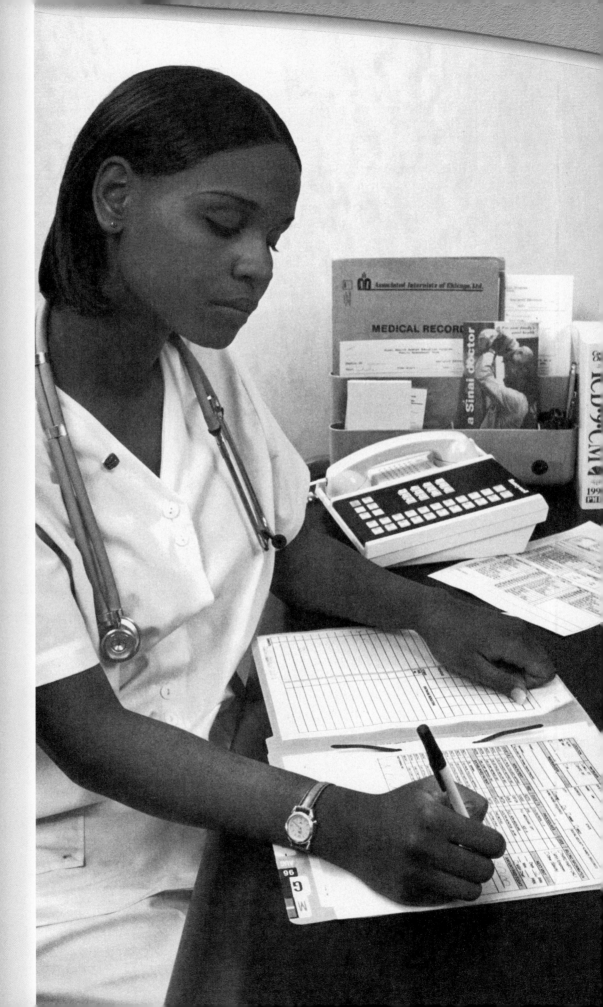

EXPLORE: VALUES, GOALS, TIME, AND STRESS

*Managing Yourself*

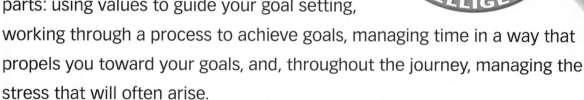

**3**

**A**chieving your most important goals depends on your ability to manage yourself. As an effective self-manager, you take charge of your life much like a CEO heads up a top-performing business. This chapter divides the indispensable skill of self-management into four parts: using values to guide your goal setting, working through a process to achieve goals, managing time in a way that propels you toward your goals, and, throughout the journey, managing the stress that will often arise.

The reality of school, workplace, and personal life will often bring problems that create obstacles and produce stress. Everyone has problems; what counts is how you handle them. Your ability to manage yourself—accompanied by a generous dose of motivation—will help you cope with what you encounter, achieve your goals, and learn lasting lessons in the process.

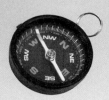

# Q & A BLUE SKY QUESTIONS DOWN-TO-EARTH ANSWERS

### How can I be comfortable talking to patients?

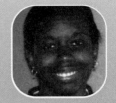

Patricia Curtis
Junior, Georgetown
University, Washington, D.C.

I plan to become a pediatric nurse with a specialty in HIV/AIDS. During my clinicals, I've had the opportunity to take care of several HIV babies. Because I'm a student and only care for one patient during clinical rotations, I've felt gratified knowing that i made their hospital stay a little more bearable by giving them the extra attention that they may need. Although I'm confident that I'll like the profession I've chosen, I still feel overwhelmed at times by the stress of preparing to become a nurse.

For one thing, I'm concerned about the difficulty I have in talking with the parents of the children I'm more comfortable than I was at the start of clinicals, but it's still an issue. I find that parents don't seem to have a lot of faith in what I'm saying. For example, I had to tell the mother of one of my patients about a procedure on her son. She was asking me a lot of questions, and I thought I did a thorough job answering her concerns. But when we finished our discussion, she still wanted to talk with the doctor.

I know I look pretty young for my age so that may be one reason why parents don't take me seriously, but I wonder if it will continue being this way once I graduate. Also, I find it difficult when parents get upset with me about a procedure that I need to do on their child. How can I communicate effectively with them?

Another stress I face in college is time management. There's always so much to do that I feel guilty relaxing or having fun. I'm doing well in my classes, but sometimes I feel like it's killing me. This semester I have two courses that require a total of 12 hours of clinical work plus 200 pages of reading a week. I also work part time as a student supervisor at the main campus library, luckily I have an understanding boss who allows me flexible hours. With regard to extracurricular activities, I'm involved in the Student Nurses Assocation, which includes volunteer work at health organizations and fundraising. Finding time for exercise seems next to impossible, but without exercise I don't have an outlet for the stress.

The nurses I work with in clinicals tell me time management continues to be a problem for them even though they are no longer in school. It's ironic that we are health care professionals and yet we have a hard time knowing how to take care of ourselves.

## PRACTICAL ANSWERS

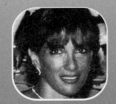

Dr. Lina Badr
Associate Professor,
University of California, Los
Angeles, California

### The key is to know that confidence comes with experience.

Being comfortable communicating with parents doesn't come with a degree. Confidence as a nurse comes with experience, which is why age gives wisdom. Feeling unsure is a good sign. This shows that you realize you have more to learn. I've seen nurses who are overly confident, and they often make mistakes because of it. When you feel incompetent you make an effort lo be more careful.

Pediatric nursing is a wonderful career choice. The HIV babies need lots of love because they can feel this at a time when they need it most. Keep in mind that the parents of a sick child are going through a very traumatic experience, too. So it's natural for them to ask lots of questions and to seek out the doctor's advice. This is their baby you're talking about, a person more precious to them than anything else on earth. Therefore, parents need you to explain things thoroughly to them. And expect to repeat those explanations several times because they may have difficulty concentrating, particularly if their child is seriously ill. Be patient with the parents and with yourself.

Time management is a crucial issue in this culture. It's no secret that American women are very stressed. I've traveled all over the world and have seen this to be true. We have many freedoms and opportunities here, but with these privileges comes so much responsibility. I used to work full-time while I was in nursing school, and I thought I would never graduate! As a professional I must continue to use my time efficiently. One of the first things I do in the morning is make a list of the things I want to achieve that day. When I finish a task, I cross it off my list. I may only complete 50 percent or 60 percent of what I set out to do, but I still have a sense of accomplishment at the end of the day.

As a student, and especially once you begin your career, avoid comparing yourself to others. We all have competencies. Some people require only four hours of sleep a night, whereas others need a full eight hours. If you need more sleep and exercise, then you must cut back on your other activities. Maybe try alternating the activities you really want to do from one semester to another. That way you'll expose yourself to a variety of experiences, but with more sanity. And remember: You're not supposed to know as much as a nurse who has been working for 20 years. You cannot rush this kind of knowledge; you have to grow into it.

# Why Is It Important to Know *What* You Value?

You make life choices—what to do, what to believe, what to buy, how to act—based on your personal **values**. Your choice to pursue a degree, for example, reflects that you value the personal and professional growth that come from a college education. Being on time for your classes shows that you value punctuality. Paying bills regularly and on time shows that you value financial stability.

**VALUES**
Principles or qualities that one considers important.

Values play a key role in your drive to achieve important goals because they help you to:

- **Understand what you want out of life.** Your most meaningful goals should reflect what you value most.

- **Build "rules for life."** Your values form the foundation for your decisions. You will return repeatedly to them for guidance, especially when you find yourself in unfamiliar territory.

- **Find people who inspire you.** Spending time with people who share similar values will help you clarify how you want to live and find support as you work toward what's important to you.

Now that you have an idea of how you can use values, focus on how to identify yours.

## Identifying and Evaluating Values

Ask yourself questions: What do you focus on in a given day? What do you consider important to be, to do, or to have? What do you wish to accomplish in your life? Answers to questions like these will point you toward your values. The exercise in the Get Analytical! box will help you think through values in more detail.

After you determine your values, evaluate them to see if they make sense for you. Many forces affect your values—family, friends, culture, media, school, work, neighborhood, religious beliefs, world events. No matter how powerful these external influences may be, whether a value feels right should be your primary consideration in deciding to adopt it.

Answering the following questions about a value will help you decide if it feels right:

- Where did the value come from?
- What other different values could I consider?
- What might happen as a result of adopting this value?
- Have I made a personal commitment to this choice? Have I told others about it?
- Do my life goals and day-to-day actions reflect this value?

Even the most solid set of values needs a reevaluation from time to time. Why? Because values often change. Life experience and education give you new perspectives that may alter what you consider important. For example, a fun-loving student who is seriously injured in an auto accident may place greater value on friends and family after the accident than he did before. If you let your values shift to fit you as you grow, you will always have a base on which to build achievable goals and wise decisions.

## How Values Affect Your Educational Experience

Well-considered values can lead to smart choices while you are in school. Your values will help you:

- **Keep going when the going gets tough.** Translate your value of education into specific actions, as a student at Palo Alto College did. "Success takes much hard work and dedication," he says. "Since I have a hard time with writing, and I can't understand algebra, I've made a commitment to write in a journal every day and attend math tutoring at least three times a week."[1]

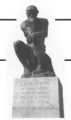

Great minds have purposes; others have wishes.

WASHINGTON IRVING

- **Choose your major and a career direction.** If you've always been an environmentalist, then you may choose to major in environmental science. If you feel fulfilled when you help people, then you might consider a career in social work.

# Explore Your Values

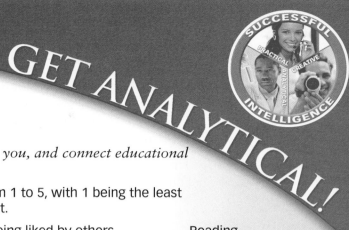

*Evaluate what you think is most important to you, and connect educational goals to your top values.*

Rate each of the values in the list on a scale from 1 to 5, with 1 being the least important to you and 5 being the most important.

| | | |
|---|---|---|
| ____ Knowing yourself | ____Being liked by others | ____Reading |
| ____Self-improvement | ____Taking risks | ____Time to yourself |
| ____Improving physical/mental health | ____Time for fun/relaxation | ____Lifelong learning |
| ____Staying fit through exercise | ____Competing and winning | ____Getting a good job |
| ____Pursuing an education | ____Spiritual/religious life | ____Making a lot of money |
| ____Good relationships with family | ____Community involvement | ____Creative/artistic pursuits |
| ____Helping others | ____Keeping up with the news | ____Other (write below) |
| ____Being organized | ____Financial stability | |

Write your top three values here:

1.
2.
3.

Values often affect your educational choices. Choose one top value that is a factor in an educational choice you have made. Explain the choice and how the value is involved. Example: A student who values mental health makes a choice to pursue a degree in psychology with a future plan to work as a school counselor.

Name an area of study that you think would help you live according to this value

_____

- **Choose friends and activities that enrich your life.** Having friends who share your desire to succeed in school will increase your motivation and reduce your stress. Joining organizations whose activities support your values will broaden your educational experience.

- **Choose what you want out of school and how hard you want to work.** What kinds of skills and knowledge do you wish to build? Do you want to focus on course work that will lead to career success? Do you want to learn about Egyptian archaeology simply because it interests you? Do you want to read every novel Toni Morrison ever wrote? Decide also how hard you are willing to work to achieve your goals. Going above and beyond will build your drive to succeed and hone your work habits—two items that will be useful in a competitive job market.

Finally, your values affect your success at school and beyond because the more ethical a student you are, the more likely you are to stay in school and to build lasting knowledge and skills.

# Academic Integrity: How Ethical Values Promote Success at School

ACADEMIC
INTEGRITY

Following a code of moral values, prizing honesty and fairness in all aspects of academic life—classes, assignments, tests, papers, projects, and relationships with students and faculty.

Having **academic integrity** promotes learning and ensures a quality education based on ethics and hard work. Read your school's code of honor, or academic integrity policy, in your student handbook. When you enrolled, you agreed to abide by it.

## Defining Academic Integrity

The Center for Academic Integrity, part of the Kenan Institute for Ethics at Duke University, defines academic integrity as a commitment to five fundamental values: honesty, trust, fairness, respect, and responsibility.[2] These values are the positive actions that define academic integrity.

- **Honesty.** Honesty defines the pursuit of knowledge and implies a search for truth in your class work, papers and lab reports, and teamwork with other students.

- **Trust.** Mutual trust—between instructor and student, as well as among students—makes possible the free exchange of ideas that is fundamental to learning. Trust means being true to your word.

- **Fairness.** Instructors must create a fair academic environment where students are judged against clear standards and in which procedures are well defined.

- **Respect.** In a respectful academic environment, both students and instructors accept and honor a wide range of opinions, even if the opinions are contrary to core beliefs.

- **Responsibility.** You are responsible for making choices that will provide you with the best education—choices that reflect fairness and honesty.

Unfortunately, the principles of academic integrity are frequently violated on college campuses. In a survey in 1999, three of four college students admitted to cheating at least once during their undergraduate careers.[3] Violations of academic integrity—turning in previously submitted work, using unauthorized devices during an exam, providing unethical aid to another student, or getting unauthorized help with a project—constitute a sacrifice of ethics that isn't worth the price.

Students who are discovered violating school policies experience a variety of consequences. In most cases, students are brought before a committee of instructors or a "jury" of students to determine whether the offense has occurred. Consequences vary from school to school and include participation in academic integrity seminars, grade reduction or course failure, suspension, or expulsion.

## Why Academic Integrity Is Worth It

Choosing to act with integrity has the following positive consequences:

- **Increased self-esteem.** Self-esteem is tied to action. The more you act in respectful and honorable ways, the better you feel about yourself, and the more likely you are to succeed.

- **Acquired knowledge.** If you cheat you might pass a test—and a course—but chances are you won't retain the knowledge and skills you need for success. Honest work is more likely to result in knowledge that lasts—and that you can use to accomplish career and life goals.

- **Effective behavioral patterns.** When you condition yourself to play fair now, you set a pattern for your behavior at work and with friends and family.

- **Mutual respect.** Respecting the work of others will lead others to respect your work.

The last two bullet points reflect the positive effect of integrity on your relationships. This is only one way in which values help you to relate to, work with, and understand the people around you successfully. Here's another way: Being open to different values, often linked with different cultures, can enhance your understanding of cultural diversity.

## Values and Cultural Diversity

At college, you may meet people who seem different in ways that you may not expect. Many of these differences stem from attitudes and behaviors that are unfamiliar to you. These attitudes and behaviors are rooted in the values that people acquire from their **culture**, either from the continuing influence of family and community in the United States or from their homeland.

Cultural misunderstandings can interfere with the relationships and friendships you form in college, career, and life. As someone who accepts and appreciates diversity, your goal is to develop the **cultural competence** to understand and appreciate these differences so that they enhance—rather than hinder—communication.[4]

Cultural understanding is a real must-have for nursing and health care. Health is an idea that comes from culture. For instance, when do you think of yourself as sick? When do you go get help? Where do you go for help first? Can you see how your answers to these questions could vary depending on your background? Think about your own culture. Many experts think the key to understanding and working with people from other cultures is understanding your own culture first.

Edward Hall, an anthropologist and an authority on cross-cultural communication, developed a simple model to help you avoid communication problems with people from other cultures. Hall linked communication styles to what he called high-context and low-context cultures:[5]

- People from *high-context* cultures rely heavily in their communication on context and situation as well as on body language and eye contact. Time (past, present, and future), fate, personal relationships and status, gender roles, trust, gestures, and sense of self and space are just some of the factors that influence communication in these cultures. High-context countries span the world and include China, Japan, Brazil, Saudi Arabia, Italy, and France.

- In contrast, people from *low-context* cultures focus on what is explicitly said or written and pay little attention to context and non-verbal cues. Countries with low-context cultures include the United States, Canada, England, Australia, Germany, and the Scandinavian countries.

CULTURE
A set of values, behaviors, tastes, knowledge, attitudes, and habits shared by a group of people.

CULTURAL COMPETENCE
The ability to understand and appreciate differences and to respond to people of all cultures in a way that values their worth, respects their beliefs and practices, and builds communication and relationships.

As you continue to read *Keys to Nursing Success*, look for examples of how cultural diversity impacts everything from teamwork and relationships, to listening, questioning, and more. Then think of the wisdom of cultural diversity consultant Helen Turnbull on turning differences into strengths:

> We must suspend our judgment. We should not judge others negatively because they are indirect, or their accents aren't clear, or their tone of voice is tentative, or they avoid eye contact. We must learn patience and suspend judgment long enough to realize these differences don't make one of us right and the other wrong. They simply mean that we approach communication from a different frame of reference and, many times, a different value system.[6]

Although clarifying your values will help you choose your educational path, goal-setting and goal-achievement skills will help you travel that path to the end. Goals turn values into tools and put them to practical use.

# How Do You *Set and Achieve* Goals?

GOAL
*An end toward which effort is directed; an aim or intention.*

When you identify something that you want, you set a **goal**. Actually *getting* what you want—from college, career, or life—demands working to *achieve* your goals. Achieving goals, whether they are short term or long term, involves following a goal-achievement plan. Think of the plan you are about to read as a map; with it helping you to establish each segment of the trip, you will be able to define your route and follow it successfully.

## Set Long-Term Goals

Start by establishing the goals that have the largest scope, the *long-term goals* you aim to attain over a period of six months, a year, or more. As a student, your long-term goals include attending school and earning a degree or certificate. Getting an education is a significant goal that often takes years to reach.

Some long-term goals have an open-ended time frame. For example, if your goal is to become a better musician, you may work at it over a lifetime. These goals also invite more creative thinking; you have more time and freedom to consider all sorts of paths to your goal. Other goals, such as completing all the courses in your major, have a shorter scope, a more definite end, and often fewer options for how to get from A to Z.

The following long-term goal statement, written by Janet Katz, a *Keys to Nusing Success* author, may take years to complete:

> My goal is improve health care by recruiting and retaining diverse students into nursing, teaching nursing students, and developing research that will help people meet their goals.

She also has long-term goals that she hopes to accomplish in no more than a year:

> Develop and publish one book. Design one community-based participation research project with Native American high school students and community members. Create materials that encourage students to enter college and nursing.

Just as Janet's goals are tailored to her personality, abilities, and interests, your goals should reflect your uniqueness. To determine your long-term goals, think about what you want to accomplish while you are in school and after you graduate. Think of ways you can link your personal values and professional aims, as in the following examples:

- **Values:** Health and fitness, helping others

  **Goal:** To become a physical therapist

- **Values:** Independence, financial success

  **Goal:** To obtain a degree in business and start a company

Basing your long-term goals on values increases your motivation. The more your goals focus on what is most important to you, the greater your drive to reach them.

## Set Short-Term Goals

*Short-term* goals are smaller steps that move you toward a long-term goal. Lasting as short as a few hours or as long as a few months, these goals help you manage your broader aspirations as they narrow your focus and encourage progress. If you had a long-term goal of graduating with a degree in nursing, for example, you may want to accomplish the following short-term goals in the next six months:

- I will learn the names, locations, and functions of every human bone and muscle.
- I will work with a study group to understand the musculoskeletal system.

These same goals can be broken down into even smaller parts, such as the following one-month goals:

- I will work with on-screen tutorials of the musculoskeletal system until I understand and memorize the material.
- I will spend three hours a week with my study partners.

In addition to monthly goals, you may have short-term goals that extend for a week, a day, or even a couple of hours in a given day. To support your monthlong goal of regularly meeting with your study partners, you may wish to set the following short-term goals:

- **By the end of today.** Call study partners to ask them about when they might be able to meet
- **One week from now.** Have scheduled each of our weekly meetings this month
- **Two weeks from now.** Have had our first meeting
- **Three weeks from now.** Type up and send around notes from the first meeting; have the second meeting

Try to pay special attention to goals that are intermediate in length—for example, one-month or one-semester goals on the way to a yearlong goal. Why? Because your motivation is at its peak when you begin to move toward a goal and when you are about to achieve that goal. If you work hard to stay motivated in the middle, you will have a more successful journey and a better result.

**FIGURE 3.1**    Goals reinforce one another

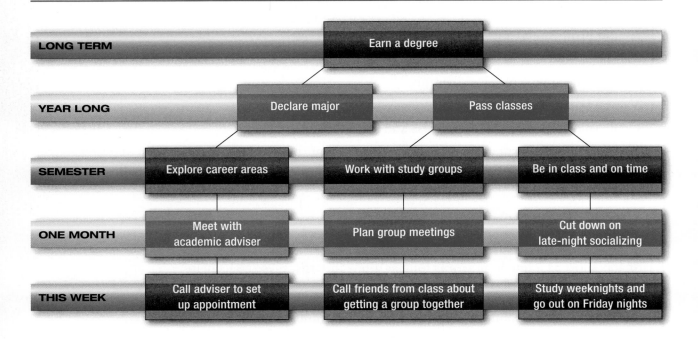

As you consider your long- and short-term goals, notice how all of your goals are linked to one another. As Figure 3.1 shows, your long-term goals establish a context for the short-term goals. In turn, your short-term goals make the long-term goals seem clearer and more reachable.

At any given time, you will be working toward goals of varying importance. Setting priorities helps you decide where and when to focus your energy and time.

## Prioritize Goals

PRIORITIZE
To arrange or deal with in order of importance.

When you **prioritize**, you evaluate everything you are working toward, decide which goals are most important, and focus your time and energy on them. What should you consider as you evaluate?

- **Your values.** Thinking about what you value will help you establish the goals that take top priority—for example, graduating in the top 25% of your class or developing a strong network of personal contacts.

- **Your personal situation.** Are you going to school and working part time? Are you taking three classes or five classes? Are you a parent with young children who need your attention? Are you an athlete on a sports team? Every individual situation requires unique priorities and scheduling.

- **Your time commitments.** Hours of your day may already be committed to class, team practices, a part-time job, or sleep. Your challenge is to make sure these commitments reflect what you value and to establish priorities for the remaining hours.

As you will see later in the chapter, setting clear priorities will help you manage your time and accomplish more.

# Map Out a Personal Goal

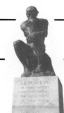

*Work backward to find an interesting path toward an important goal.*

Name one important personal goal you have for this year.

Now imagine that you have made it to the end—you already achieved your goal—and an impressed friend asks you to describe how you did it. Write your answer here, in a paragraph, as though you were telling this person about the specific steps you took to achieve your goal.

Finally, examine what you've written. You just created a potential plan! Consider putting it—or a plan similar to it—to work. As you begin, let the image of the success you created in this exercise motivate and inspire you.

---

Goals are dreams with deadlines.

DIANA SCHARF HUNT

## Work to Achieve Goals

When you've done all the work to think through a goal you want to achieve, these practical steps will help you achieve it. Remember, the more specific your plans, the more likely you are to fulfill them.

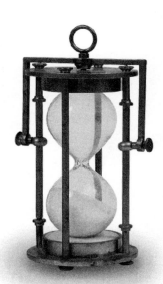

- **Define your goal-setting strategy.** *How do you plan to reach your goal?* Brainstorm different paths that might get you there. Choose one; then map out its steps and strategies. Focus on specific behaviors and events that are under your control and that are measurable.

- **Set a timetable.** *When do you want to accomplish your goal?* Set a realistic timeline that includes specific deadlines for each step and strategy you have defined. Charting your progress will help you stay on track.

- **Be accountable for your progress.** *What safeguards will keep you on track?* Define a personal reporting or buddy system that makes accountability a priority.

- **Get unstuck.** *What will you do if you hit a roadblock?* Define two ways to get help with your efforts if you run into trouble. Be ready to pursue more creative ideas if those don't work.

Through this process, you will continually be thinking about how well you are using your time. In fact, goal achievement is directly linked to effective time management.

# How Can You *Manage Your Time* Effectively?

Time is a universal resource; everyone has the same 24 hours in a day, every day. Depending on what's happening in your life, however, your sense of time may change. On some days you feel like you have hours to spare, whereas on others the clock becomes your worst enemy.

Your challenge is to turn time into a goal-achievement tool by making smart choices about how to use it. Think of each day as a jigsaw puzzle: You have all of the pieces in a pile, and your task is to form a picture of how you want your day to look. Successful time management starts with identifying your time-related needs and preferences. This self-knowledge sets the stage for building and managing your schedule, avoiding procrastination, and being flexible in the face of change.

## Identify Your Time-Related Needs and Preferences

Body rhythms and habits affect how each person deals with time. Some people are night owls; others are at their best in the morning. Some people are chronically late; others get everything done with time to spare. Individual tendencies become clear as people build up "records" of behavior.

A mismatch between your habits and your schedule causes stress and drains energy. For example, a person who loses steam in the midafternoon may struggle in classes that meet between 3 and 5 P.M. However, an awareness of your needs and preferences will help you create a schedule that maximizes your strengths and cuts down on stress. If you are a morning person, for example, look for sections of required courses that meet early in the day. If you work best at night, schedule most of your study time at a library that stays open late.

Daniel Estrada, a student at New Mexico State University, arranged his schedule to maximize his personal strengths and minimize his weaknesses. Estrada explains: "An ordinary day is getting up around 9 A.M. to get ready for my 10:30 A.M. class. I have two classes on Monday-Wednesday-Friday and three on Tuesday-Thursday. Knowing that the classes on Tuesdays and Thursdays are longer, I schedule my more difficult classes on those days and leave Monday-Wednesday-Friday for those that I find easier to work with."[7]

Take the following steps to identify your time-related needs and preferences:

### Create a Personal Time "Profile"

Ask yourself these questions: At what time of day do I have the most energy? The least energy? Do I tend to be early, on time, or late? Do I focus well for long stretches or need regular breaks? Your answers will help you find the schedule setup that works best for you.

### Evaluate the Effects of Your Profile

Which of your time-related habits and preferences will have a positive impact on your success at school? Which are likely to cause problems?

### Establish What Schedule Preferences Suit Your Profile Best

Make a list of these preferences—or even map out an ideal schedule as a way of illustrating them. For example, one student's preference list might read "Classes bunched together on Mondays, Wednesdays, and Fridays. Tuesdays and Thursdays free for studying and research. Study time primarily during the day."

Next, it's time to build the schedule that takes all of this information into account, helping you maximize your strengths and compensate for your weaker time-management areas.

## Build a Schedule

You've set up your "goal map," with all of the steps that you need to accomplish to reach your destination. With a schedule you place each step in time and, by doing so, commit to making it happen. Schedules help you gain control of your life in two ways: They provide segments of time for tasks related to the fulfillment of your goals, and they remind you of tasks, events, due dates, responsibilities, and deadlines.

### Use a Planner

A planner is the ideal practical tool for managing your time. With it, you can keep track of events and commitments, schedule goal-related tasks, and rank tasks according to priority. Time-management expert Paul Timm says that "rule number one in a thoughtful planning process is: Use some form of a planner where you can write things down."[8]

There are two major types of planners. One is a book or notebook in which to note commitments. If you write detailed daily plans, look for the kind that devotes a page to each day. If you prefer to see more days at a glance, try the kind that shows a week's schedule on a two-page spread. Some planners contain sections for monthly and yearly goals.

The other option is an electronic planner or personal digital assistant (PDA). Basic PDA functions allow you to schedule days and weeks, note due dates, make to-do lists, perform mathematical calculations, and create and store an address book. You can enter information with an on-screen or attachable keyboard or handwrite with a stylus. You can also transfer information to and from a computer.

Although electronic planners are handy and have a large data capacity, they cost more than the paper versions, and their small size means they can be easy to lose. Analyze your preferences and options, and decide which tool you are most likely to use every day. A dime-store notebook will work as well as a top-of-the-line PDA as long as you use it conscientiously.

### Keep Track of Events and Commitments

Your planner is designed to help you schedule and remember events and commitments. A quick look at your notations will remind you when items are approaching.

Putting your schedule in writing will help you anticipate and prepare for crunch times. For example, if you see that you have three tests and a presentation coming up all in one week, you may have to rearrange your schedule during the preceding week to create extra study time.

Among the events and commitments worth noting in your planner are:

- Test and quiz dates; due dates for papers, projects, and presentations
- Details of your academic schedule, including semester and holiday breaks
- Club and organizational meetings
- Personal items—medical appointments, due dates for bills, birthdays, social events
- Milestones toward a goal, such as due dates for sections of a project

Although many students don't think to do so, it's important to include class prep time—reading and studying, writing and working on assignments and projects—in the planner. According to one reasonable formula, you should schedule at least two hours of preparation for every hour of class— that is, if you take 15 credits, you'll study about 30 hours a week, making your total classroom and preparation time 45 hours. Surveys have shown, however, that most students study 15 or fewer hours per week, and some study even less—often not enough to master the material.

William Imbriale was such a student. As a freshman at Boston College, he had priorities other than studying and writing papers. "I got a D on my first philosophy paper," said William. "That woke me up, big-time." With the aid of a professor who helped him plan his time more effectively, William found ways to increase his study time and received an A− on the final paper. He says, "I felt like I earned that. The professor gave me a sense of achievement." But William was the one who did the work and put in the time.[9]

Students who hold jobs have to fit study time in where they can. Lisa Marie Webb, a University of Utah student, prepares for class while commuting from her job as a clerk at ShopKo to school and to home. Athletes, too, have to work hard to fit everything in. "I get up at 6:30, go to study hall from 7:30 to 9, have class from 9:30 to 1:15, then have practice at 2," says Ohio State defensive back A. J. Hawk. "Then we lift after practice every day through Thursday."[10] These kinds of situations demand creative time management and close attention to following your schedule.

## Schedule Tasks and Activities That Support Your Goals

Linking the events in your planner to your goals will give meaning to your efforts and bring order to your schedule. Planning study time for an economics test, for example, will mean more to you if you link the hours you spend to your goal of being accepted into business school. The simple act of relating what you do day to day to what you want in your future has enormous power to move you forward.

Here is how a student might translate his goal of entering business school into action steps over a year's time:

- *This year.* Complete enough courses to meet curriculum requirements for business school and maintain class standing
- *This semester.* Complete my economics class with a B average or higher
- *This month.* Set up economics study group schedule to coincide with quizzes and tests
- *This week.* Meet with study group; go over material for Friday's test
- *Today.* Go over Chapter 3 in econ text

The student can then arrange his time to move him in the direction of his goal. He schedules activities that support his short-term goal of doing well on the test and writes them in his planner as shown in the example just described. Achieving his overarching long-term goal of doing well in a course he needs for business school is the source of his motivation.

Before each week begins, remind yourself of your long-term goals and what you can accomplish over the next seven days to move you closer to them. Figure 3.2 shows parts of a daily schedule and a weekly schedule.

## Indicate Priority Levels

On any given day, the items on your schedule have varying degrees of importance. Prioritizing these items boosts scheduling success in two ways. First, it helps you to identify your most important tasks and to focus the bulk of your energy and time on them. Second, it helps you plan when in your day to get things done. Because many top-priority items (classes, work) occur at designated times, prioritizing helps you lock in these activities and schedule less urgent items around them.

Indicate level of importance using three different categories. Identify these categories by using any code that makes sense to you. Some people use numbers, some use letters (A, B, C), and some use different-colored pens. The three categories are as follows:

- *Priority 1* items are the most crucial. They may include attending class, completing school assignments, working at a job, picking up a child from child care, and paying bills. Enter Priority 1 items on your planner first, before scheduling anything else.

- *Priority 2* items are important but more flexible parts of your routine. Examples include library study time, completing an assignment for a school club, and working out. Schedule these around Priority 1 items.

- *Priority 3* items are least important the "it would be nice if I could get to that" items. Examples include making a social phone call, stocking up on birthday cards, and cleaning out a closet. Many people don't enter Priority 3 tasks in their planners until they know they have time for them. Others keep a separate list of these tasks so that when they have free time they can consult it and choose what they want to accomplish.

# Use Scheduling Techniques

The following strategies will help you turn your scheduling activities into tools that move you closer to your goals:

## Plan Regularly

Spending time planning your schedule will reduce stress and save you from the hours of work that might result if you forget something important. At the beginning of each week, write down specific time commitments as well as your goals and priorities. Decide where to fit activities like studying and Priority 3 items. For example, if you have a test on Thursday, you can plan study sessions on the preceding days. If you have more free time on Tuesday and Friday, you can plan workouts or other low-priority tasks. Your planner only helps you when you use it keep it with you and check it throughout the day.

FIGURE 3.2    Note daily and weekly tasks

| Monday | Tuesday | Wednesday | Thursday | Friday | Saturday | Sunday |
|---|---|---|---|---|---|---|
| 9 AM: Economics class Talk with study group members to schedule meeting. | 3–5 PM: Study econ chapter 3. | 9 AM: Economics class Drop by instructor's office hours to ask question about test | 6 PM: Go over chapter 3 7–9 PM: Study group meeting. | 9 AM: Economics class—Test 3:30 PM: Meet w/adviser to discuss GMAT and other business school requirements | Sleep in— schedule some down time | 5 PM: Go over quiz questions with study partner |

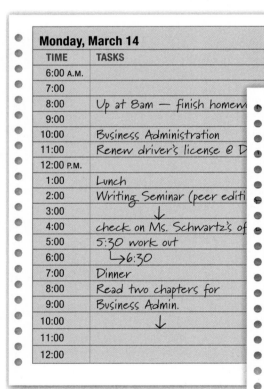

**Monday, March 14**

| TIME | TASKS | PRIORITY |
|---|---|---|
| 6:00 A.M. | | |
| 7:00 | | |
| 8:00 | Up at 8am — finish homewo... | |
| 9:00 | | |
| 10:00 | Business Administration | |
| 11:00 | Renew driver's license @ D... | |
| 12:00 P.M. | | |
| 1:00 | Lunch | |
| 2:00 | Writing Seminar (peer editi... | |
| 3:00 | ↓ | |
| 4:00 | check on Ms. Schwartz's of... | |
| 5:00 | 5:30 work out | |
| 6:00 | ↳6:30 | |
| 7:00 | Dinner | |
| 8:00 | Read two chapters for | |
| 9:00 | Business Admin. | |
| 10:00 | ↓ | |
| 11:00 | | |
| 12:00 | | |

**Monday, March 28**

| 8 | | Call: Mike Blair | 1 |
|---|---|---|---|
| 9 | BIO 212 | Finanical Aid Office | 2 |
| 10 | | EMS 262 *Paramedic | 3 |
| 11 | CHEM 203 | role-play* | 4 |
| 12 | | | 5 |
| Evening | 6pm yoga class | | |

**Tuesday, March 29**

| 8 | Finish reading assignment! | Work @ library | 1 |
|---|---|---|---|
| 9 | | | 2 |
| 10 | ENG 112 | (study for quiz) | 3 |
| 11 | ↓ | | 4 |
| 12 | | | 5 |
| Evening | | ↓ until 7pm | |

**Wednesday, March 30**

| 8 | | Meet w/adviser | 1 |
|---|---|---|---|
| 9 | BIO 212 | | 2 |
| 10 | | EMS 262 | 3 |
| 11 | CHEM 203 *Quiz | | 4 |
| 12 | | Pick up photos | 5 |
| Evening | 6pm Dinner w/study group | | |

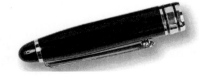

## Make and Use To-Do Lists

Use a to-do list to record the things you want to accomplish on a given day or week. Write your to-do items on a separate piece of paper so you can set priorities. Then transfer the items you plan to accomplish each day to open time periods in your planner.

To-do lists are critical time-management tools during exam week and when major projects are due. They will help you rank your responsibilities so you get things done in order of importance.

## Post Monthly and Yearly Calendars at Home

Keeping track of your major commitments on a monthly wall calendar will give you the overview you need to focus on responsibilities and upcoming events. Figure 3.3 shows a monthly calendar. If you live with family or friends, create a group calendar to stay aware of each other's plans and avoid scheduling conflicts.

## Avoid Time Traps

Try to stay away from situations that eat up time unnecessarily. Say "no" graciously if you don't have time for a project; curb excess social time that

**FIGURE 3.3**   Keep track of your time with a monthly calendar

## MARCH

| SUNDAY | MONDAY | TUESDAY | WEDNESDAY | THURSDAY | FRIDAY | SATURDAY |
|---|---|---|---|---|---|---|
| | 1 WORK | 2 Turn in English paper topic | 3 Dentist 2pm | 4 WORK | 5 | 6 |
| 7 Frank's birthday | 8 Psych Test 9am WORK | 9 | 10 6:30 pm Meeting @ Student Ctr. | 11 WORK | 12 | 13 Dinner @ Ryan's |
| 14 | 15 English paper due WORK | 16 Western Civ paper—Library research | 17 | 18 Library 6 p.m. WORK | 19 Western Civ makeup class | 20 |
| 21 | 22 WORK | 23 2 p.m. meeting, psych group project | 24 Start running program: 2 miles | 25 | 26 WORK Run 2 miles | 27 |
| 28 Run 3 miles | 29 WORK | 30 Western Civ paper due | 31 Run 2 miles | | | |

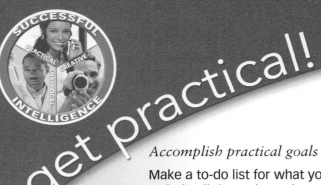

# Make a To-Do List

*Accomplish practical goals with a to-do list and reduce stress as a result.*

Make a to-do list for what you have to do on your busiest day this week. Include all the tasks and events you know about, including attending class and study time, and the activities you would like to do (working out at the gym, watching your favorite TV show) if you have extra time. Then prioritize your list using the coding system of your choice.

Date:

| | |
|---|---|
| 1. | 7. |
| 2. | 8. |
| 3. | 9. |
| 4. | 10. |
| 5. | 11. |
| 6. | 12. |

After examining this list, record your daily schedule in your planner. Include a separate list for Priority 3 items that you can fit into empty time blocks if you finish all your higher priority commitments. At the end of the day, evaluate this system. Did the list make a difference? If you liked it, use this exercise as a guide for using to-do lists regularly.

---

interferes with academics; delegate chores if you find yourself overloaded. Pay special attention to how much time you spend surfing the Internet and chatting online because these activities can waste hours.

## Schedule Downtime

**DOWNTIME**
Quiet time set aside for relaxation and low-key activity.

Leisure time is more than just a nice break—it's essential to your health and success. A little **downtime** will refresh you and actually improve your productivity when you get back on task. Even half an hour a day helps. Fill the time with whatever relaxes you—reading, watching television, chatting online, playing a game or sport, walking, writing, or just doing nothing.

## Fight Procrastination

**PROCRASTINATION**
The act of putting off a task until another time.

It's human, and common for busy students, to put off difficult or undesirable tasks until later. If taken to the extreme, however, **procrastination** can develop into a habit that causes serious problems. This excerpt from the Study Skills Library at California Polytechnic State University at San Luis Obispo illustrates how procrastination can quickly turn into a destructive pattern.

The procrastinator is often remarkably optimistic about his ability to complete a task on a tight deadline. . . . For example, he may estimate that a paper will take only five days to write; he has fifteen days; there is plenty of time, no need to start. Lulled by a false sense of security, time passes. At some point, he crosses over an imaginary starting time and suddenly realizes, "Oh no! I am not in control! There isn't enough time!"

At this point, considerable effort is directed toward completing the task, and work progresses. This sudden spurt of energy is the source of the erroneous feeling that "I work well only under pressure." Actually, at this point you are making progress only because you haven't any choice. . . . Progress is being made, but you have lost your freedom.

Barely completed in time, the paper may actually earn a fairly good grade; whereupon the student experiences mixed feelings: pride of accomplishment (sort of), scorn for the professor who cannot recognize substandard work, and guilt for getting an undeserved grade. But the net result is reinforcement: The procrastinator is rewarded positively for his poor behavior ("Look what a decent grade I got after all!"). As a result, the counterproductive behavior is repeated time and time again.[11]

Here are some reasons people procrastinate:

## Perfectionism

According to Jane B. Burka and Lenora M. Yuen, authors of *Procrastination: Why You Do It and What to Do About It*, habitual procrastinators often gauge their self-worth solely by their ability to achieve. In other words, "an outstanding performance means an outstanding person; a mediocre performance means a mediocre person."[12] To the perfectionist procrastinator, not trying at all is better than an attempt that falls short of perfection.

## Fear of Limitations

Some people procrastinate to avoid the truth about what they can achieve. "As long as you procrastinate, you never have to confront the real limits of your ability, whatever those limits are,"[13] say Burka and Yuen. If you procrastinate and fail, you can blame the failure on waiting too long, not on any personal shortcoming.

## Being Unsure of the Next Step

If you get stuck and don't know what to do, sometimes it seems easier to procrastinate than to make the leap to the next level of your goal.

Even if you're on the right track, you'll get run over if you just sit there.

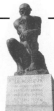

WILL ROGERS

### Facing an Overwhelming Task

Some projects are so big that they create immobilizing fear. If a person facing such a task fears failure, she may procrastinate to avoid confronting the fear.

### Avoiding Procrastination

Although it can bring relief in the short term, avoiding tasks almost always causes problems, such as a buildup of responsibilities and less time to complete them, work that is not up to par, the disappointment of others who are depending on your work, and stress brought on by the weight of the unfinished tasks. Particular strategies can help you avoid procrastination and the problems associated with it.

### Analyze the Effects of Procrastinating

What may happen if you continue to put off a responsibility? Chances are you will benefit more in the long term from facing the task head-on.

### Set Reasonable Goals

Unreasonable goals can intimidate and immobilize you. Set manageable goals and allow enough time to complete them.

### Break Tasks into Smaller Parts

If you concentrate on achieving one small step at a time, the task may become less burdensome. Setting concrete time limits for each task may help you feel more in control.

### Get Started Whether or Not You "Feel Like It"

The motivation techniques from Chapter 1 might help you take the first step. Once you start, you may find it easier to continue.

### Ask for Help

You don't have to go it alone. Once you identify what's holding you up, see who can help you face the task. Another person may come up with an innovative way that you can get moving.

### Don't Expect Perfection

No one is perfect. Most people learn by starting at the beginning, making mistakes, and learning from those mistakes. It's better to try your best than to do nothing at all.

### Reward Yourself

Find ways to boost your confidence when you accomplish a particular task. Remind yourself—with a break, a movie, some kind of treat—that you are making progress.

## Be Flexible

No matter how well you plan your time, sudden changes can upend your plans. Any change, whether minor (a room change for a class) or major (a medical emergency), can cause stress. As your stress level rises, your sense of control dwindles.

Although you can't always choose your circumstances, you have some control over how you handle them. Your ability to evaluate situations, come up with creative options, and put practical plans to work will help you manage the changes that you will inevitably encounter. Think of change as part of life, and you will be better prepared to brainstorm solutions when dilemmas arise.

Small changes—the need to work an hour overtime at your after-school job, a meeting that runs late—can result in priority shifts that jumble your schedule. For changes that occur frequently, think through a backup plan ahead of time. For surprises, the best you can do is to keep an open mind about possibilities and rely on your internal and external resources.

When change involves serious problems—your car breaks down and you have no way to get to school; you fail a class and have to consider summer school; a family member develops a medical problem and needs you more at home—use problem-solving skills to help you through. As you will see in Chapter 3.4, problem solving involves identifying and analyzing the problem, brainstorming and exploring possible solutions, and choosing the solution you decide is best. There are resources available at your college to help you throughout this process. Your academic adviser, counselor, dean, financial aid adviser, and instructors may have ideas and assistance.

Change is one of many factors associated with stress. In fact, stress is part of the normal college experience. If you take charge of how you manage stress, then you can keep it from taking charge of you.

# How Do You *Cope with the Stress of College Life?*

If you are feeling more stress in your everyday life as a student, you are not alone.[14] Stress levels among college students have increased dramatically, according to an annual survey conducted at the University of California at Los Angeles. More than 30% of the freshmen polled at 683 two- and four-year colleges and universities nationwide reported that they frequently felt overwhelmed, almost double the rate in 1985. Stress factors for college students include being in a new environment; facing increased work and difficult decisions; and juggling school, work, and personal responsibilities.

Stress refers to the way in which your mind and body react to pressure. Pressure comes from situations like heavy workloads (final exam week), excitement (being a finalist for the lead in a play), change (new school, new courses), being short on time (working 20 hours a week at a job and finding time to study), or illness (having a head cold that wipes you out for a week).

The Social Readjustment Scale, developed by psychologists T. H. Holmes and R. H. Rahe, measures the intensity of people's reaction to change and the level of stress related to it (see Figure 3.4). Holmes and Rahe found that people experience both positive and negative events as stressors. For example, whereas some events like the death of a relative are clearly

**FIGURE 3.4**   Use the Holmes-Rahe scale to find your "stress score"

To find your current "stress score," add the values of the events that you experienced in the past year. The higher the number, the greater the stress. Scoring over 300 points puts you at high risk for developing a stress-related health problem. A score between 150 and 299 reduces your risk by 30 percent, and a score under 150 means that you have only a small chance of a problem.

| EVENT | VALUE | EVENT | VALUE |
| --- | --- | --- | --- |
| Death of spouse or partner | 100 | Son or daughter leaving home | 29 |
| Divorce | 73 | Trouble with in-laws | 29 |
| Marital separation | 65 | Outstanding personal achievement | 28 |
| Jail term | 63 | Spouse begins or stops work | 26 |
| Personal injury | 53 | Starting or finishing school | 26 |
| Marriage | 50 | Change in living conditions | 25 |
| Fired from work | 47 | Revision of personal habits | 24 |
| Marital reconciliation | 45 | Trouble with boss | 23 |
| Retirement | 45 | Change in work hours, conditions | 20 |
| Changes in family member's health | 44 | Change in residence | 20 |
| Pregnancy | 40 | Change in schools | 20 |
| Sex difficulties | 39 | Change in recreational habits | 19 |
| Addition to family | 39 | Change in religious activities | 19 |
| Business readjustment | 39 | Change in social activities | 18 |
| Change in financial status | 38 | Mortgage or loan under $10,000 | 17 |
| Death of a close friend | 37 | Change in sleeping habits | 16 |
| Change to different line of work | 36 | Change in # of family gatherings | 15 |
| Change in # of marital arguments | 35 | Change in eating habits | 15 |
| Mortgage or loan over $10,000 | 31 | Vacation | 13 |
| Foreclosure of mortgage or loan | 30 | Christmas season | 12 |
| Change in work responsibilities | 29 | Minor violation of the law | 11 |

*Source:* Reprinted from *Journal of Psychosomatic Research,* 11(2), T. H. Rahe, "The social readjustment rating scale," 1967, with permission from Elsevier.

negative, other stressors, like moving to a new house or even taking a vacation, are generally positive.

At their worst, stress reactions can make you physically ill (Chapter 11 examines stress-related health issues—situations in which stress goes beyond normal levels, causing physical and emotional problems). But stress can also supply the heightened readiness you need to do well on tests, finish assignments on time, prepare for a class presentation, or meet new people. Your goal is to find a manageable balance. Figure 3.5, based on research conducted by Robert M. Yerkes and John E. Dodson, shows that stress can be helpful or harmful, depending on how much you experience.

## Successful Time Management and Goal Setting Relieve Stress

Dealing with the stress of college life is, and will continue to be, one of your biggest challenges. But here's a piece of good news: Every goal-achievement and time-management strategy you have read in this chapter

FIGURE 3.5 Stress levels can help or hinder performance

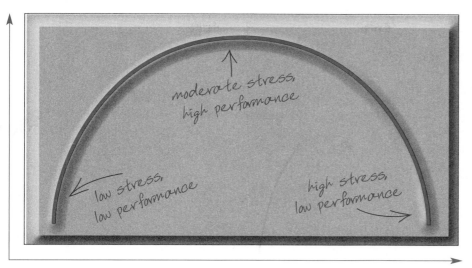

Performance or efficiency

moderate stress, high performance

low stress, low performance

high stress, low performance

Stress or anxiety

*Source:* From *Your Maximum Mind* by Herbert Benson, M.D., copyright © 1987 by Random House, Inc. Used by permission of Time Books, a division of Random House, Inc.

contributes to your ability to cope with stress. Remember that stress refers to how you react to pressure. When you set up effective plans to move toward goals, you reduce pressure. When you set a schedule that works for you and stick to it, you reduce pressure. Less pressure, less stress.

Carefully analyze the relationship between stress and your time-management habits. Often, people create extra stress for themselves without realizing it. For example, say you're a night person but have a habit of scheduling early classes. You are consistently stressed about waking up in time for them. What's wrong with this picture? Reduce your stress by finding practical ways to change your scheduling. Taking later classes will help, but if that isn't possible, cope in other ways. Get to bed earlier a few nights a week, nap in the afternoon, exercise briefly before class to restore your energy. Make sure you are not expending energy coping with stress that you can avoid with thought and planning.

## Stress-Management Strategies

Here are some practical strategies for coping with the day-to-day stress of being a college student:

- **Eat right.** The healthier you are, the stronger you are—and the more able you will be to weather tough situations like all-nighters, illnesses, and challenging academic work. Try to eat a balanced, low-fat diet and avoid overloading on junk food. Try also to maintain a healthy weight.

- **Exercise.** Physical exercise will help you manage your stress. Find a type of exercise you like and make it a regular part of your life.

- **Get sleep.** Avoid the systemwide dysfunction that sleep deprivation can create. Figure out how much sleep you need and do your best to get it. When you pull an all-nighter, make sure you play catch-up over the next couple of days.

- **Think positively.** Try to think of all you have to do as challenges, not problems.
- **Seek balance.** A balanced life includes time by yourself—for your thoughts, hopes, and plans—and time for relaxation, in whatever form you choose.
- **Address issues.** Try not to let things lie too long. Analyze stressful situations and use problem-solving strategies (see Chapter 3.5) to decide on a specific plan of action.
- **Set boundaries and learn to say no.** Try to delegate. Review obligations regularly; if you evaluate that something has become a burden, then consider dropping it from your roster of activities.
- **Surround yourself with people who are good for you.** Focus on friends who are good listeners and who will support you when things get rough. Friendship and humor go a long way toward reducing stress.

Sometimes you'll be able to pull out the strategies that fit the situation, finding ways to cope with the stress you encounter. Sometimes stress will make you feel frozen, not knowing where to turn to work your way out of it. At those times, remember: *Any step toward a goal is a stress-management strategy because it reduces pressure.* In that sense, this entire book is a stress-management strategy. Every useful tool, from test-taking hints to job-hunting strategies, will help you reduce the pressure and cover the distance toward your dreams.

As you plan your goals, think about the role luck may play in your success. If you work hard and are open to new opportunities, you may find yourself in the right place at the right time to benefit from a "lucky break." Because you are prepared, you may find a teacher who is so impressed by your tenacity and focus that she offers to become your mentor. Or, after you graduate, you may meet someone with a business opportunity that is a perfect match for your skills, and you are hired on the spot. All your hard work in the direction of your goal will prepare you to take advantage of lucky breaks that come your way.

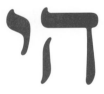

In Hebrew, this word, pronounced "chai," means "life," representing all aspects of life—spiritual, emotional, family, educational, and career. Individual Hebrew characters have number values. Because the characters in the word *chai* add up to 18, the number 18 has come to be associated with good luck. The word *chai* is often worn as a good luck charm. The phrase *l'chaim* means "to life" and good luck.

# DEVELOPING SUCCESSFUL INTELLIGENCE

## *Putting It All Together*

**The Wheel of Life.** This exercise uses a wheel—an image that has been used for centuries to promote understanding of the self and the world—to help you think about your strength and weakness in eight important goal areas. Assess your level of proficiency in self-knowledge, study skills, personal life goals, finances, health and stress management, relationships, career, and time management by filling out the wheel as directed in Figure 3.6 on p. 104.

Let this self-assessment help you make decisions about how you approach the material in this course. If you wish to improve your career preparation, for example, pay special attention to Chapter 10. If you need work on study skills, then focus specifically on the reading, note-taking, and test-taking chapters. At the end of the book you will have a chance to revisit the Wheel. If you work hard in this course, you will sense improvement in your weaker goal areas over the course of the semester. Plus, you will have developed your ability to evaluate and manage yourself—a skill that is crucial to your success in school and at work.

# TEAM BUILDING

## *Collaborative Solutions*

**Multiple Paths to a Goal.** In a group of three or four, brainstorm goals that focus on building a life skill—for example, leadership, teamwork, learning a foreign language. Write your ideas on a piece of paper. From that list, pick out one goal to explore together.

Each group member takes two minutes alone to think about this goal in terms of the first goal-achievement step on page 88—defining a strategy. In other words, answer the question: "How would I do it?" Each person writes down all of the paths they can think of.

FIGURE 3.6    Build self-knowledge with the Wheel of Life

Rate yourself in each area of the wheel on a scale of 1 to 10, 1 being least developed (near the center of the wheel) and 10 being most developed (the outer edge if the wheel). In each area, at the level of the number you choose, draw a curved line and fill in the wedge below that line. Be honest—this is for your benefit only. Finally, look at what your wheel says about the balance in your life. If this were a real wheel, how well would it roll?

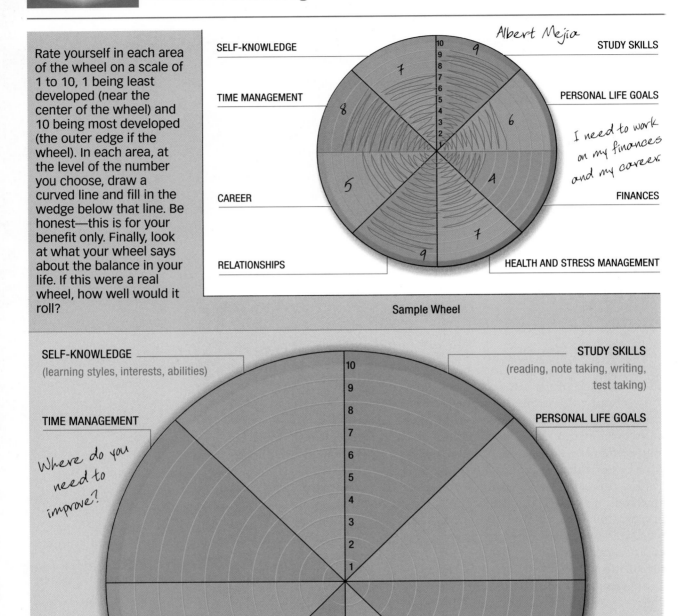

**Sample Wheel**

*Source:* Based on "The Wheel of Life" model developed by the Coaches Training Institute. © Co-Active Space 2000.

The group then gathers and everyone shares their strategies. The group evaluates strategies and chooses one that seems effective. Finally, as a group, brainstorm the rest of the goal-achievement process, based on the chosen strategy or path:

- **Set a timetable.** When do you plan to reach your goal? Discuss different time frames and how each might change the path.

- **Be accountable.** What safeguards will keep you on track? Talk about different ways to make sure you are moving ahead consistently.

- **Get unstuck.** What will you do if you hit a roadblock? Brainstorm the kinds of roadblocks that could get in the way of this particular goal. For each, come up with ways to overcome the obstacle.

At the end of the process, you will have a wealth of ideas for how to approach one particular goal—and an appreciation for how many paths you could take to get there.

# WRITING

## *Discovery Through Journaling*

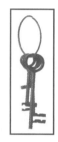

*Use the tables here to record data; answer questions and write additional thoughts on a separate piece of paper or in a journal.*

**Discover How You Spend Your Time.** In the table, estimate the total time you think you spend per week on each listed activity. Then, add the hours. If your number is over 168 (the number of hours in a week), rethink your estimates and recalculate so that the total is equal to 168.

Now spend a week recording exactly how you spend your time. The chart on page 94 has blocks showing half-hour increments. As you go through the week, write in what you do each hour, indicating when you started and when you stopped. Don't forget activities that don't feel like "activities," such as sleeping, relaxing, and watching TV. Finally, be sure to record your actual activities instead of how you want to have, or think you should have, spent your time. There are no wrong answers.

After a week, go through the chart and add up how many hours you spent on the activities for which you previously estimated your hours. Tally the hours in the boxes in the following table using straight tally marks; round off to half hours and use a short tally mark for each half hour. In the third column, total the hours for each activity. Leave the "Ideal Time in Hours" column blank for now.

Add the totals in the third column to find your grand total. Compare your grand total to your estimated grand total; compare your actual activity hour totals to your estimated activity hour totals. Use a separate sheet of paper to answer the following questions:

- What matches and what doesn't? Describe the most interesting similarities and differences.

- Where do you waste the most time? What do you think that is costing you?

Now evaluate what kinds of changes might improve your ability to achieve goals. Analyze what you do daily, weekly, and monthly. Go back to the chart and fill in the "Ideal Time in Hours" column. Consider the difference between actual hours and ideal hours. Ask questions:

- On what activities do you think you should spend more or less time?
- What are you willing to do to change, and why?

Finally, write a short paragraph describing two key time-management changes in detail. Describe what goal you are aiming for, and map out how you plan to put the changes into action.

# CAREER PORTFOLIO
## *Plan for Success*

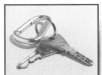

*Complete the following in your electronic portfolio or on separate sheets of paper.*

**Career Goals—Knowledge and Skills.** No matter what career goals you ultimately pursue, certain knowledge and skills are useful in any career area. Consider this list of the general skills employers look for in people they hire:

| | | |
|---|---|---|
| Acceptance | Critical thinking | Leadership |
| Communication | Flexibility | Positive attitude |
| Continual learning | Goal setting | Teamwork |
| Creativity | Integrity | |

Choose and circle three of these that you want to focus on developing this year.

Map out a plan for your progress by indicating a series of smaller goals—from short term to long term—that will lead you toward developing these skills. For each of the three skills, write what you hope to accomplish in the next year, the next six months, and the next month. For example:

## Skill: Leadership

- **Next month.** I will volunteer to lead a session with my Economics study group.
- **In six months.** I will look into leadership positions on the college newspaper.
- **By the end of the year.** I will have joined the newspaper team and expressed my interest in a leadership position.

## Suggested Readings

Allen, David. *Getting Things Done: The Art of Stress-Free Productivity*. New York: Penguin Books, 2003.

Burka, Jane B., Ph.D., and Lenora M. Yuen, Ph.D. *Procrastination*. Reading, MA: Perseus Books, 1983.

Covey, Stephen. *The Seven Habits of Highly Effective People*. New York: Simon & Schuster, 1995.

Emmett, Rita. *The Procrastinator's Handbook: Mastering the Art of Doing It Now*. New York: Walker & Co., 2000.

Gleeson, Kerry. *The Personal Efficiency Program: How to Get Organized to Do More Work in Less Time*, 2nd ed. New York: John Wiley & Sons, 2000.

Lakein, Alan. *How to Get Control of Your Time and Your Life*. New York: New American Library, 1996.

Leyden-Rubenstein, Lori. *The Stress Management Handbook*. New York: McGraw-Hill, 1999.

Sapadin, Linda, and Jack Maguire. *Beat Procrastination and Make the Grade: The Six Styles of Procrastination and How Students Can Overcome Them*. New York: Penguin USA, 1999.

Timm, Paul R. *Successful Self-Management: A Psychologically Sound Approach to Personal Effectiveness*. Los Altos, CA: Crisp Publications, 1996.

## Internet Resources

Mind Tools (section on time management): **www.mindtools.com/pages/main/newMNHTE.htm**

Top Achievement—goal-setting and self-improvement resources: **www.topachievement.com**

About.com stress-management resources: **stress.about.com**

Troubled With—information on stress management: **www.troubledwith.com**

## Endnotes

[1] Student essay submitted by the First Year Experience students of Patty Parma, Palo Alto College, San Antonio, Texas, January 2004.

[2] *A Report from the Center for Academic Integrity*, Center for Academic Integrity, Kenan Institute for Ethics, Duke University (October 1999). Retrieved March 2001, from: www.academicintegrity.org.

[3] Ibid.

[4] Background information for information on cultural diversity from Afsaneh Nahavandi and Ali Malekzadeh, *Organizational Behavior: The Person-Organization Fit.* (Upper Saddle River, NJ: Prentice Hall, 1999).

[5] Louis E. Boone, David L. Kurtz, and Judy R. Block, *Contemporary Business Communication*, 2nd ed. (Upper Saddle River, NJ: Prentice Hall, 1997), pp. 68–72.

[6] Louis E. Boone and David L. Kurtz, *Contemporary Business Communication* (Englewood Cliffs, NJ: Prentice Hall, 1994), p. 643.

[7] "What's an Ordinary Day Like When You're in College?" New Mexico State University website (June 1999). Retrieved March 2004, from: www.nmsu.edu/aggieland/students/faqordinary.html.

[8] Paul Timm, *Successful Self-Management: A Psychologically Sound Approach to Personal Effectiveness* (Los Altos, CA: Crisp Publications, 1987), pp. 22–41.

[9] Welch Suggs, "How Gears Turn at a Sports Factory: Running Ohio State's $79-million Athletics Program Is a Major Endeavor, with Huge Payoffs and Costs," *The Chronicle of Higher Education* (November 29, 2002). http://chronicle.com/weekly/v49/il4/14a03201.htm.

[10] Jeffrey R. Young, "'Homework? What Homework?' Students Seem to be Spending Less Time Studying Than They Used To," *The Chronicle of Higher Education* (December 6, 2002). Retrieved March 2004, from: http://chronicle.com/weekly/v49/i15/15a03501.htm.

[11] William E. Sydnor, "Procrastination," from the California Polytechnic State University Study Skills Library [on-line]. Based on *Overcoming Procrastination* by Albert Ellis. Available: www.sas.calpoly.edu/asc/ssl/procrastination.html (May 2003). Used with permission.

[12] Jane B. Burka and Lenora M. Yuen, *Procrastination* (Reading, MA: Perseus Books, 1983), pp. 21–22.

[13] Ibid.

[14] The following articles were used as sources in this section: Glenn C. Altschuler, "Adapting to College Life in an Era of Heightened Stress," *New York Times*, Education Life, Section 4A, August 6, 2000, p. 12; Carol Hymowitz and Rachel Emma Silverman, "Can Workplace Stress Get Worse?" *Wall Street Journal*, January 16, 2001, p. B1; Robert M. Sapolsky, "Best Ways to Reduce Everyday Levels of Stress . . . Bad Ol' Stress," *Bottom Line Personal*, January 15, 2000, p. 13; Kate Slaboch, "Stress and the College Student: A Debate" (April 4, 2001). Available: www.jour.unr.edu/outpost/voices/voi.slaboch.stress.htm (University of South Florida, The Counseling Center for Human Development, "Coping with Stress in College" (April 4, 2001). Available: http://usfweb.usf.edu/counsel/self-hlp/stress.htm; Jodi Wilgoren, "Survey Shows High Stress Levels in College Freshmen," *New York Times*, January 23, 2000, p. NA.

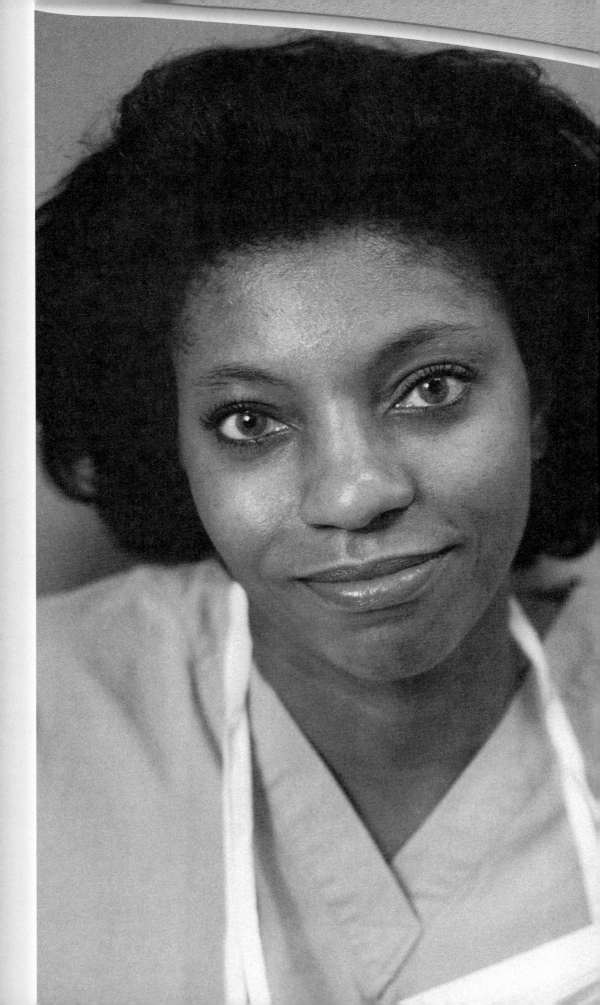

# PREPARE: LEARNING STYLES, MAJORS, AND CAREERS

*KNOWING YOUR TALENTS AND FINDING YOUR DIRECTION*

A s a college student, you are investing valuable resources—time, effort, and money—in your education. Learning is the return on your investment. How well you learn, and therefore how good a return you receive, depends in part on knowing yourself in two ways: knowing *how* you learn and knowing what you want to *do* with what you learn.

This chapter focuses first on helping you identify your learning styles because when you understand how you learn, you will be a more effective student. Then you will read about majors and careers because knowing where you want your education to take you will motivate you toward a goal.

# Q & A BLUE SKY QUESTIONS
# DOWN-TO-EARTH ANSWERS

### *How can I understand and develop my learning potential?*

I first heard about learning styles in a vocational class that I took my freshman year in college. The instructor explained that each student has their own unique way to learn. I liked the idea that learning could be a fun adventure, instead of just something you do to get a good grade.

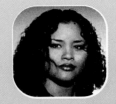

Dawn E. Bedell
Sophomore, Truman
College, Chicago, Illinois

Since then, I've noticed a few things about how I learn. For example, I usually need a little background noise to stay focused when I'm studying, so I turn on the television. And, unlike some students, I prefer straight lecture. If a teacher uses visual aids, like an overhead projector, I can't concentrate on taking notes. I also don't find graphs or charts helpful, even when they're in textbooks.

Something else that really affects my learning is the teacher's attitude. Last year I had a science teacher who seemed impatient. He acted annoyed when students asked questions, and he made me feel incapable of learning. Instead, I like teachers who joke around and who show that they care about you. For instance, I had a figure-drawing class that I thought was going to be too hard for me. The teacher saw that I was struggling, and he took the time to encourage me. I got an A in that class, and I discovered that I have a natural ability to draw.

Another interest I have is writing. I like to write poetry, and I've been keeping a journal ever since high school. My mother is a Chippewa Indian, and I'm proud of that heritage. I especially like to write about the American Indian's freedom of expression through dance. I also enjoy reading literature.

I've always done well in lab work, too. This semester I'm taking a microbiology course, and I love working with the microscopes. I wish you could see my lab book; I've made some really cool sketches of the human brain and heart. Now, I'm planning to major in forensic medicine. I knew I really liked science, and with my interest in art, the field of forensics seems to click for me. When I tell people that someday I want to do autopsies or work in a mortuary, they look at me like I'm crazy. But their reaction just confirms how we each have different interests and abilities.

Although I've noted a few things here about how I learn, it just seems like a mixed bag of likes and dislikes. I don't see any clear patterns.

# PRACTICAL ANSWERS

### *You must become a lifelong learner.*

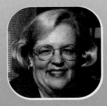

M. Kay Cresci,
PhD, RN, CCRN
Instructor, The Johns
Hopkins University School
of Nursing, Baltimore,
Maryland

As health care professionals in the information age, we must become lifelong learners. Therefore, recognizing how you learn best and your personal learning preferences can help you maximize your learning strengths. This is referred to as your learning style, or the way you take in and process information. To identify your learning style, you need to think about how you learn and your preferred learning modalities: physical, environmental, cognitive, affective, and socioeconomic. Using this information not only allows you to develop successful learning strategies but also assists you in showing teachers and mentors how to best guide you.

There are a number of instruments available for determining your learning style. The Center for Teaching and Learning at Indiana University has a website listing a number of these inventories and their authors (http://web.indstate.edu/ctl/styles/invent.html) and, where available, direct links to on-line instruments. The inventories are categorized according to major learning style approaches: instructional preferences, social interaction models, information processing, and personality levels. You may also find on-line learning style inventories through a search engine such as AltaVista (www.altavista.com). In the search box, type "learning style" within quotation marks. Many of these authors give you immediate feedback on your learning style and appropriate learning strategies to use based on that style. Felder (1993) stresses that to function effectively in any professional capacity requires that you develop your skills in most learning style modes.

In the literature, models of learning styles tend to identify four dimensions of learning: perceiving, organizing, processing, and understanding. Do you perceive information through your senses (visual) or intuitively through your thoughts and ideas (verbal)? Do you organize information using facts and observations (inductive) or through deducing outcomes from given principles (deductive)? Do you process information actively through engagement with others or reflectively through introspection? Finally, do you understand information through a logical sequence of steps or though seeing the global picture? Answering these questions can help you find clues to your learning puzzle.

Another approach to exploring learning styles is the theory of multiple intelligences by Howard Gardner (1993). He has identified eight potential ways we may process information: verbal/linguistic, logical/mathematical, visual/spatial, bodily/kinesthetic, musical, interpersonal, intrapersonal, and naturalistic. When using this theory, it's important to recognize that intelligence and learning style are not one and the same. Intelligence is the capacity or ability to learn a designated area of knowledge, whereas learning style exhibits a tendency toward learning in a specific direction.

# How Can You *Discover* Your Learning Styles?

Your style of taking in and remembering information is as unique as you are. Have you ever thought in detail about what that style is? Doing just that—working to understand your learning strengths and preferences and the primary ways in which you interact with others—will help you achieve your personal best in school and beyond.

This chapter presents two assessments designed to help you figure out how you learn and interact. The first—*Multiple Pathways to Learning*—focuses on learning strengths and preferences and is based on Professor Howard Gardner's multiple intelligences theory. The second—the *Personality Spectrum*—is based on the Myers-Briggs Type Inventory (MBTI) and helps you evaluate how you react to people and situations.

## The Value of Learning Styles Assessments

Everyone has some things that they do well and other things that they find difficult. To be a successfully intelligent learner, you need to maximize your strengths and compensate for your weaknesses. The first step toward that goal is knowing what those strengths and weaknesses *are*—and that's what these assessments will help you discover. With the information you gain from the Multiple Pathways to Learning and the Personality Spectrum, you can choose your own best ways to study, manage time, remember material, and much more.

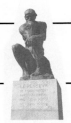

To be what we are, and to become what we are capable of becoming, is the only end of life.

ROBERT LOUIS STEVENSON

Knowing how you learn will help you set specific goals for positive change. For example, instead of saying, "I'm no good at math," you can strengthen your math skills with what you've learned from Multiple Pathways to Learning. You might draw diagrams of math problems if you are a visual learner or talk out problems with a study partner if you are an interpersonal learner. (You will learn about these and other learning styles later in the chapter.) The better you know yourself, the better you are able to handle different learning situations and challenges.

Gaining an understanding of **learning style** will also enhance your ability to see and appreciate how people differ because learning style is part of the diversity that lies within. When you sit in a classroom with 30 students, you can be sure that each person is learning the material in a unique way. The more you know about how others approach learning, the more you can use that understanding to improve communication and teamwork.

## Putting Assessment Results in Perspective

First, remember that any assessment is simply a snapshot, a look at who you are at a given moment. Your answers can, and will, change as you and the circumstances around you change. These assessments help you look at the present—and plan for the future—by asking questions: Who am I right now? How does this compare with who I want to be?

Second, there are no "right" answers, no "best" set of scores. Think of your responses in the same way you would if you were trying on a new set of eyeglasses to correct blurred vision. The glasses will not create new paths and possibilities, but they will help you see more clearly the ones that already exist.

Following each assessment is information about the typical traits of, and appropriate study strategies for, each intelligence or personality spectrum dimension. As you will see from your scores, you have abilities in all areas, though some are more developed than others. Therefore, you will find useful suggestions under all the headings. Try different techniques and keep what works for you.

## Assess Your Multiple Intelligences

**INTELLIGENCE**
As defined by Howard Gardner, an ability to solve problems or fashion products that are useful in a particular cultural setting or community.

In 1983, Howard Gardner, a Harvard University professor, changed the way people perceive **intelligence** and learning with his theory of multiple intelligences. Gardner believes there are at least eight intelligences possessed by all people and that every person has developed some intelligences more fully than others (see Figure 4.1 for descriptions). According to this theory, when you find a task or subject easy, you are probably using a more fully

## FIGURE 4.1 Each intelligence is linked to specific abilities

| INTELLIGENCE | DESCRIPTION |
| --- | --- |
| Verbal-Linguistic | Ability to communicate through language (listening, reading, writing, speaking) |
| Logical-Mathematical | Ability to understand logical reasoning and problem solving (math, science, patterns, sequences) |
| Bodily-Kinesthetic | Ability to use the physical body skillfully and to take in knowledge through bodily sensation (coordination, working with hands) |
| Visual-Spatial | Ability to understand spatial relationships and to perceive and create images (visual art, graphic design, charts and maps) |
| Interpersonal | Ability to relate to others, noticing their moods, motivations, and feelings (social activity, cooperative learning, teamwork) |
| Intrapersonal | Ability to understand one's own behavior and feelings (self-awareness, independence, time spent alone) |
| Musical | Ability to comprehend and create meaningful sound and recognize patterns (music, sensitivity to sound and patterns) |
| Naturalistic | Ability to understand features of the environment (interest in nature, environmental balance, ecosystem, stress relief brought by natural environments) |

developed intelligence. When you have trouble, you may be using a less developed intelligence.[1]

Gardner believes that the way you learn is a unique blend of intelligences, resulting from your distinctive abilities, challenges, experiences, and training. In addition, ability in the intelligences may develop or recede as your life changes. Gardner thinks that the traditional view of intelligence, based on mathematical, logical, and verbal measurements, doesn't reflect the entire spectrum of human ability:

> I believe that we should . . . look . . . at more naturalistic sources of information about how peoples around the world develop skills important to their way of life. Think, for example, of sailors in the South Seas, who find their way around hundreds, or even thousands, of islands by looking at the constellations of stars in the sky, feeling the way a boat passes over the water, and noticing a few scattered landmarks. A word for intelligence in a society of these sailors would probably refer to that kind of navigational ability.[2]

The Multiple Pathways to Learning assessment helps you determine the levels to which your eight intelligences are developed. Figure 4.2 describes specific skills associated with the eight intelligences as well as study techniques that maximize each. Finally, the Multiple Intelligence Strategies grids in Chapters 5 through 11 will demonstrate how to apply your learning styles knowledge to key college success skills.

**FIGURE 4.2**   How to put your multiple intelligences to work for you

## ABILITIES AND SKILLS ASSOCIATED WITH EACH INTELLIGENCE

### Verbal–Linguistic
- Analyzing own use of language
- Remembering terms easily
- Explaining, teaching, learning, using humor
- Understanding syntax and word meaning
- Convincing someone to do something

### Musical–Rhythmic
- Sensing tonal qualities
- Creating/enjoying melodies, rhythms
- Being sensitive to sounds and rhythms
- Using "schemas" to hear music
- Understanding the structure of music

### Logical–Mathematical
- Recognizing abstract patterns
- Reasoning inductively and deductively
- Discerning relationships and connections
- Performing complex calculations
- Reasoning scientifically

### Visual–Spatial
- Perceiving and forming objects accurately
- Recognizing relationships between objects
- Representing something graphically
- Manipulating images
- Finding one's way in space

### Bodily–Kinesthetic
- Connecting mind and body
- Controlling movement
- Improving body functions
- Expanding body awareness to all senses
- Coordinating body movement

### Intrapersonal
- Evaluating own thinking
- Being aware of and expressing feelings
- Understanding self in relation to others
- Thinking and reasoning on higher levels

### Interpersonal
- Seeing things from others' perspectives
- Cooperating within a group
- Communicating verbally and nonverbally
- Creating and maintaining relationships

### Naturalistic
- Deep understanding of nature
- Appreciation of the delicate balance in nature

## STUDY TECHNIQUES TO MAXIMIZE EACH INTELLIGENCE

### Verbal–Linguistic
- Read text; highlight no more than 10%
- Rewrite notes
- Outline chapters
- Teach someone else
- Recite information or write scripts/debates

### Musical–Rhythmic
- Create rhythms out of words
- Beat out rhythms with hand or stick
- Play instrumental music/write raps
- Put new material to songs you already know
- Take music breaks

### Logical–Mathematical
- Organize material logically
- Explain material sequentially to someone
- Develop systems and find patterns
- Write outlines and develop charts and graphs
- Analyze information

### Visual–Spatial
- Develop graphic organizers for new material
- Draw mind maps
- Develop charts and graphs
- Use color in notes to organize
- Visualize material (method of loci)

### Bodily–Kinesthetic
- Move or rap while you learn; pace and recite
- Use "method of loci" or manipulatives
- Move fingers under words while reading
- Create "living sculptures"
- Act out scripts of material, design games

### Intrapersonal
- Reflect on personal meaning of information
- Visualize information/keep a journal
- Study in quiet settings
- Imagine experiments

### Interpersonal
- Study in a group
- Discuss information
- Use flash cards with others
- Teach someone else

### Naturalistic
- Connect with nature whenever possible
- Form study groups of people with like interests

Adapted from Lazear, *Seven Pathways of Learning*, 1994.

## Assess Your Personality with the Personality Spectrum

Personality assessments help you understand how you respond to the world around you—including information, thoughts, feelings, people, and events. The assessment used in this chapter is based on one of the most widely used personality inventories in the world, the Myers-Briggs Type Inventory, developed by Katharine Briggs and her daughter, Isabel Briggs Myers. It also relies on the work of David Keirsey and Marilyn Bates, who combined the 16 Myers-Briggs types into four temperaments and developed an assessment called the Keirsey Sorter based on those temperaments.

The Personality Spectrum assessment adapts and simplifies their material into four personality types—Thinker, Organizer, Giver, and Adventurer—and was developed by Dr. Joyce Bishop. The Personality Spectrum helps you identify the kinds of interactions that are most, and least, comfortable for you. Figure 4.3, on page 116, shows techniques that improve performance, learning strategies, and ways of relating to others for each personality type.

# What Are the Benefits of Knowing *How You Learn?*

Generally, self-knowledge helps you make choices that boost your strong areas and help you to manage weaker ones. For example, understanding what you value can help you choose friends who cheer on your successes as well as friends who broaden your horizons with their different perspectives. Likewise for learning style: When you know your multiple intelligences and personality traits, you can choose strategies that will help you learn more, remember better, and use your knowledge more successfully—in any academic or workplace situation.

## Study Benefits

Knowing how you learn helps you choose study techniques that capitalize on your strengths. For example, if you learn successfully from a linear, logical presentation, you can look for order (for example, a chronology or a problem–solution structure) as you review notes. If you are a strong interpersonal learner, you can try to work in study groups whenever possible.

Learning style also points you toward strategies that help with tasks and topics that don't come so easily. An Adventurer who does *not* respond well to linear information, for example, has two choices when faced with logical presentations. She can apply her strengths to the material—for example, she might find a hands-on approach. Or she can work on her ability to handle the material by developing study skills that work well for linear learners.

When you study with others, understanding of diverse learning styles will help you assign tasks effectively and learn more comprehensively. An interpersonal learner might take the lead in teaching material to others; an Organizer might be the schedule coordinator for the group; a musical learner might present information in a new way that helps solidify concepts.

**FIGURE 4.3**   How to put your Personality Spectrum to work for you

## CHARACTERISTICS OF EACH PERSONALITY TYPE

### Thinker

- Solving problems
- Developing models and systems
- Analytical and abstract thinking
- Exploring ideas and potentials
- Ingenuity
- Going beyond established boundaries
- Global thinking—seeking universal truth

### Organizer

- Responsibility, reliability
- Operating successfully within social structures
- Sense of history, culture, and dignity
- Neatness and organization
- Loyalty
- Orientation to detail
- Comprehensive follow-through on tasks
- Efficiency
- Helping others

### Giver

- Honesty, authenticity
- Successful, close relationships
- Making a difference in the world
- Cultivating potential of self and others
- Negotiation; promoting peace
- Openness
- Helping others

### Adventurer

- High ability in a variety of fields
- Courage and daring
- Hands-on problem solving
- Living in the present
- Spontaneity and action
- Ability to negotiate
- Nontraditional style
- Flexibility
- Zest for life

## STUDY TECHNIQUES TO MAXIMIZE PERSONALITY TYPES

### Thinker

- Find time to reflect independently on new information
- Learn through problem solving
- Design new ways of approaching issues
- Convert material into logical charts
- Try to minimize repetitive tasks
- Look for opportunities to work independently

### Organizer

- Try to have tasks defined in clear, concrete terms so that you know what is required
- Look for a well-structured, stable environment
- Request feedback
- Use a planner to schedule tasks and dates
- Organize material by rewriting and organizing class or text notes, making flash cards, or carefully highlighting

### Giver

- Study with others
- Teach material to others
- Seek out tasks, groups, and subjects that involve helping people
- Find ways to express thoughts and feelings clearly and honestly
- Put energy into your most important relationships

### Adventurer

- Look for environments that encourage nontraditional approaches
- Find hands-on ways to learn
- Seek people whom you find stimulating
- Use or develop games and puzzles to help memorize terms
- Fight boredom by asking to do something extra or perform a task in a more active way

Joyce Bishop, *Keys to Success,* © 2001.

# Classroom Benefits

Your college instructors will most likely have a range of teaching styles (an instructor's teaching style often reflects his or her dominant learning style). Your particular learning style may work well with some instructors and be a mismatch with others. After several class meetings, you should be able to assess an instructor's teaching styles (see Figure 4.4). Then you can use what you know to maximize styles that suit you and compensate for those that don't.

Although presentation styles vary, the standard lecture is still the norm in most classrooms. For this reason, the traditional college classroom is generally a happy home for the verbal or logical learner and the Thinker and Organizer. However, many students learn best when interacting more than a lecture allows. What can you do if your styles don't match up with those of your instructor?

## Play to Your Strengths

For example, an Organizer with an instructor who delivers material in a random way might rewrite notes in an outline format to bring structure to concepts and insert facts where they fit best. Likewise, a Giver taking a straight lecture course with no student-to-student contact might meet with a study group to go over the details and fill in factual gaps.

## Work to Build Weaker Areas

As a visual learner reviews notes from a structured lecture course, he could outline them, allot extra time to master the material, and work with a study group. A Thinker, studying for a test from notes delivered by an Adventurer

| FIGURE 4.4 | Instructors often rely on one or more teaching styles |
| --- | --- |

| TEACHING STYLE | WHAT TO EXPECT IN CLASS |
| --- | --- |
| LECTURE, VERBAL FOCUS | Instructor speaks to the class for the entire period, with little class interaction. Lesson is taught primarily through words, either spoken or written on the board, overhead projector, handouts, or text. |
| GROUP DISCUSSION | Instructor presents material but encourages class discussion. |
| SMALL GROUPS | Instructor presents material and then breaks class into small groups for discussion or project work. |
| VISUAL FOCUS | Instructor uses visual elements such as diagrams, photographs, drawings, transparencies. |
| LOGICAL PRESENTATION | Instructor organizes material in a logical sequence, such as by time or importance. |
| RANDOM PRESENTATION | Instructor tackles topics in no particular order, and may jump around a lot or digress. |

instructor, could find hands-on ways to review the material (for example, for a science course, working in the lab).

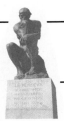

Learning is not attained by chance, it must be sought for with ardor and attended to with diligence.

ABIGAIL ADAMS

### Ask Your Instructor for Additional Help

If you are having trouble with course work, communicate with your instructor through e-mail or face to face during office hours. This is especially important in large lectures where you are anonymous unless you speak up. The visual learner, for example, might ask the instructor to recommend graphs or figures that illustrate the lecture.

Instructors are unique. No instructor can give each of a diverse group of learners exactly what each one needs. The flexibility that you need to mesh your learning style with instructors' teaching styles is a tool for career and life success. Just as you can't handpick your instructors, you will rarely, if ever, be able to choose your supervisors or their work styles.

## Workplace Benefits

Knowing how you learn brings you these benefits in your career:

- **Better performance through self-awareness.** Because your learning styles are essentially the same as your working styles, knowing how you learn will help you identify career and work environments that suit you. Knowing your strengths will help you use and highlight them on the job. When a task involves one of your weaker skills, you can either take special care to accomplish it or suggest someone else who is a better fit.

- **Better teamwork.** The more attuned you are to abilities and personality traits, the better you will be at identifying the tasks you and others can best perform in team situations. For example, a Giver might enjoy helping new hires get used to the people and environment. Or a supervisor directing an intrapersonal learner might offer the chance to take material home to think about before a meeting.

- **Better career planning.** The more you know about how you learn and work, the more you will be able to focus on career paths that could work well for you. For the following student, strength in both logical-mathematical and interpersonal intelligence has guided him toward specific jobs and activities while in school and has helped him choose career goals:

A family joke around the Patterson household centers on the roots of eldest son Cody's love affair with mathematics. Like any young child, the story goes, Cody would grow impatient when forced to wait in line in a public place. In an attempt to distract her fidgeting son, his mother, Janalyn, would dig in her purse for her pocket calculator. Once in his hands, the calculator's blinking electronic numerals would mesmerize young Cody, and the wait was soon forgotten. . . . Patterson, 21, laughed as he recalled the hours spent punching buttons on that little gadget. "A lot of guys grew up with G.I. Joes and action figures," he said with a smile. "I grew up with calculators."[3]

Whether or not his mother's calculator did indeed encourage a life dedicated to mathematical pursuits, there is no doubt that Patterson was born with a gift for numbers. He worked as a teaching assistant for an upper-level analysis course, a "math problem" writer for math competitions, and a help session leader for advanced math courses, and he has served as a Math Camp counselor and vice president of the Pi Mu Epsilon math honor society. "I'd like to be a college teacher and help students like me who have had opportunities to hit the big time," Patterson said, "and find some other students who are trying to find their place in academics, get them interested in math, and make believers out of them."

A better understanding of your learning strengths and preferences and personality traits will aid you in an upcoming educational challenge: choosing the right major.

# Why Do You Need *Science* and *Math* to Be a Nurse?

If you lack a realistic view of what nurses do, you might ask yourself why you need to take courses in math and science to be a nurse. As a prenursing student you may be taking chemistry and math. Perhaps you understand the need for chemistry because you know that chemical reactions underlie physiological reactions. The kidneys, for instance, spend most of their time regulating ions. Or, you may know that medications interact with receptors on cells to set off various chemical processes that can cause both positive and negative effects and that muscle cells are regulated by the inflow and outflow of calcium, sodium, and potassium. But, you might wonder, what is the purpose of math and other science courses that seem less obviously related to health and illness? The following example illustrates the reason math skills as well as science are important.

Matt is an emergency nurse in a large urban hospital. He is taking care of a 23-year-old who has been in a motor vehicle accident. The patient is very badly hurt and needs immediate surgery for internal trauma. Matt needs to give her antibiotics, along with other medications, before she goes to surgery. Matt will be giving the antibiotics intravenously (into a vein with a needle).

In the pharmacy, the antibiotic, powder or solution, is mixed with a specific volume of fluid and sent to Matt. Matt gets the antibiotics pre-mixed, and the rate of administration to give the correct dose is written on the intravenous medication bag. Matt is having a hectic day—another big trauma case is coming through the doors—and so he decides to hang the medications right away.

Unfortunately, Matt administers the medication without checking the original order or the pharmacy math calculations and gives the young patient the wrong dose. Luckily, he catches the error and corrects it before the patient goes to surgery with either too little antibiotic (no therapeutic effect) or too much antibiotic (potential harmful effect).

In school Matt took math and science prerequisites, and in nursing school he learned how to calculate medication dosages. Therefore, he could

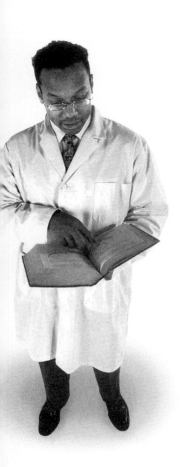

have easily figured the rate the intravenous antibiotic needed to run to give the correct dose. If only he had used those skills. After this experience, and while he is filling out the incident report, he vows to check each medication every time. Matt also knows from biochemistry that a chemical reaction of the antibiotic occurs in the kidneys, so it is important to be very careful because giving the drug incorrectly could cause kidney damage.

Next time Matt receives a drug from the pharmacy he checks it by recalculating the equations. Noticing a mistake, he calls the pharmacy, and the pharmacist also rechecks it. The medication is corrected before it is sent to the emergency department. Matt rechecks it a second time before he administers it. He also thinks about possible side effects and what he needs to monitor while the patient is under his care.

This example is not intended to imply that pharmacists often make mistakes, but rather that anyone can make a mistake. A nurse's job, along with the rest of the health care team, is to do the very best to prevent mistakes. This is the most dramatic reason a strong background in science and math is crucial to being a nurse. Science gives you the skills you need to provide safe, rational, and effective nursing care. Just as an air traffic controller must understand trajectories and math, or where the planes are going in the air, so nurses need to understand what keeps people going. Both have people's lives in their hands.

Science and math also teach you how to think critically (for more on critical thinking, see Chapter 5) and how to observe, how to reason, and how to problem-solve. Nurses use reasoning and problem-solving skills every day. Understanding how to do this requires knowing why you do it. Understanding about chemicals and cell receptors, and about the number of milliliters an intravenous line needs to run to give a certain number of micrograms, are essential keys to success in nursing. Remember, too, nurses work with the whole person. They take care of bodies and minds, and science teaches you about how the mind works, too. This can help you problem-solve questions about why a person behaves the way he or she does. For instance, why does your patient continue to drink alcohol even though his liver is in poor condition? Why doesn't a client with diabetes take her medicine?

If you deal with psychiatric problems, you will also need science to help you understand treatments and to explore topics such as the effect of sleep deprivation or poor nutrition on a patient's brain and therefore behavior.

This is what nurses do. They apply the knowledge learned in school, on the job, and in continuing education classes to real-life situations. If you want to do safe, high-quality work you must be well educated. Theory and its connecting principles are key to being a good nurse in your area of practice. And don't let anyone tell you otherwise!

Within the United States, there is great variation among high school students' science scores, often depending on the state in which they live. If you come from Iowa or Utah, your high school is probably doing very well in preparing you in math and science. Or you may live in a state where students have poorer scores; if so, your high school may not have prepared you to meet the challenge of prenursing and nursing courses. You will have some catching up to do, but that's not an impossible feat. Students from every state in the union have been attending college and graduating with nursing honors. And you can, too.

# How Can You *Choose* a Nursing Major?

The **major:** It may not be around the corner, but it's probably not that far away. At some point in the next two years (if you are in a four-year college), after you complete your general education requirements, you will apply to nursing school. If you are in prenursing now, you have already declared your major. Through this act you largely determine the courses you take, what you learn, and with whom you spend your school time.

Taking a practical approach to declaring your major now can help you avoid becoming overwhelmed by the task. Think of it as a long-term goal made up of multiple steps (short-term goals) that begin with knowing your learning styles, interests, and talents; exploring options; and establishing your academic schedule. Even if you have declared your major, you can go through the following steps to reconfirm your choice.

> MAJOR
> An academic subject area chosen as a field of specialization, requiring a specific course of study.

## Short-Term Goal #1: Use Learning Styles Assessments to Identify Interests and Talents

Considering what you like and what you do well can lead to a fulfilling area of study. When you identify your interests and talents and choose a nursing major that focuses on them, you are likely to have a positive attitude and perform at your highest level.

You may have sensed a career direction since you were young. This was the case with University of Illinois student Brian DeGraff, whose interests were mechanical: "I am amazed by how things work. The way a car can turn a tank of greasy, smelly, toxic liquid into my ride to school. People always say stop and smell the roses, but I'd rather stop and wonder why the roses smell. It was this passion that drove me to want to be an engineer; it's the best way I can imagine to spend my life figuring out how things work."[4]

Likewise, it is not uncommon to meet nurses who always knew they wanted to be a nurse. But this is not always true either. Some of us decide much later in life. You have plenty of time.

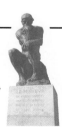

> You have to have confidence in your ability, and then be tough enough to follow through.
>
> ROSALYNN CARTER

To pinpoint the areas that spark your interest, and to see if they point toward nursing, use your Multiple Intelligences and Personality Spectrum assessment results to answer the following questions:

- What courses have I enjoyed the most in college and high school? What do these courses have in common?
- What subjects am I drawn to in my personal reading?
- What activities do I look forward to most?
- In what skills or academic areas do I perform best? Am I a "natural" in any area?

*(continued)*

- What do people say I do well?
- What are my dominant learning styles?

## Short-Term Goal #2: Explore Academic Options

Next, find out about the academic choices available at your school. Plan to achieve the following minigoals to reach this short-term goal:

### Learn What's Possible

Consult your college catalog for guidelines on declaring (and changing) your major. Find answers to these questions:

- When do I have to declare a major? (generally at the end of the second year for four-year programs; earlier for associate or certificate programs)
- What are my options in majoring? (double majors, minors, interdisciplinary majors)
- What other majors besides nursing are offered at my school?
- What minimum grade point average (GPA), if any, does the department require before it will accept me as a major?
- What GPA must I maintain in the courses included in the major?
- What preparatory courses (prerequisites) are required?
- What courses will I be required to take and in what sequence? How many credits do I need to graduate in the major?
- Will I have to write a thesis to graduate in this major?

### Work Closely with Your Adviser

Early on, find the nursing adviser on your campus and get acquainted. Begin discussing your major early on with your adviser; he or she can help you evaluate different options.

For any given major, your adviser may be able to tell you about both the corresponding department at your school and the possibilities in related career areas. You may also discuss the possibility of a double major (completing the requirements for two different majors) or designing your own major, if your school offers an opportunity to do so.

### Visit the Department, School, or College

Analyze your comfort with the nursing department as well as with the material. When Ashiana Esmail decided to major in ethnic studies at the University of California at Berkeley, she did so in part because she wanted a close-knit department where faculty knew her and could be her advocates. Being involved like this "was better than an A+" in helping to build academic momentum, she explains.[5]

To learn more, ask the department secretary for information. Then sit in on several classes to get a feel for the instructors and the work. Consider asking an instructor for an appointment to discuss the major.

### Speak to People with Experience in the Major

Ask students who are a year or two ahead of you to describe their experiences with the courses, the workload, and the instructors.

## Consider Creative Options for Majoring

Think beyond the traditional majoring path, and investigate the possibilities at your school. For instance, you may be a nursing major because everyone told you that you'd never get a job, or make money, as a writer—what you really wanted to study in college. Rather than choosing one or the other, combining them may be a possibility. You can continue as a nursing major and take plenty of writing and literature courses as electives. Plan on continuing your study of literature as a lifelong pursuit *and* working as a nurse. Your various interests are not mutually exclusive; they can actually enhance each other. Creativity helps you in nursing, and nursing can help in your other pursuits. Echo Heron, RN, has written several bestsellers about her experiences in critical care. Nursing is *the* place to learn about human nature and to participate in plenty of fascinating stories.

## Consider a Double Major

If, for example, you want to major in nursing and business, ask your academic adviser if it is possible to meet the requirements for both departments. Usually nursing school is very tough, and obtaining a second major may not be optimal.

Kyle, a nursing student, was studying business before he decided to become a nurse. He knew he was interested in business and helping people. His goal now was to become a certified registered nurse anesthetist (CRNA) and open his own business. CRNAs can practice on their own, and it is not uncommon for a group to open a practice together. Kyle is a very bright student, and after a rough first semester in nursing school he has excelled with his double major.

# Short-Term Goal #3: Establish Your Academic Schedule

Effective time management will enable you to fulfill the requirements of your major and complete all additional credits.

## Look at your Time Frame

How many years do you plan to study as an undergraduate or graduate student? Do you plan to attend graduate school? If so, do you plan to go there directly after graduation or take time off?

## Set Timing for Short-Term Goals

Within your time frame, pinpoint when to accomplish the important short-term goals that lead to graduation. What are the deadlines for completing core requirements, declaring a major, writing a thesis? Although you won't need to plan out your entire college course load at the beginning of your first semester, drafting a tentative **curriculum**—both within and outside your major—can help clarify where you are heading.

CURRICULUM
The particular set of courses required for a degree.

## Identify Dates Connected to Your Goal Fulfillment

Pay attention to academic dates (you will find an academic calendar in each year's college catalog and on the college's website). Such dates include registration dates, final date to declare a major, final date to drop a course, and so forth. Plan ahead so you don't miss a deadline.

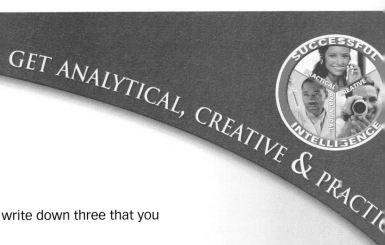

# Link Your Interests to Intriguing Majors Including Nursing

Looking at a list of the majors your school offers, write down three that you want to consider:

1. _____
2. _____
3. _____

Now look at the list again. Other than what you just wrote, what majors catch your eye? Write down three intriguing majors—*without* thinking about what you would do with them or whether they are practical choices.

1. _____
2. _____
3. _____

Choose one major from the second list and explore it. Talk to your adviser about the major. Read about it in your college catalog. Consider a minor in the subject. Speak to an instructor in the department about related careers. You will have taken a casual interest and turned it into a viable academic option.

## Be Flexible as You Come to a Decision

As with any serious challenge that involves defining your path, flexibility is essential. Many students change their minds as they consider majors; some declare a major and then change it one or more times before finding a good fit. Just act on any change right away—once you have considered it carefully—by informing your adviser, completing any required paperwork, and redesigning your schedule to reflect your new choices.

Some people may change their mind several times before honing in on a major that fits. Although this may add to the time you spend in college, being happy with your decision is important. For example, a student majoring in science education may begin student teaching only to discover that he or she really doesn't feel comfortable in front of students.

If this happens to you, don't be discouraged. You're certainly not alone. Changing a major is much like changing a job. Skills and experiences from one job will assist you in your next position, and some of the course from your first major may apply—or event transfer as credits—to your next major. Talk with your academic adviser about any desire to change majors. Sometimes an adviser can speak to department heads to get the maximum number of credits transferred to your new major.

Whatever you decide, realize that you do have the right to change your mind. Continual self-discovery is part of the journey. No matter how many detours you make, each interesting class you take along the way helps point you toward a major that feels like home.

# How Can Multiple Intelligences Help You *Explore Majors and Careers?*

All that you have learned in this chapter about your learning styles and strengths has practical application as you begin thinking about your future at school and in the workplace. A strength in one or more intelligences may lead you to a major, an internship, and even a lifelong career.

Figure 4.5 lists some possibilities for the eight intelligence types. This list is by no means complete. Rather, it represents only a fraction of the available opportunities. Use what you see here to inspire thought and spur investigation.

## Career Exploration Strategies

Whatever your major, nursing or not, you will benefit from starting to think about careers early on. Use the following strategies to explore what's out there.

### Keep What You Value in Mind

Ask yourself what careers support the principles that guide your life. How important to you are service to others, financial security, a broad-based education, time for family?

### Follow Your Passion

Find something you love doing more than anything else in the world, and then find a way to make money doing it. If you are sure of what you love to do but cannot pinpoint a career niche, open yourself to your instructors' advice.

# How Can You *Identify and Manage* Learning Disabilities?

Some learning disabilities cause reading problems, some create difficulties in math, and some make it difficult for students to process the language they hear. The following will help you understand learning disabilities and, should you be diagnosed with one, give you the tools to manage your disability successfully.

## Identifying a Learning Disability

The National Center for Learning Disabilities (NCLD) defines learning disabilities in terms of what they are and what they are not:[6]

- They are neurological disorders that interfere with one's ability to store, process, and produce information.
- They do *not* include mental retardation, autism, behavioral disorders, impaired vision, hearing loss, or other physical disabilities.

*(continued)*

FIGURE 4.5

## Multiple intelligences may open doors to majors, internships, and careers

| MULTIPLE INTELLIGENCE | CONSIDER MAJORING IN . . . | THINK ABOUT AN INTERNSHIP AT A . . . | LOOK INTO A CAREER AS . . . |
|---|---|---|---|
| Bodily-Kinesthetic | Massage Therapy<br>Physical Therapy<br>Kinesiology<br>Construction Engineering<br>Chiropractic<br>Sports Medicine<br>Anatomy<br>Dance<br>Theater | Sports Physician's Office<br>Athletic Club<br>Physical Therapy Center<br>Chiropractor's Office<br>Construction Company<br>Surveying Company<br>Dance Studio<br>Athletic Trainer<br>Drafting Firm<br>Theater Company | Carpenter<br>Draftsperson<br>Recreational Therapist<br>Physical Therapist<br>Mechanical Engineer<br>Massage Therapist<br>Dancer or Acrobat<br>Exercise Physiologist<br>Actor |
| Intrapersonal | Psychology<br>Sociology<br>English<br>Finance<br>Liberal Arts<br>Biology<br>Computer Science<br>Economics | Research and<br>   Development Firm<br>Accounting Firm<br>Computer Company<br>Publishing House<br>Pharmaceutical Company<br>Engineering Firm<br>Biology Lab | Research Scientist<br>Motivational Speaker<br>Engineer<br>Physicist<br>Sociologist<br>Computer Scientist<br>Economist<br>Author<br>Psychologist |
| Interpersonal | Psychology<br>Sociology<br>Education<br>Real Estate<br>Public Relations<br>Nursing<br>Business<br>Hotel/Restaurant<br>   Management<br>Rhetoric/Communications | Hotel or Restaurant<br>Travel Agency<br>Real Estate Agency<br>Public Relations Firm<br>Human Resources<br>Customer Service<br>Teaching Assistant<br>Marketing/Sales<br>Group Counseling<br>Social Service | Social Worker<br>PR Rep/Media Liaison<br>Human Resources<br>Travel Agent<br>Sociologist<br>Anthropologist<br>Counselor<br>Therapist<br>Teacher<br>Nurse |
| Naturalistic | Forestry<br>Astronomy<br>Geology<br>Biology<br>Zoology<br>Atmospheric Sciences<br>Oceanography<br>Agriculture<br>Animal Husbandry<br>Environmental Law<br>Physics | Museum<br>National Park<br>Oil Company<br>Botanical Gardens<br>Environmental Law Firm<br>Outward Bound<br>Adventure Travel Agency<br>Zoo<br>Camp Counselor<br>Biological Research Firm | Forest Ranger<br>Botanist or Herbalist<br>Geologist<br>Ecologist<br>Marine Biologist<br>Archaeologist<br>Astronomer<br>Adventure Travel Agent<br>Wildlife Tour Guide<br>Landscape Architect |

*(continued)*

| MULTIPLE INTELLIGENCE | CONSIDER MAJORING IN . . . | THINK ABOUT AN INTERNSHIP AT A . . . | LOOK INTO A CAREER AS . . . |
|---|---|---|---|
| Musical | Music<br>Musical History<br>Musical Theory<br>Performing Arts<br>Composition<br>Voice<br>Liberal Arts<br>Entertainment Law | Performance Hall<br>Radio Station<br>Record Label<br>Ballet or Theater Company<br>Recording Studio<br>Children's Music Camp<br>Orchestra or Opera Company<br>Musical Talent Agency<br>Entertainment Law Firm | Lyricist or Composer<br>Singer or Musician<br>Voice Coach<br>Music Teacher or Critic<br>Record Executive<br>Conductor<br>Radio DJ<br>Sound Engineer<br>Entertainment Lawyer |
| Logical-Mathematical | Math<br>Accounting<br>Physics<br>Economics<br>Medicine<br>Banking/Finance<br>Astronomy<br>Computer Science<br>Systems Theory<br>Law<br>Chemistry<br>Engineering | Law Firm<br>Health Care Office<br>Real Estate Brokerage<br>Accounting Firm<br>Animal Hospital<br>Science Lab<br>Consulting Firm<br>Pharmaceutical Firm<br>Bank | Doctor, Dentist, or<br>Veterinarian<br>Accountant<br>Pharmacist<br>Chemist<br>Physicist<br>Systems Analyst<br>Investment Banker<br>Financial Analyst<br>Computer Scientist |
| Verbal-Linguistic | Communications<br>Marketing<br>English/Literature<br>Journalism<br>Foreign Languages<br>Linguistic Theory<br>Political Science<br>Advertising/PR | Newspaper/Magazine<br>Network TV Affiliate<br>Publishing House<br>Law Firm<br>PR/Marketing Firm<br>Speech Therapist<br>Ad Agency<br>Training Company<br>Human Resources<br>Customer Service | Author<br>Playwright<br>Journalist<br>TV/Radio Producer<br>Literature Teacher<br>Speech Pathologist<br>Business Executive<br>Copywriter or Editor |
| Visual-Spatial | Visual Arts<br>Architecture<br>Interior Design<br>Multimedia Design<br>Film Theory<br>Photography<br>Art History | Art Gallery<br>Museum<br>Photography Studio<br>Design Firm<br>Advertising Agency<br>Theatrical Set Designer<br>Multimedia Firm<br>Architecture Firm<br>Film Studio | Graphic Artist<br>Photographer<br>Architect<br>Cinematographer<br>Art Therapist<br>Designer<br>Cartoonist/Illustrator<br>Art Museum Curator<br>Art Teacher |

- They do *not* include attention-deficit disorder and attention-deficit/hyperactivity disorder (disorders involving consistent and problematic inattention, hyperactivity, and/or impulsivity), although these problems may accompany learning disabilities.[7]
- They often run in families and are lifelong, although people with learning disabilities can use specific strategies to manage and even overcome areas of weakness.
- They must be diagnosed by professionals in order for the disabled person to receive federally funded aid.

How can you determine if you should be evaluated for a learning disability? According to the NCLD, persistent problems in any of the following areas may indicate a learning disability:[8]

- Reading or reading comprehension
- Math calculations, understanding language and concepts
- Social skills or interpreting social cues
- Following a schedule, being on time, meeting deadlines
- Reading or following maps
- Balancing a checkbook
- Following directions, especially on multistep tasks
- Writing, sentence structure, spelling, and organizing written work

Details on specific learning disabilities appear in Figure 4.6. For an evaluation, contact your school's learning center or student health center for a referral to a licensed professional.

## Managing a Learning Disability

If you are diagnosed with a learning disability, focused action will help you manage it and maximize your ability to learn and succeed:

### Be Informed About Your Disability

Search the library and the Internet—try NCLD at www.ncld.org or LD Online at www.ldonline.org (other websites are listed at the end of the chapter). Or call NCLD at 1-888-575-7373. Make sure you understand your Individualized Education Program (IEP), the document describing your disability and recommended strategies.

### Seek Assistance from Your School

Speak with your adviser about specific accommodations that will help you learn. Services mandated by law for students who are learning disabled include extended time on tests; note-taking assistance (for example, having a fellow student take notes for you); assistive technology devices (tape recorders or laptop computers); modified assignments; alternative assessments and test formats. Other services are tutoring, study skills assistance, and counseling.

### Be a Dedicated Student

Be on time and attend class. Read assignments before class. Sit where you can avoid distractions. Review notes soon after class. Spend extra time on assignments. Ask for help.

FIGURE 4.6

## What different learning disabilities are and how to recognize them

| DISABILITY/CONDITION | WHAT ARE THE SIGNS? |
| --- | --- |
| Dyslexia and related reading disorders | Problems with reading (including spelling, word sequencing, and comprehension) and processing (translating written language to thought or thought to written language) |
| Dyscalculia (developmental arithmetic disorders) | Difficulties in recognizing numbers and symbols, memorizing facts, aligning numbers, understanding abstract concepts like fractions, and applying math to life skills (time management, gauging distance, handling money, etc.) |
| Developmental writing disorders | Difficulties in composing complete sentences, organizing a writing assignment, or translating thoughts coherently to the page |
| Handwriting disorders (dysgraphia) | Disorder characterized by writing disabilities, including writing that is distorted or incorrect. Sufferers have poor handwriting that is difficult to read because of inappropriately sized and spaced letters. The use of wrong or misspelled words is also common |
| Speech and language disorders | Problems with producing speech sounds, using spoken language to communicate, and/or understanding what others say |
| LD-related social issues | Problems in recognizing facial or vocal cues from others, controlling verbal and physical impulsivity, and respecting others' personal space |
| LD-related organizational issues | Difficulties in scheduling and in organizing personal, academic, and work-related materials |

*Source:* LD Online: Learning Disabilities Information and Resources, www.ldonline.org (accessed March 17, 2004). © 2001 WETA.

## Build a Positive Attitude

See your accomplishments in light of how far you have come. Rely on people who support you. Know that the help you receive will give you the best possible chance to learn and grow.

# *Sabiduría*

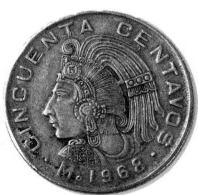

In Spanish, the term *sabiduría* represents the two sides of learning: knowledge and wisdom. *Knowledge* involves gaining information, understanding concepts, building what you know about how the world works. *Wisdom* is the collected meaning and significance gained from knowledge. The learning and life experiences you gain in college will build your personal *sabiduría*, which, in turn, will help you make wise personal, educational, and career choices.

Think of this concept as you acquire knowledge in your classes. Try to transform the facts and concepts you study into the building blocks of wisdom.

# Building World-Class Skills

*for College, Career, and Life Success*

## Create Your Future

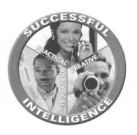

## DEVELOPING SUCCESSFUL INTELLIGENCE

### *Putting It All Together*

**Learn from the experiences of others**. Look back to Dawn E. Bedell's question about learning on page 110. After you've read her story, relate her experience to your own life by completing the following:

**Step 1. Think it through:** *Analyze your experience and compare it to Dawn's.* What is a consistent learning challenge for you as a student, and how does this relate to Dawn's experience? How might this be explained by your learning styles?

**Step 2. Think out of the box:** *Imagine ways of advising.* You are an adviser to a student identical to yourself. Be a harsh adviser: How would you criticize your performance as a student? Then be a wise adviser, focused on tapping into learning styles information: How would you identify challenges and suggest ways to handle them?

**Step 3. Make it happen:** *Head off your own challenges with practical strategies.* You have named a consistent challenge—and you have imagined what you would say as your own adviser. Now identify steps that will help you face your challenge (choosing particular courses, meeting with an adviser or instructor who can give you ideas, approaching work in particular ways).

## TEAM BUILDING

### *Collaborative Solutions*

**Ideas About Personality Types.** Divide into groups according to the four types of the Personality Spectrum: Thinker-dominant students in one group, Organizer-dominant students in another, Giver-dominant students in a third, and

Adventurer-dominant students in the fourth. If you have scored the same in more than one of these types, join whatever group is smaller. With your group, brainstorm the following lists for your type:

1. The strengths of this type
2. The struggles it brings
3. The stressors (things that cause stress) for this type
4. Career areas that tend to suit this type
5. Career areas that are a challenge for this type
6. People who annoy this type the most (often because they are strong in areas where this type needs to grow)

If there is time, each group can present this information to the entire class; this will boost understanding and acceptance of diverse ways of relating to information and people.

# WRITING

## Discovery Through Journaling

*Record your thoughts on a separate piece of paper or in a journal.*

**Strengths and Weaknesses**. What have the personal assessments in this chapter taught you about your strengths? Choose what you consider your greatest strength, and discuss how you plan to use it to your advantage this semester. What areas of weakness did the assessments highlight? Choose a weakness that has given you difficulty in school, and brainstorm ways to compensate for it this semester. Finally, brainstorm ideas for how you will deal this semester with the kinds of people who challenge you the most.

# CAREER PORTFOLIO

## Plan for Success

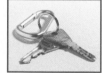

*Complete the following in your electronic portfolio, if you can use a graphics program, or on separate sheets of paper.*

**Self-Portrait**. Because self-knowledge helps you make the best choices about your future, a self-portrait is an important step in your career exploration. Use this exercise to synthesize everything you have been exploring about yourself into one comprehensive "self-portrait." Design your protrait in "think link" style, using words and visual shapes to describe your dominant Multiple Intelligences and Personality Spectrum dimensions, values, abilities, career interests, and anything else that is an important part of who you are.

A think link is a visual construction of related ideas, similar to a map or web, that represents your thought process. Ideas are written inside geometric shapes, often boxes or circles, and related ideas and facts are attached to those ideas by lines that connect the shapes. See the note-taking section in Chapter 6 for more about think links.

Use the style shown in the example in Figure 4.7 or create your own. For example, in this exercise you may want to create a "wheel" of ideas coming off your central shape, entitled "Me." Then, spreading out from each of those ideas (interests, learning style, etc.), draw lines connecting all of the thoughts that go along with that idea. Connected to "Interests," for example, might be "singing," "stock market," and "history."

You don't have to use the wheel image. You might want to design a treelike think link or a line of boxes with connecting thoughts written below the boxes, or anything else you like. Let your design reflect who you are, just as what you write does.

**FIGURE 4.7** One example of a self-portrait

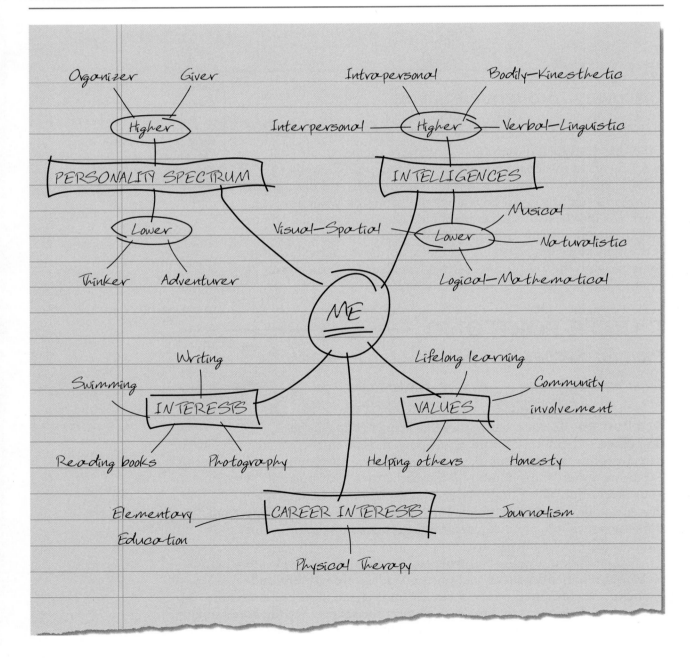

## Suggested Readings

Cobb, Joyanne. *Learning How to Learn: A Guide for Getting into College with a Learning Disability, Staying in, and Staying Sane.* Washington, DC: Child Welfare League of America, 2001.

College Board, ed. *The College Board Index of Majors and Graduate Degrees 2001.* New York: College Entrance Examination Board, 2000.

Gardner, Howard. *Intelligence Reframed: Multiple Intelligences for the 21st Century.* New York: Basic Books, 2000.

Fogg, Neeta, et al. *The College Majors Handbook with Real Career Paths and Payoffs: The Actual Jobs, Earnings, and Trends for Graduates of 60 College Majors.* Indianapolis, IN: Jist Works, 2004.

Keirsey, David. *Please Understand Me II: Temperament, Character, Intelligence.* Del Mar, CA: Prometheus Nemesis Book Company, 1998.

Pearman, Roger R., and Sarah C. Albritton. *I'm Not Crazy, I'm Just Not You: The Real Meaning of the 16 Personality Types.* Palo Alto, CA: Consulting Psychologists Press, 1997.

Phifer, Paul. *College Majors and Careers: A Resource Guide for Effective Life Planning,* 4th ed. Chicago: Ferguson Publishing, 1999.

Sclafani, Annette. *College Guide for Students with Learning Disabilities.* New York: Laurel Publications, 2003.

## Internet Resources

Attention Deficit Disorder Association: **www.add.org**

Children and Adults with Attention Deficit/Hyperactivity Disorder: **www.chadd.org**

International Dyslexia Association: **www.interdys.org**

Keirsey Sorter and other Myers-Briggs information: **www.keirsey.com**

Learning Disabilities Online: **www.ldonline.org**

National Center for Learning Disabilities: **www.ncld.org**

Prentice Hall Student Success Supersite Majors Exploration: **www.prenhall.com/success/ MajorExp/index.html**

## Endnotes

[1] Howard Gardner, *Multiple Intelligences: The Theory in Practice* (New York: HarperCollins, 1993), pp. 5–49.

[2] Ibid., p. 7.

[3] Kara Bounds Socol, "Cody Patterson '03: Math Student Benefits from Private Gifts," Texas A&M website. Available: http://giving.tamu.edu/ content/impactofgiving/studentstories/studentget. php?get=6.

[4] Students Speak: Excerpts from Your Educational Experience Essays, the University of Illinois (October 2, 2001). Retrieved March 2004 from: http://ae3.cen.uiuc.edu/stessay/StudentsSpeak.

[5] Terry Strathman, "L & S Colloquium on Undergraduate Education: What Do Students Want?" (April 15, 2002). Retrieved March 2004 from: http://ls.berkeley.edu/undergrad/colloquia/ 02–02.html.

[6] National Center for Learning Disabilities, "LD at a Glance" (May 2003). Available: www.ncld.org/ LDInfoZone/InfoZone_FactSheet_LD.cfm.

[7] National Center for Learning Disabilities, *Adult Learning Disabilities: A Learning Disability Isn't Something You Outgrow. It's Something You Learn to Master* (pamphlet). New York: National Center for Learning Disabilities.

[8] National Center for Learning Disabilities, "LD Advocates Guide" (May 2003). Available: www. ld.org/Advocacy/tutorial_talking_about.cfm.

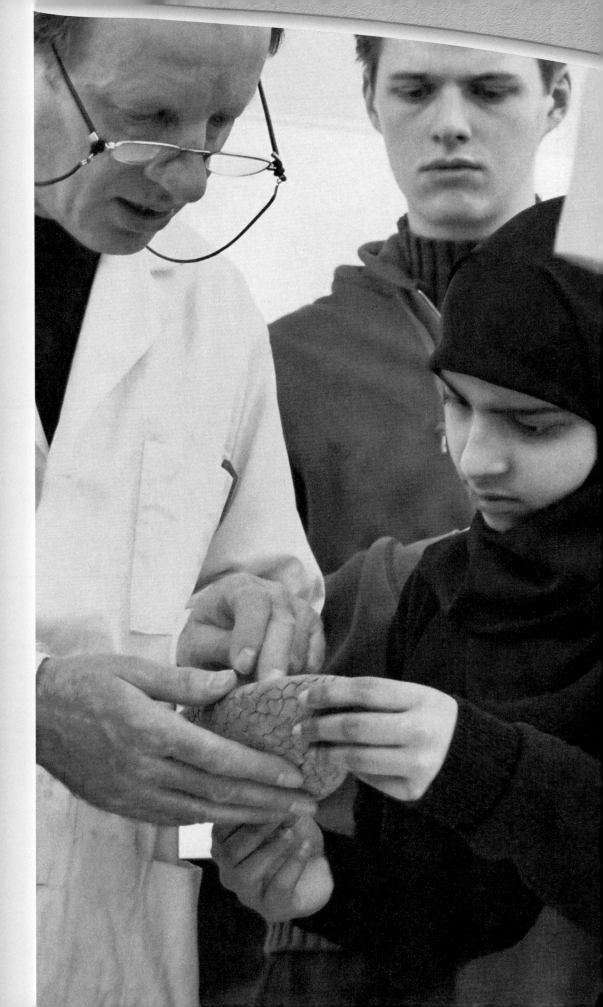

# 5

To survive and to thrive in college and beyond, you will need to use your thinking power to do more than remember formulas for a test. When problems or decisions arise on the road toward goals large and small, how can you work through them successfully? The answer lies in how you combine your analytical, creative, and practical thinking skills—in other words, how you use your successful intelligence. As you remember from Chapter 1, successful intelligence is "the kind of intelligence used to achieve important goals."[1]

Thinking, like note taking or car repair, is a skill that can be developed with practice. This chapter will help you build your ability to analyze information, come up with creative ideas, and put a practical plan into action. With these skills you can become a better thinker, problem solver, and decision maker, able to reach the goals that mean the most to you.

## IN THIS CHAPTER ...

*you will explore answers to the following questions:*

- What is successfully intelligent thinking? 137
- How can you improve your analytical thinking skills? 140
- How can you improve your creative thinking skills? 146
- How can you improve your practical thinking skills? 151
- How can you put analytical, creative, and practical thinking together in nursing? 155
- How are critical thinking and the scientific method used in evidence-based practice? 162

## What will it be like after I finish nursing school and become a real nurse?

Even though I'm in my last rotation of nursing clinicals, I have a lot of apprehension about beginning my career as a nurse. I still feel fuzzy about what to expect, and I don't think I'm alone in the way feel. I've talked to many other nursing students and they also feel nervous about starting their first real job. I mean, it's one thing to be a student but it's something else to be a nurse on the floor. In about six months I'll be a professional and that's scary.

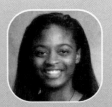

Crystal Johnson
Senior, Emory University,
Atlanta, Georgia

I think part of the reason I feel less than confident is that I don't see how the theory I'm learning in class applies to clinical work. What I've learned in the textbooks sometimes doesn't seem practical in real-life situations. Maybe I'm looking at it the wrong way, but the two often appear incompatible. For example, I've learned about family-centered care, which is a theory that says to keep the patient at the center by allowing the patient to have input in their treatment. But in my clinical experience, I've noticed that few nurses seem to follow that procedure. Most nurses tell the patient what to do without inviting feedback. Seeing these inconsistencies leaves me feeling a little confused about my future role as a nursing professional.

## PRACTICAL ANSWERS

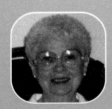

Barbara Andre, RN,
CCRN, CRNA
Retired. Westlake
Community Hospital
Melrose Park, Illinois

### You will grow in professionalism and learn over the course of your career.

Your question about theory versus the real would is a good one. Theory is essential to providing quality patient care. You need to know the theory behind nursing practices in order to set your own goals for what kind of nurse you want to be. Theory gives you the ideal situation. Of course, we all know there are few ideal situations in the real world!

As a nurse, you will create your own method of doing things, and your motives should be to aim for the ideal.

You do want to communicate with your patients and involve them in their own health care. For instance, if they are reluctant to learn how to give their own inhalation treatments, you could give them the option of doing it while sitting up in a chair or waiting until they go back to bed. This may help them feel a little more in charge and motivate them. However, you may be very busy with other, more critical patients, making it necessary for you to give the treatment when you have a free moment. But your goal will be to try your best to work it into your schedule because you know how important it will be for your patients to follow through on their own when they get home. You want them to become self-motivated.

Feeling comfortable communicating with and involving patients in their care comes with experience. I have found that older nurses are very willing to share their knowledge and experience with new gradutes—if they ask. I worked with one new graduate who pretended she knew everything. She isolated herself and made mistakes. The first lesson to learn on any new job is to ask questions. Most hospitals provide training programs that introduce new nurses to the job. The theory you are learning in school can help you to understand why certain situations have been adapted or altered to fit a particular hospital setting.

Therefore, if you are taught to do something one way in school but then asked to do it another way in clinicals, find out why. There is probably a good reason for the change. A bruised ego is easier to heal than a reprimand for doing it wrong. The safety of the patient always comes before pride, not only in theory but in practice. Occasionally you may discover an error in another nurse's judgment. Or your theory may reveal a better way to carry out a procedure. Other nurses are more likely to listen to you if you submit your ideas to them humbly.

It's perfectly normal to feel apprehensive about your future role as a nurse, but rest assured that gradually you'll grow in confidence and professionalism. The theory you are learning in class coupled with practical work experience will help you succeed in your nursing career.

# What Is *Successfully Intelligent* Thinking?

Robert Sternberg uses this story to illustrate the impact of successful intelligence:

> Two boys are walking in a forest. They are quite different. The first boy's teachers think he is smart, his parents think he is smart, and as a result, he thinks he is smart. He has good test scores, good grades, and other good paper credentials that will get him far in his scholastic life.
>
> Few people consider the second boy smart. His test scores are nothing great, his grades aren't so good, and his other paper credentials are, in general, marginal. At best, people would call him shrewd or street smart.
>
> As the two boys walk along in the forest, they encounter a problem—a huge, furious, hungry-looking grizzly bear, charging straight at them. The first boy, calculating that the grizzly bear will overtake them in 17.3 seconds, panics. In this state, he looks at the second boy, who is calmly taking off his hiking boots and putting on his jogging shoes.
>
> The first boy says to the second boy, "You must be crazy. There is no way you are going to outrun that grizzly bear!"
>
> The second boy replies, "That's true. But all I have to do is outrun you!"[2]

This story shows that successful problem solving and decision making require more than "book smarts." When confronted with a problem, using only analytical thinking put the first boy at a disadvantage. The second boy, in contrast, thought in different ways; he analyzed the situation, creatively considered the options, and took practical action. He asked and answered questions. He knew his purpose. And he lived to tell the tale.

## Successfully Intelligent Thinking Is Balanced

Some tasks require only one thinking skill, or ability, at a time. You might use analytical thinking to complete a multiple-choice quiz, creative thinking to figure out how to get a paper done the same day you work a long shift,

**FIGURE 5.1**   Successful intelligence depends on three thinking skills

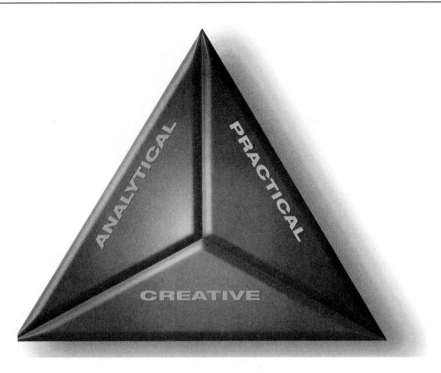

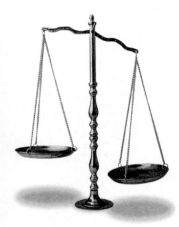

or practical thinking to put together a desk marked "some assembly required." However, when you need to solve a problem or make a decision, your analytical, creative, and practical thinking skills build on one another to move you forward.[3] Envision it this way: Just as a pyramid needs three sides to stand, successful thinkers need all three thinking skills to develop the best solutions and decisions (see Figure 5.1).

Each thinking skill adds an important dimension to accomplishing goals. Developing a balanced set of skills and knowing how and when to use each of them gives you more thinking power than having a strong aptitude in any one ability.[4] This kind of flexible thinking will help you connect your academic tasks to life goals—and show you where your hard work can take you (see Figure 5.2).

## Successfully Intelligent Thinking Means Asking and Answering Questions

What is thinking? According to experts, it is what happens when you ask questions and move toward the answers.[5] "To think through or rethink anything," says Dr. Richard Paul, director of research at the Center for Critical Thinking and Moral Critique, "one must ask questions that stimulate our thought. Questions define tasks, express problems and delineate issues. . . . Only students who have questions are really thinking and learning."[6]

As you answer questions, you transform raw data into information that you can use. A *Wall Street Journal* article, "The Best Innovations Are Those That Come from Smart Questions," relays the story of a cell biology student,

| DISCIPLINE | ANALYTICAL THINKING | CREATIVE THINKING | PRACTICAL THINKING |
|---|---|---|---|
| **Behavioral Science** | Comparing one theory of child development with another | Devising a new theory of child development | Applying child development theories to help parents and teachers understand and deal with children more effectively |
| **Literature** | Analyzing the development of the main character in a novel | Writing alternative endings to the novel | Using the experience of the main character to better understand and manage one's own life situations |
| **History** | Considering similarities and differences between World War I and World War II | Imagining yourself as a German citizen, dealing with economic depression after WWI | Seeing what WWI and WWII lessons can be applied to current Middle East conflicts |
| **Sports** | Analyzing the opposing team's strategy on the soccer field | Coming up with innovative ways to move the ball downfield | Using tactics to hide your strategy from an opposing team—or a competing company |

*Source:* Adapted from Robert J. Sternberg, *Successful Intelligence.* Plume: New York, 1997, p. 149.

William Hunter, whose professor told him that "the difference between good science and great science is the quality of the questions posed." Later, as a doctor and the president and CEO of a pharmaceutical company, Dr. Hunter asked questions about new ways to use drugs. His questions led to the development of a revolutionary product—a drug-coated coronary stent that prevents scar tissue from forming. Through seeking answers to probing questions, Dr. Hunter reached a significant goal.[7]

You use questions to analyze ("How bad is my money situation?"), come up with creative ideas ("What ways could I earn money?"), and apply practical solutions ("How can I get a job on campus?"). Later in the chapter, in the sections on analytical, creative, and practical thinking, you will find examples of the kinds of questions that drive each skill.

Like any aspect of thinking, questioning is not often a straightforward process. Sometimes the answer doesn't come right away. Often the answer leads to more—and more specific—questions.

## Successfully Intelligent Thinking Requires Knowing Your Purpose

To ask useful questions, you need to know *why* you are questioning. In other words, you need to define your purpose. Not knowing your purpose may lead you to ask questions that take you in irrelevant directions and waste your time. For example, if an assignment asks you to analyze the effectiveness of John F. Kennedy's foreign policy during his presidency, asking questions about his personal life may lead you off the track.

A general question can be your starting point for defining your purposes: "What am I trying to accomplish, and why?" Then, within each stage of the process, you will find more specific purposes, or subgoals, that help you generate analytical, creative, or practical questions along the way.

## Successfully Intelligent Thinking Is Yours to Build

You can improve, now and throughout your life, your ability to think. Studies have shown that the brain continues to develop throughout your life if you continue to learn new things.[8] Puzzle master Nob Yoshigahara has said, "As jogging is to the body, thinking is to the brain. The more we do it, the better we become."[9]

The mini-assessments within this chapter will help you to get an idea of how you perceive yourself as an analytical, creative, and practical thinker. Every other chapter's set of *Get Analytical, Get Creative*, and *Get Practical* exercises then helps you to build your skills in those areas. Finally, the *Developing Successful Intelligence*: *Putting It All Together* exercises at the ends of chapters encourage you to both build and combine your skills. *Your work throughout the book is geared toward building your successful intelligence.*

Begin by exploring the analytical thinking skills that you'll need to solve problems and make decisions effectively.

# How Can You Improve Your *Analytical Thinking* Skills?

Analytical thinking—also known as critical thinking—is the process of gathering information, analyzing it in different ways, and evaluating it for the purposes of gaining understanding, solving a problem, or making a decision. It is as essential for real-life problems and decisions as it is for thinking through the hypothetical questions on your chemistry homework.

The first step in analytical thinking, as with all aspects of successful intelligence, is to define your purpose. What do you want to analyze, and why? Perhaps you need to analyze the plot of a novel to determine its structure; maybe you want to analyze your schedule to figure out whether you are arranging your time and responsibilities effectively.

Once you define your purpose, the rest of the analytical process involves gathering the necessary information, analyzing and clarifying the ideas, and evaluating what you've found.

## Gather Information

Information is the raw material for thinking. Choosing what to gather requires a careful analysis of how much information you need, how much time to spend gathering it, and whether the information is relevant. Say, for instance, that your assignment is to write a paper on one style of American jazz music. If you gathered every available resource on the topic, it might be next semester before you got to the writing stage.

Here's how you might use analysis to gather information for that paper effectively:

- Reviewing the assignment, you learn that the paper should be 10 pages and cover at least three influential musicians.
- At the library and online, you find lots of what appears to be relevant information.
- You choose a jazz movement, find five or six comprehensive pieces on it, and then select three in-depth sources on each of three musicians.

In this way you achieve a subgoal—a selection of useful materials—on the way to your larger goal of writing a well-crafted paper.

## Analyze and Clarify Information

Once you've gathered the information, the next step is to analyze it to determine whether the information is reliable and useful in helping you answer your questions.

### Break Information into Parts

When analyzing information, you break information into parts and examine the parts so that you can see how they relate to each other and to information you already know. The following strategies help you break information down into pieces and set aside what is unclear, unrelated, or unimportant, resulting in a deeper and more reliable understanding.

**Separate the ideas.** If you are reading about the rise of the bebop movement, you might name events that influenced it, key musicians, facts about the sound, and ideas behind it.

**Compare and contrast.** Look at how things are similar to, or different from, each other. You might explore how three bebop musicians are similar in style. You might look at how they differ in what they want to communicate with their music.

**Examine cause and effect.** Look at the possible reasons why something happened (possible causes) and its consequences (effects, both positive and negative). You might examine the causes that led up to the bebop sound as well as its effects on other nonjazz musical styles.

An important caution: Analyze carefully to seek out *true causes*—some apparent causes may not be actual causes (often called "false causes"). For example, events in the musical world and general society took place when the first musicians were developing the bebop style. Some may have led directly to the new style; some may simply have occurred at the same time.

**Look for themes, patterns, and categories.** Note connections that arise out of how bits of information relate to one another. A theme of freedom versus structure, for example, might emerge out of an examination of bebop versus swing jazz. A pattern of behavior might develop as you look at how different musicians broke off from the swing movement. Musicians with different styles might fall into the bebop category based on their artistic goals.

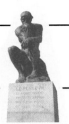

> Too often we enjoy the comfort of opinion without the discomfort of thought.

JOHN F. KENNEDY

Once the ideas are broken down, you can examine whether examples support ideas, separate fact from opinion, consider perspective, and investigate hidden assumptions.

## Examine Whether Examples Support Ideas

When you encounter an idea or claim, examine how it is supported with examples or evidence (facts, expert opinion, research findings, personal experience, and so on). Ideas that aren't backed up with solid evidence or made concrete with examples are not useful. Be critical of the information you gather; don't take it at face value.

For example, an advertisement for a weight-loss pill, claiming that it allows users to drop a pound a day, quotes "Anne" who says that she lost 30 pounds in 30 days. The word of one person, who may or may not be telling the truth, is not adequate support. But a claim that water once existed on Mars, backed up by measurements and photography from one of the Mars Exploration Rovers, may prove more reliable.

## Distinguish Fact from Opinion

A *statement of fact* is information presented as objectively real and verifiable ("It's raining outside right now"). In constrast, a *statement of opinion* is a belief, conclusion, or judgment that is inherently difficult, and sometimes impossible, to verify ("This is the most miserable rainstorm ever"). Figure 5.3 defines important characteristics of fact and opinion. Finding credible, reliable information with which to answer questions and come up with ideas enables you to separate fact from opinion. Even though facts may seem more solid, you can also make use of opinions if you determine they are backed up with facts. However, it is important to examine opinions for their underlying perspectives and assumptions.

## Examine Perspectives and Assumptions

*Perspective* is a characteristic way of thinking about people, situations, events, and ideas. Perspectives can be broad, such as a generally optimistic or pessimistic view of life. Or they can be more focused, such as an attitude about whether students should commute or live on campus.

Perspectives are associated with *assumptions*—judgments, generalizations, or biases influenced by experience and values. For example, the perspective that there are many different successful ways to be a family leads to assumptions such as "Single-parent homes can provide nurturing environments" and "Same-sex couples can rear well-adjusted children." Having a particular experience with single-parent homes or same-sex couples can build or reinforce a perspective.

## FIGURE 5.3    Examine how fact and opinion differ

| OPINIONS INCLUDE STATEMENTS THAT . . . | FACTS INCLUDE STATEMENTS THAT . . . |
|---|---|
| . . . *show evaluation.* Any statement of value indicates an opinion. Words such as *bad, good, pointless,* and *beneficial* indicate value judgments. Example: "Jimmy Carter is the most successful peace negotiator to sit in the White House." | . . . *deal with actual people, places, objects, or events.* Example: "In 1978, Jimmy Carter's 13-day summit meeting with Egyptian President Anwar Sadat and Israeli Prime Minister Menachem Begin led to a treaty between the two countries." |
| . . . *use abstract words.* Words that are complicated to define, like *misery* or *success,* usually indicate a personal opinion. Example: "The charity event was a smashing success." | . . . *use concrete words or measurable statistics.* Example: "The charity event raised $5,862." |
| . . . *predict future events.* Statements that examine future occurrences are often opinions. Example: "Mr. Barrett's course is going to set a new enrollment record this year." | . . . *describe current events in exact terms.* Example: "Mr. Barrett's course has 378 students enrolled this semester." |
| . . . *use emotional words.* Emotions are by nature unverifiable. Chances are that statements using such words as *delightful* or *miserable* express an opinion. Example: "That class is a miserable experience." | . . . *avoid emotional words and focus on the verifiable.* Example: "Citing dissatisfaction with the instruction, 7 out of the 25 students in that class withdrew in September." |
| . . . *use absolutes.* Absolute *qualifiers,* such as *all, none, never,* and *always,* often point to an opinion. Example: "All students need to have a job while in school." | . . . *avoid absolutes.* Example: "Some students need to have a job while in school." |

Source: Adapted from Ben E. Johnson, *Stirring Up Thinking.* New York: Houghton Mifflin, 1998, pp. 268–70.

Assumptions often hide within questions and statements, blocking you from considering information in different ways. Take this classic puzzler as an example: "Which came first, the chicken or the egg?" Thinking about this question, most people assume the egg is a chicken egg. If you think past that assumption and come up with a new idea—such as the egg is a dinosaur egg—then the obvious answer is that the egg came first!

Examining perspectives and assumptions is important for two reasons. First, they often affect your perception of the validity of materials you read and research. Second, your own perspectives and assumptions can cloud your interpretation of the information you encounter.

## Perspectives and Assumptions in Information

Being able to determine the perspectives that underlie materials will help you separate **biased** from unbiased information. For example, the conclusions in two articles on federal versus state government control of education may differ radically if one appears in a politically conservative publication and one appears in a liberal publication. Comparing those articles will require that you understand and take into account the conservative and liberal perspectives on government's role in education.

BIASED
Leaning in a particular direction; influenced by a point of view.

Assumptions often affect the validity of materials you read and research. A historical Revolutionary War document that originated in the colonies, for example, may assume that the rebellion against the British was entirely justified and leave out information to the contrary. Clearly understanding such a document means separating the assumptions from the facts.

## Personal Perspectives and Assumptions

Your own preferences, values, and prejudices—which influence your perspective—can affect how accurately you view information. A student who thinks that the death penalty is wrong, for example, may have a hard time analyzing the facts and arguments in an article that supports it. Or, in a research situation, he might use only materials that agree with his perspective.

Consider the perspectives and assumptions that might follow from your values. Then, when you have to analyze information, try to set them aside. "Anticipate your reactions and prejudices and then consciously resist their influence," says Colby Glass, professor of information research and philosophy at Palo Alto College.[10]

In addition to helping you analyze accurately, opening yourself to new perspectives will help you build knowledge. The more you know, the more information you have to work with as you move through life and encounter new problems and decisions. Come to school ready to hear and read new ideas, think about their merits, and make informed decisions about what you believe. Says Sternberg, "We need to . . . see issues from a variety of viewpoints and, especially, to see how other people and other cultures view issues and problems facing the world."[11]

## Evaluate Information

You've gathered and analyzed your information. You have examined its components, its evidence, its validity, its perspective, and any underlying assumptions. Now, based on an examination of evidence and careful analysis, you *evaluate* whether an idea or piece of information is good or bad, important or unimportant, right or wrong. You then set aside what is not useful and use the rest to form an opinion, possible solution, or decision.

For example, you're working on a group presentation on the effects of television watching on young children. You've gathered information that relates to your topic, come up with an idea, and analyzed whether the information supports this idea. Now you evaluate all of the evidence, presenting what's useful in an organized, persuasive way. Another example: In creating a résumé, you decide which information to include that will generate the most interest in potential employers and present you in the best light possible.

See Figure 5.4 for some questions you can ask to build and use analytical thinking skills.

Analytical thinking is only part of the picture. Pursuing your goals, in school and in the workplace, requires not just analyzing information but also thinking creatively about how to use it.

| | |
|---|---|
| **FIGURE 5.4** | Ask questions like these in order to analyze |

| | |
|---|---|
| To gather information, ask: | ● What requirements does my goal have? |
| | ● What kinds of information do I need to meet my goal? |
| | ● What information is available? |
| | ● Where and when is it available? Where and when can I access it? |
| | ● Of the sources I found, which ones will best help me achieve my goal? |
| To analyze, ask: | ● What are the parts of this information? |
| | ● What is similar to this information? What is different? |
| | ● What are the reasons for this? Why did this happen? |
| | ● What ideas or themes emerge from this material? |
| | ● How would you categorize this information? |
| | ● What conclusions can you make about this information? |
| To see if examples support an idea, ask: | ● What examples, or evidence, support the idea? |
| | ● Does the evidence make sense? |
| | ● Does the evidence support the idea/claim? |
| | ● Is this evidence key information that I need to answer my question? |
| | ● Are there examples that might disprove the idea/claim? |
| To distinguish fact from opinion, ask: | ● Do the words in this information signal fact or opinion? (See Figure 5.3) |
| | ● What is the source of this information? Is the source reliable? |
| | ● How does this information compare to other facts or opinions? |
| | ● If this is an opinion, is it supported by facts? |
| | ● How can I use this fact or opinion? |
| To examine perspectives and assumptions, ask: | ● Who is the author? What perspectives might this person have? |
| | ● What might be emphasized or left out as a result of the perspective? |
| | ● How could I consider this information from a different perspective? |
| | ● What assumptions might lie behind this statement or material? |
| | ● How could I prove, or disprove, an assumption? |
| | ● What contradictory assumptions might be equally valid? |
| | ● How might a personal perspective or assumption affect the way I see this material? |
| To evaluate, ask: | ● Do I agree with this information? |
| | ● Does this information fit what I'm trying to prove or accomplish? |
| | ● Is this information true or false, and why? |
| | ● How important is this information? |
| | ● Which ideas or pieces of information would I choose to focus on? |

Adapted from www.ed.final.gov/trc/tutorial/taxonomy.html (Richard Paul, *Critical Thinking: How to Prepare Students for a Rapidly Changing World*, 1993) and from www.kcmetro.edu/longview/ctac/blooms.htm, Barbara Fowler, Longview Community College, "Bloom's Taxonomy and Critical Thinking."

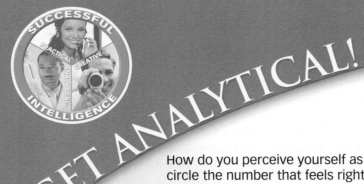

# Assess Analytical Thinking Skills

How do you perceive yourself as an analytical thinker? For each statement, circle the number that feels right to you, from 1 for "least like me" to 5 for "most like me."

1. I tend to perform well on objective tests.　　　　　　　　1  2  3  4  5

2. People say I'm a "thinker," "brainy," "studious."　　　　　1  2  3  4  5

3. I am not comfortable with gray areas—I prefer　　　　　1  2  3  4  5
   information to be laid out in black and white.

4. In a group setting, I like to tackle the details of a problem.　1  2  3  4  5

5. I sometimes overthink things and miss my moment of　　1  2  3  4  5
   opportunity.

Total your answers here: _____

If your total ranges from 5 to 12, you consider your analytical thinking skills to be *weak*.

If your total ranges from 13 to 19, you consider your analytical thinking skills to be *average*.

If your total ranges from 20 to 25, you consider your analytical thinking skills to be *strong*.

# How Can You Improve Your *Creative Thinking* Skills?

Some researchers define creativity as combining existing elements in an innovative way to create a new purpose or result. For example, 3M researcher Spencer Silver, in 1970, created a weak adhesive; four years later, another 3M scientist, Arthur Fry, used it for a hymnal marker. Stick-on notes are now an office staple. Others see creativity as the art of generating ideas from taking a fresh look at how things are related (noting what ladybugs eat inspired organic farmers to bring them in to consume crop-destroying aphids).[12] Still others, including Sternberg, define it as the ability to make unusual connections—to view information in quirky ways that bring about unique results.

To think creatively is to generate new ideas that often go against conventional wisdom and may bring change. Consider how, in the 1940s, mathematician Grace Murray Hopper pioneered the effort to create com-

FIGURE 5.5 Creativity connects analytical and practical thinking

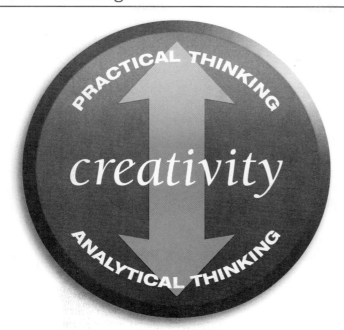

puter languages that nonmathematicians could understand; her efforts opened the world of computers to a wide audience.

Creativity is not limited to inventions. For example, Smith College junior Meghan E. Taugher used her creative mind in two ways. First, she and her study group, as part of their class on electrical circuits, devised a solar-powered battery for a laptop computer. "We took the professor's laptop, put all the parts together, and sat outside watching it with a little device to see how much power it was saving. When it fully charged the battery, it was one of those times I felt that what I was learning was true, because I was putting it to use in real life."[13] Second, her experience led her to generate an idea of a new major and career plan—engineering.

Creativity forms a bridge between analytical and practical thinking (see Figure 5.5). You need to think analytically to evaluate the quality of your creative ideas. You also need to think practically to implement them.

Where does creativity come from? Some people, through luck or natural inclination, seem to come up with inspired ideas more often than others. However, creative thinking, like analytical thinking, is a skill that can be developed. Creativity expert Roger von Oech says that mental flexibility is essential. "Like race-car drivers who shift in and out of different gears depending on where they are on the course," he says, you can enhance your creativity by learning to "shift in and out of different types of thinking depending on the needs of the situation at hand."[14]

The following strategies will help you make those shifts and build your ability to think creatively. Note that, because creative ideas often pop up at random, writing them down as they arise will help you remember them. Keep a pen and paper by your bed, your PDA in your pocket, and/or a notepad in your car so you can grab ideas before they fade from your mind.

## Brainstorm

Brainstorming—letting your mind free-associate to come up with different ideas or answers—is also referred to as *divergent thinking:* You start with a question and then let your mind diverge—go in many different directions—in search of solutions. Think of brainstorming as *deliberate* creative thinking: You go into it fully aware that you are attempting to create new ideas. When you brainstorm, generate ideas without thinking about how useful they are; evaluate their quality later. Brainstorming works well in groups because group members can become inspired by, and make creative use of, one another's ideas.[15]

One way to inspire ideas when brainstorming is to think of similar situations—in other words, to make analogies. For example, the discovery of Velcro is a product of **analogy:** When imagining how two pieces of fabric could stick to each other, the inventor thought of the similar situation of a burr sticking to clothing.

When you are brainstorming ideas, don't get hooked on finding the one right answer. Questions may have many "right answers"—or many answers that have degrees of usefulness. The more possibilities you generate, the better your chance of finding the best one. Also, don't stop the process when you think you have the best answer. Keep going until you are out of steam. You never know what may come up in those last gasps of creative energy.[16]

## Shift Your Perspective

Just because everyone believes something doesn't make it so; just because something "has always been that way" doesn't make it good. Changing how you look at a situation or problem can inspire creative ideas. Here are some ways to do it:

### Challenge Assumptions

In the late 1960s, conventional wisdom said that school provided education and television provided entertainment. Jim Henson, a pioneer in children's television, asked, "Why can't we use TV to educate young children?" From that question, the characters of *Sesame Street*—and a host of other educational programs—were born.

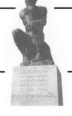

It is better to have enough ideas for some of them to be wrong, than to be always right by having no ideas at all.

EDWARD DE BONO

### Take a New and Different Look

Try on new perspectives by asking others for their views, reading about new ways to approach situations, or deliberately going with the opposite of your first instinct.[17] Then use those perspectives to inspire creativity. For your English lit course, analyze a novel from the point of view of one of the

**FIGURE 5.6**   Try these perception puzzles

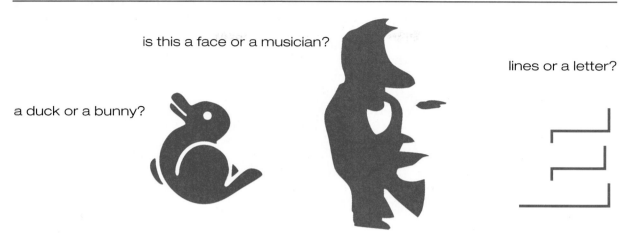

is this a face or a musician?

lines or a letter?

a duck or a bunny?

Face puzzle: "Sara Nadar" illustration from *Mind Sights by Roger Shepard.* Copyright © 1990 by Roger Shepard. Reprinted by permission of Henry Holt & Company.

main characters. For political science, craft a position paper for a presidential or senatorial candidate. Perception puzzles are a fun way to experience how looking at something in a new way can bring a totally different idea (see Figure 5.6).

## Ask "What If" Questions

Set up hypothetical environments in which new ideas can grow: "What if I knew I couldn't fail?" "What if I had unlimited money or time?" Ideas will emerge from your what-if questions. For example, the founders of Seeds of Peace, faced with generations of conflict in the Middle East, asked, What if Israeli and Palestinian teens met at a summer camp in Maine so the next generation has greater understanding and respect than the last? And what if follow-up programs and reunions are set up to cement friendships so relationships change the politics of the Middle East? Based on the ideas that came up, they created an organization to prepare teenagers from the Middle East with the leadership skills needed to coexist peacefully.

# Set the Stage for Creativity

Use these strategies to give yourself the best possible chance at generating creative ideas.

## Choose—or Create—Environments That Free Your Mind

Find places that energize you. Play music that moves you. Paint your study walls your favorite color. Seek out people who inspire you. Sternberg agrees: "Find the environment that rewards what you have to offer," he says, "and then make the most of your creativity and of yourself in that environment."[18]

## Be Curious

Try something you consider new and different—take a course that is completely unlike your major, try a new sport or game, listen to a new genre of music, read a magazine or book that you've never seen before.

Seeking out new experiences and ideas will broaden your knowledge, giving you more raw material with which to build creative ideas.[19]

### Give Yourself Time to "Sit" with a Question

American society values speed, so much so that to say someone is "quick" is to consider that person intelligent.[20] Equating speed with intelligence can stifle creativity because many creative ideas come when you allow time for thoughts to percolate. Take breaks when figuring out a problem. Take the pressure off by getting some exercise, napping, talking with a friend, working on something else, doing something fun. Creative ideas often come when you give your brain permission to "leave the job" for a while.[21]

### Believe in Yourself as a Creative Thinker

Although it is normal to want critical approval and success for your creative efforts, you may not get it right away, especially if your ideas break new ground. When Gustav Mahler's Symphony No. 2—the Resurrection Symphony—was performed in 1910, critics walked out of the concert hall because of its innovative sound. Today, the Resurrection Symphony is considered one of the formative compositions of this era. Like Mahler, you must believe in your creative expression, no matter what others say. Critics, after all, can be wrong or simply a step or two behind.

## Take Risks

Creative breakthroughs can come from sensible risk taking.

### Fly in the Face of Convention

Entrepreneur Michael Dell turned tradition on its ear when he took a "tell me what you want and I will build it for you" approach to computer marketing instead of a "build it and they will buy it" approach. The possibility of failure did not stop him from risking money, time, energy, and reputation to achieve a truly unique and creative goal.

### Let Mistakes Be Okay

Open yourself to the learning that comes from not being afraid to mess up. Sternberg reports that "in the course of their schooling . . . children learn that it's not all right to make mistakes. As a result, they become afraid to err and thus to risk the kind of independent, if sometimes flawed, thinking that can promote creative ideas.[22] When Dr. Hunter—successful inventor of the drug-coated coronary stent—and his company failed to develop a particular treatment for multiple sclerosis, he said, "You have to celebrate the failures. If you send the message that the only road to career success is experiments that work, people won't ask risky questions, or get any dramatically new answers."[23]

As with analytical thinking, asking questions powers creative thinking. See Figure 5.7 for examples of the kinds of questions you can ask to get your creative juices flowing.

When you are working to solve a problem or decision, creative thinking allows you to generate possible solutions and choices. However, choices aren't enough, and potential solutions must be tried out. You need practical thinking to make the best solution or choice happen.

**FIGURE 5.7** Ask these questions to jump-start creative thinking

| To brainstorm, ask: | • What do I want to accomplish? |
| --- | --- |
| | • What are the craziest ideas I can think of? |
| | • What are ten ways that I can reach my goal? |
| | • What ideas or strategies have worked before and how can I apply them? |
| | • How else can this be done? |

| To shift your perspective, ask: | • How has this always been done—and what would be a different way? |
| --- | --- |
| | • What is another way to look at this situation? |
| | • How can I approach this task from a completely new angle? |
| | • How would others do this? How would they view this? |
| | • What if . . . ? |

| To set the stage for creativity, ask: | • Where and with whom do I feel relaxed and inspired? |
| --- | --- |
| | • What music helps me think out of the box? |
| | • When in the day or night am I most likely to experience a flow of creative ideas? |
| | • What do I think would be new and interesting to try, to see, to read? |
| | • What is the most outrageous outcome of a situation that I can imagine? |

| To take risks, ask: | • What is the conventional way of doing this? What would be a totally different way? |
| --- | --- |
| | • What would be a risky approach to this problem or question? |
| | • What choice would people caution me about and why? |
| | • What is the worst that can happen if I take this risk? What is the best? |
| | • What have I learned from this mistake? |

# How Can You Improve Your *Practical Thinking* Skills?

Practical thinking—also called "common sense" or "street smarts"—refers to how you adapt to your environment, or shape or change your environment to adapt to you, to pursue important goals. A basic example: Your goal is to pass your required freshman composition course. You are a visual learner in a verbally focused classroom. To achieve your goal, you can build your verbal skills (adapt to your environment) or ask the instructor and your study group to help you present information in visual terms (change your environment to adapt to you)—or both.

Why do you need to think practically? Because many academic problems can be solved with analytical thinking alone, it's easy to get the impression that strong analytical thinking skills translate into life success. However, real-world problems are different from many academic problems: They are often less clear, related closely to your life and needs, and answerable in more than one way. Plus, stakes are often higher—in other words,

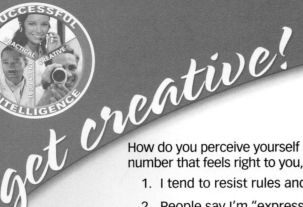

## Assess Creative Thinking Skills

How do you perceive yourself as a creative thinker? For each statement, circle the number that feels right to you, from 1 for "least like me" to 5 for "most like me."

1.  I tend to resist rules and regulations.                                1 2 3 4 5

2.  People say I'm "expressive," "full of ideas," "innovative."           1 2 3 4 5

3.  I break out of my routine and find new experiences.                   1 2 3 4 5

4.  In a group setting, I like to toss ideas into the ring.               1 2 3 4 5

5.  If you say something is too risky, I'm all for it.                     1 2 3 4 5

Total your answers here: _____

If your total ranges from 5 to 12, you consider your creative thinking skills to be *weak*.

If your total ranges from 13 to 19, you consider your creative thinking skills to be *average*.

If your total ranges from 20 to 25, you consider your creative thinking skills to be *strong*.

the way you solve a financial dilemma has a more significant impact on your life than how you work through a geometry proof. Successfully solving real-world problems demands a practical approach.[24]

Practical thinking allows you to bridge the gap between what makes a successful student and what brings real-world success. In other words, even if you ace the courses for your math and education double major, you also need to be able to apply what you learned in a specific job.

The accomplishments of David Hosei, a student at Indiana University, show how practical thinking makes things happen. As a finance and entrepreneurship major, Hosei has built extensive knowledge in business and money matters. Pursuing a goal to help others, Hosei formed HELP (Help Educate Lots of People), a nonprofit organization, to teach peers about money management. In addition, he organizes an annual fund-raiser—the IU Battle of the Bands—to raise money for Jill's House, a refuge for families seeking cancer treatments at a local medical center.[25]

### Experience Helps Develop Practical Thinking Skills

You gain much of your ability to think practically—your common sense—from personal experience, rather than from formal lessons. This knowledge is an important tool in achieving goals.[26]

What you learn from experience answers "how" questions—how to talk, how to behave, how to proceed.[27] For example, after completing a few papers for a particular course, you may pick up cues about how to impress that in-

FIGURE 5.8 One way to map out what you learn from experience

Goal: You want to talk to the soccer coach about your status on the team.

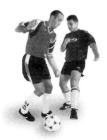 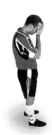 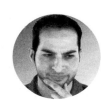 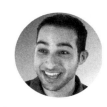 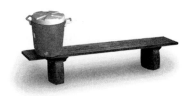

IF the team has had a good practice and IF you've played well during the scrimmage and IF the coach isn't rushing off somewhere, THEN grab a moment with him right after practice ends.

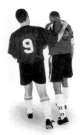 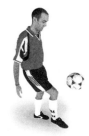 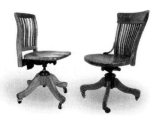

IF the team is having a tough time and IF you've been sidelined and IF the coach is in a rush and stressed, THEN drop in on his office hours tomorrow.

structor. Following a couple of conflicts with a partner, you may learn how to avoid sore spots when the conversation heats up. See Figure 5.8 for ways in which this kind of knowledge can be shown in "if-then" statements.

There are two keys to making practical knowledge work for you. First, make an active choice to learn from experience—to pay attention to how things work at school, in personal relationships, and at work. Second, make sure you apply what you learn, assuring you will not have to learn the same lessons over and over again. As Sternberg says, "What matters most is not how much experience you have had but rather how much you have profited from it—in other words, how well you apply what you have learned."[28]

## The Emotional Intelligence Connection

Part of what you learn from experience involves *emotional intelligence*. Based on the work of psychologist Daniel Goleman, your emotional intelligence quotient (EQ) is the set of personal and social competencies that involve knowing yourself, mastering your feelings, and developing social skills.[29] *Social competence*—involving skills such as sensing other people's feelings and needs, getting your message across to others, managing conflict, leading and bonding with people—usually is built through experience rather than by reading theory or a how-to manual.

Emotional intelligence has a significant effect on your ability to communicate and maneuver in a social environment in a way that helps you achieve your goals. It will be examined in greater detail in the section on communication in Chapter 9.

# Practical Thinking Means Action

Learning different ways to take action and stay in motion builds your practical thinking ability. Strategies you learn throughout this course will keep you moving toward your goals:[30]

- **Stay motivated.** Use techniques from Chapter 1 to persevere when you face a problem. Get started on achieving results instead of dwelling on exactly how to start. Translate thoughts into concrete actions instead of getting bogged down in "analysis paralysis."

- **Make the most of your personal strengths.** What you've learned in Chapter 2 will help you see what you do best—and use those strengths as you apply practical solutions.

- **When things go wrong, accept responsibility and reject self-pity.** You know from Chapter 1 that failure is an excellent teacher. Learn from what happened, act on what you have learned, and don't let self-pity stall your momentum.

- **Focus on the goal and avoid distractions.** Keep your eye on the big picture and complete what you've planned, rather than getting lost in the details. Don't let personal problems or other distractions take you off the track.

- **Manage time and tasks effectively.** Use what you know from Chapter 2 to plan your time in a way that promotes goal accomplishment. Avoid the pitfalls of procrastination. Accurately gauge what you can handle—don't take on too many projects, or too few.

- **Believe in yourself.** Have faith in your ability to achieve what you set out to do.

See Figure 5.9 for some questions you can ask to apply practical thinking to your problems and decisions.

**FIGURE 5.9** Ask questions like these to activate practical thinking

| | |
|---|---|
| To learn from experience, ask: | • What worked well, or not so well, about my approach? My timing? My tone? My wording? |
| | • What did others like or not like about what I did? |
| | • What did I learn from that experience, conversation, event? |
| | • How would I change things if I had to do it over again? |
| | • What do I know I would do again? |
| To apply what you learn, ask: | • What have I learned that would work here? |
| | • What have I seen others do, or heard about from them, that would be helpful here? |
| | • What does this situation have in common with past situations I've been involved in? |
| | • What has worked in similar situations in the past? |
| To boost your ability to take action, ask: | • How can I get motivated and remove limitations? |
| | • How can I, in this situation, make the most of what I do well? |
| | • If I fail, what can I learn from it? |
| | • What steps will get me to my goal, and what trade-offs are involved? |
| | • How can I manage my time more effectively? |

# Assess Practical Thinking Skills

How do you perceive yourself as a practical thinker? For each statement, circle the number that feels right to you, from 1 for "least like me" to 5 for "most like me."

1. I can find a way around any obstacle.          1  2  3  4  5

2. People say I'm a "doer," the "go-to," person, "organized."          1  2  3  4  5

3. When I have a vision, I translate it into steps from A to B to C.          1  2  3  4  5

4. In a group setting, I like to set up the plan.          1  2  3  4  5

5. I don't like to leave loose ends dangling—I'm a finisher.          1  2  3  4  5

Total your answers here:          _____

If your total ranges from 5 to 12, you consider your practical thinking skills to be *weak*.

If your total ranges from 13 to 19, you consider your practical thinking skills to be *average*.

If your total ranges from 20 to 25, you consider your practical thinking skills to be *strong*.

***Your skills at a glance:*** In the sections of the triangle, write your assessment scores from *Get Analytical (p. 146); Get Creative (p. 152)*, and *Get Practical (here)*. Looking at the scores together will give you an idea of how you perceive your skills in all three aspects of successful intelligence, and it will help you think about where you may want to build strength.

# How Are *Analytical, Creative, and Practical Thinking* Used *Together* in Nursing?

Problem solving and decision making are probably the two most crucial and common thinking processes used in nursing. Each requires various mind actions. They overlap somewhat because every problem that needs solving requires you to make a decision. Each process is considered separately here. You will notice similarities in the steps involved in each.

Although both of these processes have multiple steps, you will not always have to work your way through each step. As you become more comfortable with solving problems and making decisions, your mind will automatically click through the steps you need whenever you encounter a problem or decision. Also, you will become more adept at evaluating which problems and decisions need serious consideration and which can be taken care of more quickly and simply. As you become an expert nurse, learning these skills will take many years of experience and reflection—so, start now!

Problem solving and decision making follow similar paths. Both require you to identify and analyze a situation, generate possibilities, choose one, follow through on it, and evaluate its success. Figure 5.10 gives an overview of the paths, indicating how you think at each step.

How do you choose which path to follow? Understanding the differences will help. First of all, problem solving generally requires more focus on coming up with possible solutions; when you face a decision, your choices are often determined. Second, problem solving aims to remove or counteract negative effects; decision making aims to fulfill a need. See Figure 5.11 for some examples. Remember, too, that whereas all problem solving requires you to make a decision—when you decide on a solution—only some decision making requires you to solve a problem.

**FIGURE 5.10**  Solve problems and make decisions using successful intelligence

| PROBLEM SOLVING | THINKING SKILL | DECISION MAKING |
|---|---|---|
| Define the problem—recognize that something needs to change, identify what's happening, look for true causes | **STEP 1** DEFINE | Define the decision—identify your goal (your need) and then construct a decision that will help you get it |
| Analyze the problem—gather information, break it down into pieces, verify facts, look at perspectives and assumptions, evaluate information | **STEP 2** ANALYZE | Examine needs and motives—consider the layers of needs carefully, and be honest about what you really want |
| Generate possible solutions—use creative strategies to think of ways you could address the causes of this problem | **STEP 3** CREATE | Name and/or generate different options—use creative questions to come up with choices that would fulfill your needs |
| Evaluate solutions—look carefully at potential pros and cons of each, and choose what seems best | **STEP 4** ANALYZE (EVALUATE) | Evaluate options—look carefully at potential pros and cons of each, and choose what seems best |
| Put the solution to work—persevere, focus on results, and believe in yourself as you go for your goal | **STEP 5** TAKE PRACTICAL ACTION | Act on your decision—go down the path and use practical strategies to stay on target |
| Evaluate how well the solution worked—look at the effects of what you did | **STEP 6** ANALYZE (REEVALUATE) | Evaluate the success of your decision—look at whether it accomplished what you had hoped |
| In the future, apply what you've learned—use this solution, or a better one, when a similar situation comes up again | **STEP 7** TAKE PRACTICAL ACTION | In the future, apply what you've learned—make this choice, or a better one, when a similar decision comes up again |

FIGURE 5.11 Examine how problems and decisions differ

| SITUATION | YOU HAVE A PROBLEM IF . . . | YOU NEED TO MAKE A DECISION IF . . . |
|---|---|---|
| You are planning your summer activities | Your low GPA means you need to attend summer school—and you've already accepted a summer job. | You've been accepted into two summer abroad internship programs. |
| You want to go to nursing school at a private university | The private college costs twice as much as the state university. | You can't afford the private school. |
| You are doing clinical rotations as a student nurse and working with experienced nurses on the units | You are feeling intimidated by some of the nurses you are working with. | You have a choice which nurses you work with during clinical. |

## Solving a Problem

A problem exists when a situation has negative effects. Recognizing that there is a problem—being aware of those effects—is essential before you can begin to solve it. In other words, your first move is to go from the effects—"I'm unhappy/uneasy/angry"—to determining why: "My work schedule is overwhelming me." "I'm over my head in this nursing course." "My patient is out of control." Then you begin the problem-solving process in earnest.

What happens if you *don't* act in a successfully intelligent way? Take, for example, a nurse having an issue with a nurse manager. He may get into an argument with the nurse manager during work time. He may start showing up late to work. He may not make an effort with his patient assignments. All of these choices will most likely have bad consequences for him.

Now look at how this nurse might work through this problem using his analytical, creative, and practical thinking skills. Figure 5.12 shows how his effort can pay off.

As you go through the problem-solving process, keep these tips in mind.

### Use Probing Questions to Define Problems

Focus on causes. If you are not happy in a class or work environment, for example, you could ask questions like these:

- What do I think about when I feel unhappy?
- Do my feelings involve my instructor or nurse manager? The other nurses on my unit?
- Are these the types of patients I want to take care of? Is the patient load too much?

Chances are that how you answer one or more of these questions may lead to a clear definition—and ultimately to the right solution.

**FIGURE 5.12** Working through a problem relating to a nurse manager

**DEFINE PROBLEM HERE:**

I don't like my
nurse manager

**ANALYZE THE PROBLEM**

We have different views about patient care and really
different personality types. I don't feel respected or
heard. I feel unmotivated to come to work or do a good
job since it never gets noticed.

*Use boxes below to list possible solutions:*

| POTENTIAL POSITIVE EFFECTS | SOLUTION #1 | POTENTIAL NEGATIVE EFFECTS |
|---|---|---|
| *List for each solution:* | Talk with the nurse manager | *List for each solution:* |
| Could work things out and learn about myself and others—professional growth. | | Nothing will change and I will feel worse. The manager will get angry and take it out on me. |
| | **SOLUTION #2** | |
| Not have to deal with manager. Learn new things. | Transfer to another unit | Might not like manager on another unit either. Just avoiding the problem. |
| | **SOLUTION #3** | |
| Give myself a chance to think about things. | Take a long vacation | I am not dealing with problem and using up vacation time. |

*Now choose the solution you think is best—circle it and make it happen.*

| ACTUAL POSITIVE EFFECTS | PRACTICAL ACTION | ACTUAL NEGATIVE EFFECTS |
|---|---|---|
| *List for chosen solution:* | Asked another nurse to come in as a facilitator when I first went to talk to the nurse manager. | *List for chosen solution:* |
| Love my new nurse manager. Manager was defensive at first, but then happy I came into talk. We worked things out and now I get more good feedback. | | A few of the other nurses angry. I was very stressed out and lost several nights of sleep. |

**FINAL EVALUATION: Was it a good or bad solution?**

This was the hardest, but best, choice. I really didn't want to deal with the problem because I dislike any conflict. But I knew as a nurse I had to learn to deal with difficulty—something I was already good at doing with patients and doctors. So I decided to work on this with the nurse manager and use it to grow professionally.

## Analyze Carefully

Gather all the information you can, so you can consider the situation comprehensively. Consider what you can learn from how the problem is similar to, or different from, other problems. Clarify facts. Note your own perspective, and ask others for theirs. Make sure you are not looking at the problem through the lens of an assumption.

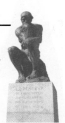

---

No problem can stand the assault of sustained thinking.

VOLTAIRE

---

## Generate Possible Solutions Based on Causes, Not Effects

Addressing a cause provides a lasting solution, whereas "fixing" an effect cannot. Say your shoulder hurts when you use your computer. Getting a friend to massage it is a nice but temporary solution because the pain returns whenever you go back to work. Changing the height of your keyboard and mouse is a better idea because it eliminates the cause of your pain.

# Making a Decision

Psychologists who have studied decision making have learned that many random factors influence the choices people make. For example, you may choose a major, not because you love the subject, but because you think your parents will approve of it. The goal is to make well-considered decisions despite factors that may derail your thinking.

What happens when you make important decisions quickly, without using your analytical, creative, and practical thinking skills? Consider a nurse trying to decide whether to transfer from her current unit to another. If she stays at her current unit because the other nurses say, "You can't leave us with all the work!" or transfers because she doesn't like her relationship with the nurse manager, she may question her choice later—most likely because she didn't consider cause and effect carefully when deciding.

Now look at how this student might make a successfully intelligent decision. Figure 5.13 shows how she worked through the analytical, creative, and practical parts of the process.

As you use the steps in Figure 5.13 to make a decision, remember these hints.

## Look at the Given Options—Then Try to Think of More

Some decisions have a given set of options. For example, your school may allow you to major, double major, or major and minor. However, when you are making your decision, you may be able to brainstorm with an adviser to come up with more options—such as an interdisciplinary major you create on your own.

**FIGURE 5.13**

## Making a decision about whether to change from the cardiac to the pediatric unit

| DEFINE THE DECISION | EXAMINE NEEDS AND MOTIVES |
|---|---|
| Whether or not to transfer to a different unit | I would like to work with different patients. I have worked on the cardiac unit for five years and am interested in working with children on a pediatrics unit. The nurses I work with now really don't want me to leave them short staffed. |

*Use boxes below to list possible choices:*

| POTENTIAL POSITIVE EFFECTS | CHOICE #1 | POTENTIAL NEGATIVE EFFECTS |
|---|---|---|
| *List for each solution:* | Stay on cardiac unit | *List for each solution:* |
| Perfect my knowledge and skills in in this area—make other nurses happy. | | Not learning new things. Not doing what I want to do, but being dictated by others' needs. |

| POTENTIAL POSITIVE EFFECTS | CHOICE #2 | POTENTIAL NEGATIVE EFFECTS |
|---|---|---|
| Learn new things. Take advantage of reason I went into nursing: flexibility. | Transfer to pediatric unit | Letting other nurses down. Losing the skills I have learned on cardiac unit. |

| POTENTIAL POSITIVE EFFECTS | CHOICE #3 | POTENTIAL NEGATIVE EFFECTS |
|---|---|---|
| Give nurse manager a chance to find a new nurse to take my place. | Stay on cardiac unit but tell them I will transfer in one year | People will treat me poorly knowing I am leaving. I am delaying my goals. |

*Now choose the one you think is best—circle it and make it happen.*

| ACTUAL POSITIVE EFFECTS | PRACTICAL ACTION | ACTUAL NEGATIVE EFFECTS |
|---|---|---|
| *List for chosen solution:* | Took position on pediatric unit with 3-week notice to cardiac unit. | *List for chosen solution:* |
| Love my new nurse manager and co-workers. Love working with children. Feel I did what was best for my career. | | A few of the other nurses are angry with me. |

**FINAL EVALUATION: Was it a good or bad choice?**

It was a good choice, but difficult because I worried about what others thought. I didn't want to be seen as selfish or as leaving the other nurses with more work. But I went into nursing to be able to do lots of different things. I had been on the cardiac unit for five years, which was a good and fair commitment. I am very happy with my decision.

### Think About How Your Decision Affects Others

For example, the student thinking about a transfer considers the impact on friends and family. What she concludes about that impact may inform when she transfers and even the school she chooses.

### Gather Perspectives

Talk with others who have made similar decisions. There are more ways of doing things than one brain can possibly imagine on its own.

### Look at the Long-Term Effects

For important decisions, do a short-term evaluation and another evaluation after a period of time. See whether your decision has sent you down a path that has continued to bring positive effects.

## Ethical Dilemmas: Is There One Right Way to Respond?

Ask yourself these questions: Is there an absolute truth? Who decides what is true and what is not true? Remember when you consider these questions that some people believe the position of the stars at the time of their birth determines their future; others that the Bible holds literal truths; and still others that women and girls do not need an education. How can you decide on the perplexing issues in nursing science? Can you decide what is the right thing for everyone? When you take ethics in nursing school, you will learn how decisions are made based on ethical models. But discussion of the problem is most important.

## Keeping Your Balance

No one has equal strengths in analytical, creative, and practical thinking. Adjusting your expectations to match what you can accomplish is a key principle of successful intelligence. It requires that you

- Use what you've learned in this chapter and the rest of the text to maximize your analytical, creative, and practical abilities.
- Reflect on what you do well and focus on strengthening weaker skills.
- Combine all three thinking skills to accomplish your goals, knowing when and how to apply your analytical, creative, and practical abilities.
- Believe in your skills as a thinker.

"Successfully intelligent people," says Sternberg, "defy negative expectations, even when these expectations arise from low scores on IQ or similar tests. They do not let other people's assessments stop them from achieving their goals. They find their path and then pursue it, realizing that there will be obstacles along the way and that surmounting these obstacles is part of the challenge."[31] Let the obstacles come, as they will for everyone, in all aspects of life. You can face and overcome them with the power of your successfully intelligent thinking.

# How Are *Critical Thinking* and the *Scientific Method* Used in Evidence-Based Practice?

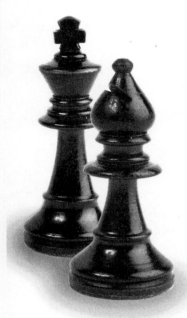

Evidence-based practice (EBP) is founded on a process of inquiry in which we try to gain a better understanding of the world—from stars and meteors to the human brain and behavior to entire ecosystems. Inquiry is based on a standard set of rules known as the *scientific method*. The scientific method is important because it provides a regulated process for conducting research:

- Essential questioning: asking questions
- Possible answers: forming hypotheses
- Testing hypotheses: looking for answers

The scientific method is a process that other nurse researchers can then follow and repeat to reproduce and validate your results. Repetition of research studies gives the results more strength by increasing the amount of supporting evidence. For instance, you'd like to know that a medication you give a patient to fight a bacterial infection has been researched using a standard method, tested repeatedly, and has strong evidence supporting its effectiveness. Furthermore, you would want to be confident that it works on the specific bacteria your patient has and that it doesn't have any dangerous side effects.

The main ingredient of the scientific method is the ability to think, which sounds pretty easy, perhaps like breathing. But you can learn to improve your thinking as you progress through college course work. Even thinking about your own thinking, called *reflection*, can help you. Reflection helps you understand your own biases, or your particular way of looking at phenomena, so you can find out how your previous views might be getting in the way when what you need is a fresh perspective.

Observation is a critical skill in inquiry, and you can learn to become an astute observer through practicing the journal exercises in Chapters 1 and and 2. Another thinking skill you can learn is making connections between what you already know and what you are learning. This skill will help you put information together to make new discoveries or to come up with new solutions to old problems.

Inquiry in nursing relies on asking critical questions. Questions help direct your inquiry; they help you decide where to go for information, what tests to perform, or what experiments to design. The more you improve your thinking through practice and experience, the better you will be at coming up with questions about the world, or your area of practice, and finding methods for answering those questions.

EBP is used in nursing and throughout health care. It uses evidence gained from the scientific process (also referred to as research findings and data) to make decisions about the best kind of treatments. EBP is important for many reasons, but two are:

- Safety
- Effectiveness

Here is an example: Consider when the drug Vioxx came on the market a few years ago. It was hailed as an excellent drug for arthritis and other pain conditions. It was approved by the FDA, but no large-scale testing had been done. Some health care organizations, for instance Group Health Cooperative, refused to pay for its use by its members. Group Health Cooperative had a mission to provide health care that was evidenced based, and the drug Vioxx had not been shown to be any more affective than other similar types of drugs. But, most important, its safety was not fully established.

As you may have heard, the drug was pulled from the market when some people taking it had severe heart problems. Currently, investigations are proceeding to determine if the drug was actually the cause of the heart problems, but the point is that people were being prescribed and taking a drug before strong evidence, gathered through research, supported its effectiveness and safety.

This example is only one that supports the use of EBP. If you think about it, it may seem just good common sense to have solid evidence before asking people to use and pay for a new treatment. Especially, if the old ones, tried and true, were working.

# *Krinein*

The word "critical" is derived from the Greek word *krinein*, which means to separate in order to choose or select. Successful intelligence requires that you separate, evaluate, and select ideas and information as you think through problematic situations. Says Sternberg, "It is more important to know when and how to use these aspects of successful intelligence than just to have them."[32]

Think of this concept as you use your analytical, creative, and practical thinking skills to solve problems, make decisions, innovate, and question. Consider information carefully, and separate out and select the best approaches. Successful intelligence gives you the power to choose how to respond to information, people, and events in ways that help you reach your goals.

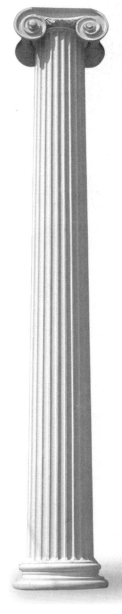

## Create Your Future

# DEVELOPING SUCCESSFUL INTELLIGENCE
### *Putting It All Together*

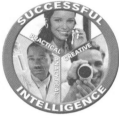

**Make an Important Decision.** Put the decision-making process to work on something that matters to you. You will apply your analytical, creative, and practical thinking skills. Use a separate sheet of paper for steps 2 and 3.

**Step 1. Analyze:** *Define the decision.* Write an important long-term goal that you have, and define the decision that will help you fulfill it. Example: "My goal is to become a nurse. My decision: What to specialize in."

**Step 2. Analyze:** *Examine needs and concerns.* What do you want? What are your needs, and how do your values come into play? What needs of others will you need to take into account? What roadblocks might be involved? List everything you come up with. For example, the prospective nurse might list needs like "I need to feel that I'm helping people. I intend to help with the nursing shortage. I need to make a good living."

**Step 3. Be creative:** *Generate options.* Ask questions to imagine what's possible. Where might you work? What might be the schedule and pace? Who might work with you? What would you see, smell, and hear on your job? What would you do every day? List, too, all of the options you know of. The prospective nurse, for example, might list ER, pediatrics, surgery, oncology, geriatrics, and so on. Brainstorm other options that might not seem so obvious.

**Step 4. Analyze:** *Evaluate options.* Think about how well your options will fulfill your needs. For two of your options, write potential positive and negative effects (pros and cons) of each.

**Option 1:**    Potential pros: _____

                  Potential cons: _____

**Option 2:**    Potential pros: _____

                  Potential cons: _____

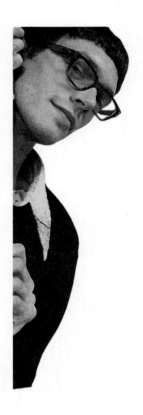

**Step 5. Get practical:** *Imagine acting on your decision.* Describe one practical course of action, based on your thinking so far, that you might follow. List the specific steps you would take. For example, the prospective nurse might list actions that help him determine what type of nursing suits him best, such as interning, summer jobs, academic goals, and talking to working nurses.

Finally, over time, plan to put your decision into action. Eventually you will need to complete the two final steps of the process. **Step 6** is to evaluate the decision: How did it work out? Analyze whether you, and others, got what you needed. **Step 7** is to apply practically what you've learned from the decision to other decisions you make in the future.

# TEAM BUILDING
## *Collaborative Solutions*

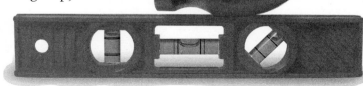

**Powerful Group Problem Solving.** On a 3 × 5 card or a plain sheet of paper, each student in the class writes a school-related problem—this could be a fear, a challenge, a sticky situation, or a roadblock. Students hand these in without names. The instructor writes the list up on the board.

Divide into groups of two to four. Each group chooses one problem to work on (try not to have two groups working on the same problem). Use the empty problem-solving flowchart (Figure 5.14) on p. 166 to fill in your work.

**Step 1. Analyze:** *Define the problem.* As a group, look at the negative effects and state your problem specifically. Then, explore and write down the causes.

**Step 2. Analyze:** *Examine the problem.* Pick it apart to see what's happening. Gather information from all group members, verify facts, go beyond assumptions.

**Step 3. Create:** *Generate possible solutions.* From the most likely causes of the problem, derive possible solutions. Record all the ideas that group members offer. After 10 minutes or so, each group member should choose one possible solution to evaluate independently.

**Step 4. Analyze:** *Evaluate each solution.* In thinking independently through the assigned solution, each group member should (a) weigh the positive and negative effects, (b) consider similar problems, and (c) describe how the solution affects the causes of the problem. Evaluate your assigned solution. Is it a good one? Will it work?

**Step 5. Get practical:** *Choose a solution.* Group members then come together, share observations and recommendations, and then take a vote: Which solution is the best? You may have a tie or may want to combine two different solutions. Try to find the solution that works for most of the group. Then, together, come up with a plan for how you would put your solution to work.

**Step 6. Analyze:** *Evaluate your solution.* As a group, share and discuss what you had individually imagined the positive and negative effects of this solution would be. Try to come to an agreement on how you think the solution would work out.

FIGURE 5.14 Work through a problem using this flowchart

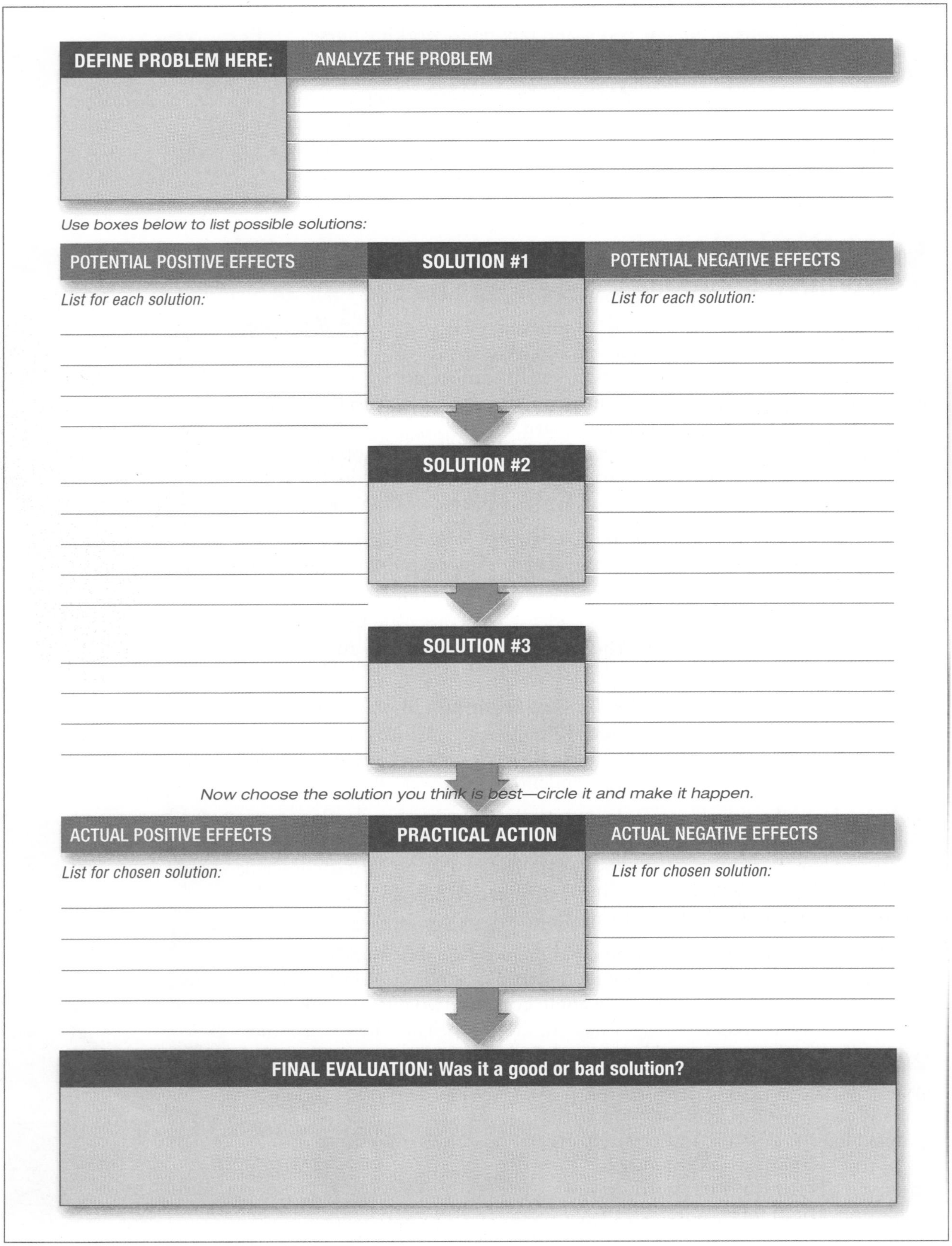

**DEFINE PROBLEM HERE:** ANALYZE THE PROBLEM

Use boxes below to list possible solutions:

| POTENTIAL POSITIVE EFFECTS | SOLUTION #1 | POTENTIAL NEGATIVE EFFECTS |
| --- | --- | --- |
| List for each solution: | | List for each solution: |

SOLUTION #2

SOLUTION #3

Now choose the solution you think is best—circle it and make it happen.

| ACTUAL POSITIVE EFFECTS | PRACTICAL ACTION | ACTUAL NEGATIVE EFFECTS |
| --- | --- | --- |
| List for chosen solution: | | List for chosen solution: |

**FINAL EVALUATION: Was it a good or bad solution?**

# WRITING

## Discovery Through Journaling

*Record your thoughts on a separate piece of paper or in a journal.*

**Wiser Choices.** Think about a choice you made that, looking back, you wish you had handled differently. First, describe what the decision was, what option you chose, and what the consequences were. Then, write about what you would do if you could make the decision again. What did you learn from your experience that you can apply to other decisions? How could being analytical, creative, and practical have helped you reach a more effective outcome?

# CAREER PORTFOLIO

## Plan for Success

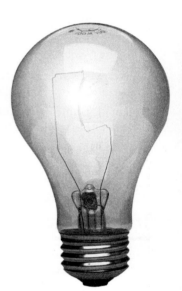

**Generating Ideas for Internships.** People often put more time and effort into deciding what cell phone to buy than they do with life-altering decisions like how to prepare for career success. Pursuing internships is part of a comprehensive career decision-making process. It's a practical way to get experience, learn what you like and don't like, and make valuable connections.

Fill in the following:

## Career areas that I'm considering. Why?

1. Because:

2. Because

3. Because:

## People whom I want to interview about their fields/professions. Why?

1. Because:

2. Because:

3. Because:

Next, take practical steps to investigate internships. Talk to the people you listed. Contact companies you would like to work for and see what internship opportunities are available. Talk with someone in your school's career office. If a company doesn't offer internships, ask them if you might be the pioneer intern.

Finally, after you have gathered some useful information, use a separate sheet of paper to creatively envision your internship experience. Describe it: What would it look like? What would you do each day? Each week? Where would you go? With whom would you work? What would you contribute with your gifts and talents? Make it happen with your successful intelligence.

## Suggested Readings

Cameron, Julia, with Mark Bryan. *The Artist's Way: A Spiritual Path to Higher Creativity,* 10th ed. New York: G.P. Putnam's Sons, 2002.

de Bono, Edward. *Lateral Thinking: Creativity Step by Step.* New York: Perennial Library, 1990.

Goleman, Daniel. *Emotional Intelligence: Why It Can Matter More Than IQ.* New York: Bantam, 1995.

Moscovich, Ivan. *1000 Playthinks.* New York: Workman Publishing, 2001.

Noone, Donald J., Ph.D. *Creative Problem Solving.* New York: Barron's, 1998.

Sark. *Make Your Creative Dreams Real: A Plan for Procrastinators, Perfectionists, Busy People, and People Who Would Rather Sleep All Day.* New York: Fireside Press, 2004.

von Oech, Roger. *A Kick in the Seat of the Pants.* New York: Harper & Row, 1986.

von Oech, Roger. *A Whack on the Side of the Head.* New York: Warner Books, 1998.

## Internet Resources

Creativity at Work (resources for workplace creativity): **www.creativityatwork.com**

Creativity for Life (tips and strategies for creativity): **www.creativityforlife.com**

Roger von Oech's Creative Think Web site: **www. creative-think.com**

## Endnotes

[1] Robert J. Sternberg, *Successful Intelligence* (New York: Plume, 1997), p. 12.

[2] Ibid., p. 127.

[3] Matt Thomas, "What Is Higher-Order Thinking and Critical/Creative/Constructive Thinking?" The Center for Studies in Higher-Order Literacy (April 2004). Available: http://members.aol.com/MattT10574/HigherOrderLiteracy.htm#What.

[4] Sternberg, p. 128.

[5] Vincent Ruggiero, *The Art of Thinking*, 2001, quoted in "Critical Thinking," Oregon State University. Retrieved April 2004, from: http://success.oregonstate.edu/study/learning.cfm.

[6] Richard Paul, "The Role of Questions in Thinking, Teaching, and Learning," The Center for Thinking and Learning (1995). Retrieved April 2004, from: www.criticalthinking.org/University/univclass/roleofquest.html.

[7] "The Best Innovations Are Those That Come from Smart Questions," *Wall Street Journal*, April 12, 2004, B1.

[8] Lawrence F. Lowery, "The Biological Basis of Thinking and Learning," 1998, Full Option Science System at the University of California at Berkeley (1998). Retrieved April 2004, from: http://lhsfoss.org/newsletters/archive/pdfs/FOSS_BBTL.pdf.

[9] Ivan Moscovich, *1000 Playthinks* (New York: Workman Publishing), p. 7.

[10] Colby Glass, "Strategies for Critical Thinking" (March 1999). Retrieved April 2003, from: www.accd.edu/pac/philosop/phil1301/ctstrategies.htm.

[11]Sternberg, p. 49.

[12]Charles Cave, "Definitions of Creativity" (August 1999). Retrieved April 2003, from: http://members.ozemail.com.au/~caveman/Creative/Basics/definitions.htm.

[13]Elizabeth F. Farrell, "Engineering a Warmer Welcome for Female Students: The Dicipline Tries to Stress Its Social Relevance, an Important Factor for Many Women," *The Chronicle of Higher Education* (February 22, 2002). Retrieved March 2004, from: http://chronicle.com/weekly/v48/i24/24a03101.htm.

[14]Roger von Oech, *A Kick in the Seat of the Pants* (New York: Harper & Row, 1986), pp. 5–21.

[15]Dennis Coon, *Introduction to Psychology: Exploration and Application*, 6th ed. (St. Paul: West, 1992), p. 295.

[16]Roger von Oech, *A Whack on the Side of the Head* (New York: Warner Books, 1990), pp. 11–168.

[17]J. R. Hayes, *Cognitive Psychology: Thinking and Creating* (Homewood, IL: Dorsey, 1978).

[18]Sternberg, p. 219.

[19]Adapted from T. Z. Tardif and R. J. Sternberg, "What Do We Know About Creativity?" in *The Nature of Creativity*, ed. R. J. Sternberg. (London: Cambridge University Press, 1988).

[20]Sternberg, p. 212.

[21]Hayes.

[22]Sternberg, p. 202.

[23]"The Best Innovations Are Those That Come from Smart Questions," *Wall Street Journal*, April 12, 2004, p. B1.

[24]Sternberg, pp. 229–30.

[25]"Amazing Student, David Hosei—Entrepreneur with a Heart," Indiana University Web site, 2003 [on-line]. Available: http://excellence.indiana.edu/hosei/ (March 2004).

[26]Sternberg, p. 236.

[27]Robert J. Sternberg and Elena L. Grigorenko, "Practical Intelligence and the Principal," Yale University: Publication Series No. 2, 2001, p. 5.

[28]Sternberg, p. 241.

[29]Daniel Goleman, *Emotional Intelligence: Why It Can Matter More Than IQ* (New York: Bantam, 1995).

[30]Sternberg, pp. 251–69.

[31]Sternberg, p. 19.

[32]Sternberg, p. 128.

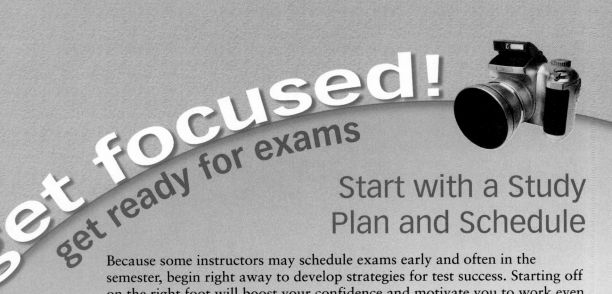

# get focused!
## get ready for exams

## Start with a Study Plan and Schedule

Because some instructors may schedule exams early and often in the semester, begin right away to develop strategies for test success. Starting off on the right foot will boost your confidence and motivate you to work even harder. The saying that "success breeds more success" couldn't be more true as you begin college.

The material in this Study Break is designed to help you organize yourself as you prepare for exams. As you learn to create a pretest study plan and schedule, you will also build your ability to use your time efficiently.

When you reach Chapter 7, "Test Taking: Showing What You Know," you will study test taking in depth, including test preparation, test anxiety, general test-taking strategies, strategies for handling different types of test questions, and learning from test mistakes.

### Decide on a Study Plan

Start your test preparation by deciding what you will study. Go through your notes, texts, related primary sources, and handouts, and set aside materials you don't need. Then prioritize the remaining materials. Your goal is to focus on information that is most likely to be on the exam. Use the test preparation tips on pages 243 to 247 and the material on studying your text in Chapter 5 to boost your effectiveness as you prepare.

### Create a Study Schedule and Checklist

Next, use the time-management and goal-setting skills from Chapter 2 to prepare a schedule. Consider all of the relevant factors—your study materials, the number of days until the test, and the time you can study each day. If you establish your schedule ahead of time and write it in a planner, you are more likely to follow it.

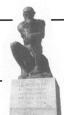

Let our advance worrying become advance thinking and planning.

WINSTON CHURCHILL

A checklist like the one here will help you organize and stay on track as you prepare. Use a checklist to assign specific tasks to particular study times and sessions. That way, not only do you know when you have time to study, but you also have defined goals for each study session. Make extra copies of the checklist so you can fill out a new one each time you have an exam.

## Decide How Well These Techniques Work for You

After you've used these studying and scheduling techinques to prepare for a few exams, answer the following questions:

- How did this approach help you organize your time before an exam?
- How did this approach help you organize your study material so you remembered to cover every topic?
- Can you think of ways to change the checklist to improve your test-prep efficiency? If you can, list the ways here and incorporate them into the checklist.

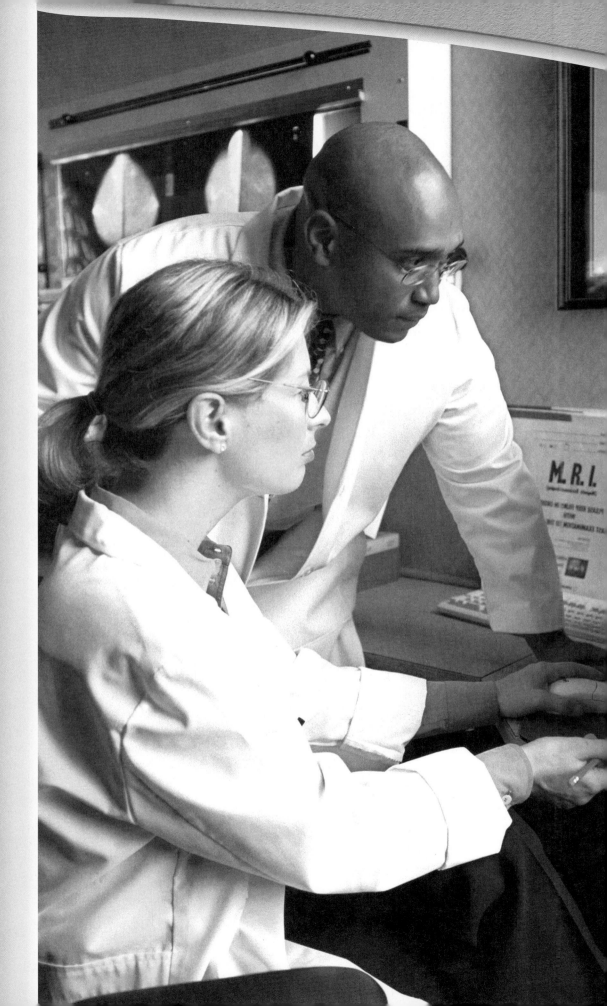

# 6

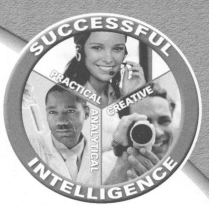

Your ability to read—and to understand, analyze, and use what you read—is the cornerstone of college learning. However, your background as a reader may not have prepared you for the amount and the complexity of the reading you will be assigned in college. It isn't just students with learning disabilities who face challenges. Almost all students need to adjust their habits to handle the increased demands of a college reading load.

Taking a step-by-step approach linked to analytical, creative, and practical thinking techniques will help you get what you need from the materials you read and study. This chapter introduces you to strategies to increase your speed, efficiency, and depth of understanding. When you use these strategies to learn more and retain more of what you learn, every hour you spend with your books will be more valuable.

# Q & A BLUE SKY QUESTIONS
# DOWN-TO-EARTH ANSWERS

## *Is community health nursing as respected as hospital nursing?*

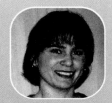

Toni M. Riehm
Senior, Indiana University
South Bend,
South Bend, Indiana

As a nontraditional student, I've been taking college courses for nine years on a part-time basis. I've worked on and off during this time, but for the most part, I've been a stay-at-home mom. In thinking about preparing for a future career, I wanted a degree that would allow me diversity in the job market and fulfillment as a person. Nursing offers much flexibility and personal rewards like no other career. The BSN program requires prerequisite classes in fields such as humanities and the sciences. Taking these courses enabled me to take about six to eight credit hours per semester while my children were small, and now that they are more independent, I can manage clinicals..

I'm very happy about my choice to become a nurse. There are many disciplines within the nursing profession to choose from, and I see nursing as very purposeful because of the opportunity to assist people in achieving their optimal level of health. Sometimes you're helping patients face dramatic life changes because their current illness is forcing them to live a new way. Other times you're helping people at the end of their lives to make that transition as gracefully as possible. In my clinical practice, I like taking a holistic approach to caring for people. Nursing teaches me to assist them with not only their immediate sickness but with how their health concerns affect their whole life.

In light of all these positives, I sometimes struggle to balance the completion of a bachelor's degree in nursing with all of my other responsibilities. This semester, in particular, has been very stressful. Last year my mother was diagnosed with lung cancer. She lived in Florida so I spent much of the summer there and then went back again this fall to be with her when she died. Juggling the needs of my family with the responsibilities of being a nursing student took a lot out of me. I continue to deal with the loss I'm experiencing, and so much of what I'm feeling has to be put on hold.

I realize many students encounter difficult situations like mine in which family priorities have to be balanced with the demands of school. I've also noticed that dedicated nursing students are high achievers who are dissatisfied if they aren't producing their best work. This is my dilemma now, too. My test scores have dropped some recently, which bothers me because I know I am capable of doing better. With so many life happenings going on, however, my mind is scattered on other things in addition to my classwork. There have even been times I've wanted to quit, but I know the regret I'd feel if I did that. My family has seen all the hard work I've put in so far, and my close friends and instructors have given me so much support along the way. I also think it's been a good example for my children to learn that making an effort and struggling to achieve do produce results. How can I manage all my responsibilities and still achieve my goals in pursuing my nursing degree?

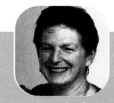

Susanna Cunningham,
BSN, PhD, FAAN
Professor of Biobehavioral
Nursing and Health
Systems,
University of Washington,
Seattle, Washington

### Don't let stereotypes influence you

We have students here who are doing similar kinds of balancing acts. Managing our lives requires creative thinking of the highest order. The students who seem to do the best job at making these kinds of life decisions are those who sort through their priorities. Then they slowly step through what they know they have to do. When I was in my postdoctoral program I made the decision to treat school like a job. I constrained it to certain hours and made my family the priority.

Although I have a doctoral degree, my secondary degree is in vacationing. I just returned from two weeks of scuba diving in Maui with my adult children. You need to play with your family. Trying new things leads us into different thinking processes. You don't have to get A's to prove you're smart. You're already a long way in achieving your goals, and you've proven that you have the skills for a successful nursing career. You'll do better later once you've given yourself time to recover. I consider it an act of courage when a student takes time to deal with personal issues rather than ignore them. The more important issue is, "What am I learning?" If you're going to class and focusing on the material in front of you, then you're learning and that's what matters.

Our brain is a miraculous organ. It has the ability to process information on various levels even when we're off doing something else. For example, I like to do crossword puzzles. If I can't figure out several words on a given day, I'll put it aside. I've noticed that when I come back to it another day with fresh spirit, the words often pop out. We as a society seem to think that doing more and running faster is a virtue, which is a strange thought. As nurses, we need to model self-care. Depending on your program's requirements, perhaps you could take only one or two classes the next quarter or even postpone school for a semester. In any case, slowing down is a smart decision.

Another strategy is to integrate what you're learning into family time. When I had statistics, I included my kids by having them draw diagrams. By teaching your kids what you're learning, you also refine your thoughts on the subject. The most creative people in science, and in other fields as well, are those who have taken ideas from different worlds and put them together in a new way. They can look at a problem from one field and put it with what they know from another field and find that it fits.

Losing our parents is a universal experience that often causes us to sit back and evaluate life more deeply. You need to honor the loss of your mother. I hope you're talking and thinking about her. Perhaps seeing a school counselor or enlisting the support of other students who are facing similar challenges can help. In so doing, you not only help yourself, you also demonstrate healthy ways to cope with loss for your children. So my main message to you is this: Be kind to yourself. Why should you be disheveled in the time you're alive? This is your life. It's not your boss's, or your professor's, or your spouse's; it's yours. Make the most of it.

# What Will *Help You Understand* What You Read?

Reading is an analytical process that requires you, the reader, to make meaning from written words. You do this by connecting what you know to what you read. Your understanding is affected by your familiarity with a subject, your cultural background and life experiences, and even the way you interpret words and phrases. Because these factors are different for every person, your reading experiences are uniquely your own.

Reading comprehension refers to your ability to understand what you read. True comprehension goes beyond parroting facts and figures to being able to apply concepts to new ideas and situations. Improving your reading comprehension is especially important in college because assignments are generally longer and more difficult, and you usually have to complete them on your own. In addition, what you learn from introductory-level texts is the foundation for your understanding of advanced course material. Following are general comprehension boosters to keep in mind as you work through this chapter and tackle early-semester reading assignments.

## Read as Much as You Can

More than any other factor, what you already know influences comprehension by giving you a frame of reference for what you read.

## Think Analytically

Ask yourself questions: Do I understand the sentence, paragraph, or chapter I just read? Are the ideas and supporting examples clear? Could I explain the material to someone else? Could I apply the concepts to another topic or situation?

## Build Vocabulary

The larger your vocabulary, the more material you will understand without checking a dictionary or guessing.

## Look for Order and Meaning in Seemingly Chaotic Reading Materials

The information in this chapter on the SQ3R reading technique contains patterns that will help you learn new material.

## Think Positively

Instead of telling yourself that you cannot understand, tell yourself *I can learn this material. I am able to complete every reading assignment.*

# How Can You *Set the Stage* for Reading?

On any given day during college, you may face reading assignments like these:

- A textbook chapter on the history of South African apartheid (World History)
- An original research study on the relationship between sleep deprivation and the development of memory problems (Psychology)

*(continued)*

# Be the Author of Your Life

*get creative!*

*Think about a book that made a difference for you.*

Henry David Thoreau, a nineteenth-century American author, poet, and philosopher, made the following observation: "How many a man has dated a new era in his life from the reading of a book." What do you think Thoreau meant by this statement?

Think of a book that influenced your education—or life—and describe why it is important.

If you could write a book that would help others succeed in college, what would be the book's message? Why do you think your book would be important for others to read?

- Chapter 4 to 6 in John Steinbeck's classic novel *The Grapes of Wrath* (American Literature)
- A technical manual on the design of computer antivirus programs (Computer Science—Software Design)

This material is rigorous by anyone's standards. In fact, many students are surprised at how much reading there is in college and that they may be expected to learn material never covered in class.

To get through it all—and master what you read—you need a systematic approach that taps into your analytic and practical thinking skills. Without one, you may face problems similar to those of this student at a large northeastern university. He explains: "I did not get off to a great start because I had never really learned to study this enormous amount of material in a systematic way. I tended to do one subject for a big span of time and then neglect it for a week. Then I moved on to another subject, and forgot about that for a week. So there was no continuity within each course. That had a lot to do with it. Finally I figured it out. This year, I'm pushing myself to spend a little bit of time every day on each subject."[1]

## Take an Active Approach to Difficult Texts

Generally, the further you advance in your education, the more likely you are to encounter unfamiliar concepts and terms. This happens often when assignments involve *primary sources*—original documents rather than another writer's interpretation of these documents—or when they are from academic journals and scientific studies that don't define terms or supply examples. Primary sources include historical documents, works of literature (novels, poems, and plays), scientific studies including lab reports and accounts of experiments, and journal articles.

The following strategies may help you approach difficult material actively and positively:

### Approach Reading Assignments with an Open Mind

Avoid judging material as impossible or boring before you start.

### Know That Some Texts Require Extra Work and Concentration

Set a goal to make your way through the material and learn. Do whatever it takes. Consult resources—instructors, students, reference materials—for help.

### Own Frequently Used Reference Materials

Purchase a dictionary, a writer's style handbook, an atlas, and references in your major. "If you find yourself going to the library to look up the same reference again and again, consider purchasing that book for your personal library," advises library expert Sherwood Harris.[2]

## Choose the Right Setting

Finding the best places and times to study will maximize your focus and discipline. Here are some suggestions:

### Select the Right Location

Many students study at a library desk. Others prefer an easy chair or even the floor. Choose a spot that's comfortable but not so cushy that you fall asleep. Make sure you have adequate lighting and aren't too hot or cold. If you prefer to read alone, find an out-of-the-way spot at the library or an after-class hour in an empty classroom where interruptions are less likely. Even if you don't mind activity nearby, try to minimize distractions.

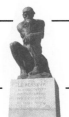

Reading is a means of thinking with another person's mind; it forces you to stretch your own.

CHARLES SCRIBNER JR.

### Select the Right Time

Choose a time when you feel alert and focused. If possible, complete assignments just before or after the related class. Eventually, you will associate preferred places and times with focused reading. Recall from Chapter 2 what you learned about creating a schedule that suits your natural body rhythms—your goal is to study when your energy is high. Although night owls may be productive after 10 o'clock at night, morning people will be fuzzy during late-night sessions.

## Deal with Internal Distractions

Internal distractions—personal worries, anticipation of upcoming events, or even hunger—can get in the way of work. Try taking a break to tend to an issue that's bothering you, or use exercise, music, or silence to relax and refocus. If you're hungry, get a snack and come back to work.

Students with young children have an added factor when deciding when, where, and how to study. Figure 6.1 explores ways that these students can maximize their study efforts.

**FIGURE 6.1** Use these tools to manage children while studying

**Keep them up to date on your schedule.**

Let them know when you have a big test or project due and when you are under less pressure, and what they can expect of you in each case.

**Explain what your education entails.**

Tell them how it will improve your life and theirs. This applies, of course, to older children who can understand the situation and compare it with their own schooling.

**Find help.**

Ask a relative or friend to watch your children or arrange for a child to visit a friend. Consider trading babysitting hours with another parent, hiring a sitter to come to your home, or using a day-care center.

**Keep them active while you study.**

Give them games, books, or toys. If there are special activities that you like to limit, such as watching videos or TV, save them for your study time.

**Offset study time with family time and rewards.**

Children may let you get your work done if they have something to look forward to, such as a movie night or a trip for ice cream.

**Study on the phone.**

You might be able to have a study session with a fellow student over the phone while your child is sleeping or playing quietly.

**SPECIAL NOTES FOR INFANTS**

Study at night if your baby goes to sleep early, or in the morning if your baby sleeps late.

Study during nap times if you aren't too tired yourself.

Lay your notes out and recite information to the baby. The baby will appreciate the attention, and you will get work done.

Put baby in a safe and fun place while you study, such as a playpen, motorized swing, or jumping seat.

# Define Your Purpose for Reading

It's study time and you are about to crack open a book. Before you start, define your purpose by asking yourself, "Why am I reading this?" You might answer by completing this sentence: "In reading this material, I intend to define/learn/answer/achieve . . ."

Defining your purpose helps you choose reading strategies and decide how much time and effort to spend. You will approach each of the four following purposes in different ways. Keep in mind that you may have one or more purposes for any "reading event."

## Purpose 1: Read for Understanding

Studying involves reading to comprehend general ideas and specific facts or examples. Facts and examples help explain or support ideas, and ideas provide a framework for remembering facts and examples.

- **General ideas.** Reading for general ideas requires rapid reading of headings, subheadings, and summary statements to gain an overview—in other words, skimming the material (see page 186).
- **Specific facts or examples.** At times, your focus may be on specific pieces of information—names and dates, chronologies, and so on. At other times, your search may center on examples that support general ideas—for example, the causes of economic recession. In both cases, scanning will help you find information rapidly (see page 181).

## Purpose 2: Read to Evaluate Analytically

Analytical evaluation involves considering ideas and asking questions that test the writer's argument and assumptions. Analytical reading brings an understanding of the material that goes beyond basic information recall (see pages 204–205 for more on analytical reading).

## Purpose 3: Read for Practical Application

When you read a computer manual or an instruction sheet for conducting a chemistry experiment, your goal is to learn how to do something. Reading and action usually go hand in hand.

## Purpose 4: Read for Pleasure

Some materials are read for entertainment, such as *Sports Illustrated* magazine, the latest John Grisham courtroom thriller, or a Jane Austen novel.

Different subjects present different reading challenges. Subjects vary—a calculus text and a world religions text have little in common—and your learning styles and preferences may make you more comfortable with some subjects than others. Math and science readings present unique challenges to many students. Try some of the following analytical, creative, and practical thinking techniques to meet the challenge:

- **Interact with the material critically as you go.** Math and science texts move sequentially (later chapters build on concepts introduced in previous chapters) and are often problem-and-solution based. Keep a pad nearby to solve problems and take notes. Draw sketches to help visualize material. Try not to move on until you understand the example and how it relates to the central ideas. Write down questions to ask your instructor or classmates.

- **Note formulas.** Make sure you understand the principle behind every **formula**—why it works—before memorizing it. Read the assigned material to prepare for homework.

- **Use memory techniques.** Science textbooks are packed with specialized vocabulary that you will be expected to know. Mnemonic devices, flash cards, and rehearsing aloud or silently aid memorization (for more on memory techniques, see Chapter 7). Selective highlighting and summarizing your readings in table format will also help.

FORMULA
A general fact, rule, or principle usually expressed in mathematical symbols.

## Develop Strategies to Manage Learning Disabilities

Students with reading-related learning disabilities may need to engage their practical thinking skills to manage reading assignments. Roxanne Ruzic of CAST explored the strategies used by students with learning disabilities at an urban college in the Northeast. For two students, here is what worked:

- Danielle received an A in her art history survey course, in part because she chose some courses with heavy reading requirements and some with light requirements. This allowed her to complete all her assignments on time. In addition, she frequently sought instructors' advice about what they wanted her to learn from assigned texts and used tutors whenever she needed extra help.

- Chloe received an A in her introduction to psychology course, in part because she met twice weekly with a tutor who helped her prioritize her reading assignments and keep on top of her work. She also learned to tailor the amount of time she spent on different text sections to the importance of the sections on upcoming tests. Finally, when she felt comfortable with text concepts, she read them quickly or skipped them entirely, but when she had trouble with the material, she did extra reading or sought help.[3]

If you have a learning disability, think of these students as you investigate the services your college offers through reading centers and tutoring programs. Remember: The ability to succeed is often linked to the willingness to ask for help.

## Build Reading Speed

Although comprehension is more important than reading quickly, a reasonable increase in reading speed saves time and effort. Although the average American adult reads between 150 and 350 words per minute, faster readers are capable of speeds up to 1,000 words per minute.[4] Raising your reading speed above 350 words per minute involves "skimming" and "scanning." The following suggestions also increase speed without sacrificing comprehension:

- Try to read groups of words rather than single words.
- Avoid pointing your finger to guide your reading; use an index card to move quickly down the page.
- When reading narrow columns, focus your eyes in the middle of the column. With practice, you'll be able to read the entire column width as you read down the page.
- Avoid subvocalization—speaking the words or moving your lips—when reading.

A key component to building speed is practice and more practice, says reading expert Steve Moidel. To achieve your goal of reading between 500 and 1,000 words per minute, Moidel suggests that you start practicing at three times the rate you want to achieve, a rate that is much faster than you can comprehend.[5] For example, if your goal is 500 words per minute, speed up to 1,500 words per minute. Reading at such an accelerated rate pushes your eyes and mind to adjust to the faster pace. When you slow down to 500 words per minute—a pace you can actually manage—your rate will feel comfortable even though it is much faster than your original speed. Self-paced computer software is available to help you gain speed.

## Expand Your Vocabulary

A strong vocabulary increases speed and comprehension. The best way to build your vocabulary is to learn new and unfamiliar words as you encounter them. This involves the following steps.

### Analyze Word Parts

**ROOT**
*The central part or basis of a word, around which prefixes and suffixes can be added to produce different words.*

Often, if you understand part of a word, you can figure out the entire word. This is true because many English words are made up of a combination of Greek and Latin prefixes, **roots,** and suffixes. *Prefixes* are word parts that are added to the beginning of a root. *Suffixes* are added to the end of the root.

Figure 6.2 contains some common prefixes, roots, and suffixes. Knowing these verbal building blocks can dramatically increase your vocabulary. Figure 6.3 shows how one root can be the stem of many words.

| FIGURE 6.2 | Knowing common prefixes, roots, and suffixes expands your vocabulary |
|---|---|

| PREFIX | PRIMARY MEANING | EXAMPLE |
|---|---|---|
| a-, ab- | from | abstain, avert |
| con-, cor-, com- | with, together | convene, correlate, compare |
| il- | not | illegal, illegible |
| sub-, sup- | under | subordinate, suppose |

| ROOT | PRIMARY MEANING | EXAMPLE |
|---|---|---|
| -chron- | time | synchronize |
| -ann- | year | biannual |
| -sper- | hope | desperate |
| -voc- | speak, talk | convocation |

| SUFFIX | PRIMARY MEANING | EXAMPLE |
|---|---|---|
| -able | able | recyclable |
| -meter | measure | thermometer |
| -ness | state of | carelessness |
| -y | inclined to | sleepy |

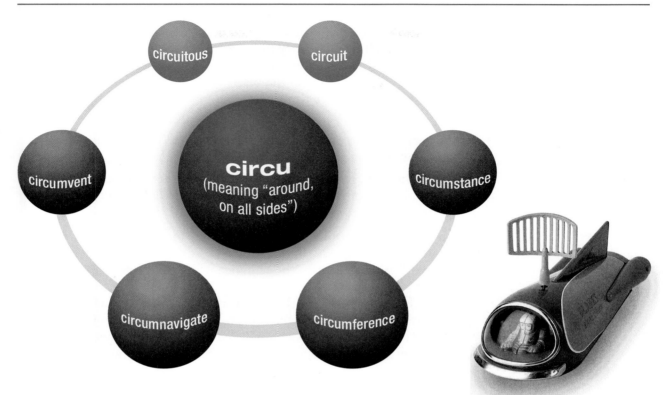

**FIGURE 6.3**  Knowing a single root can help you build different words

circuitous

circuit

**circu**
(meaning "around, on all sides")

circumvent

circumstance

circumnavigate

circumference

Using prefixes, roots, and suffixes, you can piece together the meaning of new words. For example, the word *prologue* is made up of the prefix *pro* (before) and the root *logue* (to speak). Thus prologue refers to words spoken or written before the main text.

## Use Words in Context

Although a definition tells you what a word means, it may not include a *context*—the part of a statement that surrounds a word and affects its meaning. Using a word in context after defining it helps anchor the information in memory. Here are strategies for using context to solidify new vocabulary words.

- Use a new word in a sentence immediately after reading a definition while the meaning is fresh.

- Reread, a few times, the sentence where you originally saw the word to make sure you understand how the word is used.

- Use the word over the next few days whenever it may apply. Try it while talking with friends, writing e-mails or notes, or in your own thoughts.

- Solidify your understanding by going back to sentences you previously didn't understand. For example, most children learn the Pledge of Allegiance by rote without understanding what *allegiance* means. When they finally learn the definition, the pledge itself will help them connect "allegiance" with the concept of loyalty.

- Talk about it. If after looking up a word you still have trouble with its meaning, ask an instructor or a friend to help you figure it out.

## Use a Dictionary

Dictionaries provide broad information such as word origin, pronunciation, parts of speech, and multiple meanings. Get a good-quality college dictionary, and consult it when you encounter unfamiliar words. Many textbooks include a *glossary* that defines terms found in the text. Electronic dictionaries are handy, although definitions are less complete. Dictionaries are also available on the Internet.

You may not always have time to use the following suggestions, but when you can, they will help you make the most of your dictionary.

- **Read every meaning of a word, not just the first.** Think critically about which meaning suits the context; then choose the one that is the best fit.
- **Use the definition.** Imagine, for example, that you read the following sentence and do not know the word *indoctrinated: The cult indoctrinated its members to reject society's values.*

In the dictionary, you find several definitions, including "brainwashed" and "instructed." You decide that the one closest to the correct meaning is "brainwashed." With this term, the sentence reads: *The cult brainwashed its members to reject society's values.*

You have laid the groundwork for effective studying. You are now ready for the SQ3R process, which will give you tools for learning and mastering textbook material. As you will see next, SQ3R engages all three aspects of successful intelligence: analytical, creative, and practical.

# What *Special Strategies* Can You Use with Nursing and Science Texts?

Readings in nursing and science courses will differ from those in liberal arts courses in three ways:

1. *The amount of new vocabulary you will need to learn is greater.* Any science you study will have new terms to describe phenomena unique to that discipline. For example, in biology words such as *chloroplasts, isotonic, plasmolysis,* and *vestigial* are used. In nursing, acronyms are the rule rather than the exception. A patient has an AMI (anterior myocardial infarction), requires q 1 ABGs (arterial blood gases monitored every hour), and is on an IABP (intra-aortic balloon pump) in preparation for a PTCA (percutaneous transluminal angioplasty) or a CABG (coronary artery bypass graft).

2. *Content is generally not written in a narrative style.* Therefore, following the flow of the text is more challenging. Science books, if written in typical technical writing style, can be dry and a drudgery to plow through. Fortunately, many technical and textbook writers are able to present scientific information in lively and interesting ways. It is hoped that these writers will be the ones you are required to read. If not, just take extra time for your reading and ask for help interpreting the "foreign" language you are learning.

3. *Content is concentrated and text is full of information, diagrams, and formulas.* Science and nursing texts are concentrated, usually lacking any story or, as just stated, lacking easy narrative flow. In addition, you are required to read and understand symbols, math formulas and equations, diagrams of models, and graphs, which are used to explain the material. You will be memorizing new terms and models to learn more complex concepts. Graphics, that is, not written text, are often used to represent ideas.

Along with your readings from textbooks, you will read from research journals and possibly other science-oriented publications such as *Scientific American, Natural History,* or *The Journal of Nursing Scholarship.* Books may hold up-to-date information but not the most current, cutting-edge information. From the time an author submits a manuscript for a textbook, it can take a year or more for the book to be printed. For basic, or beginning, science courses, such as geology, physiology, or chemistry, the age of a textbook matters less than for courses dealing with information on technology or breakthrough discoveries, such as new cancer treatments.

The most up-to-date information is found in journals that publish research findings. Journals are designed to disseminate new and relevant information to the scientific community of a particular field. In nursing there is the *Journal of Advanced Nursing Science* and *The Journal of Nursing Scholarship;* in medicine, *JAMA* and the *New England Journal of Medicine;* in life sciences, *Nature.* These are all examples of discipline-specific journals that publish research articles.

Journals serve the function of letting other researchers, or would-be researchers, see what their colleagues are doing. Repetition of studies is an important step in validating results before they are put into practice or applied to further study. Many research studies are designed to replicate research found in journals.

Another purpose of journals is to provide critical reviews of the research being submitted for publication. Journals have reviewers who are asked to read and comment on an article before it is published. This review process helps ensure that published research is of high quality. However, not all published research is of the highest quality, which is one very good reason why you will be learning to review research articles yourself. You have to understand the concepts of research and research methodology before you continue in a science career because once in the field you must be able to review the research you read critically before you put it into practice.

How will you use research journals? For researching—but this is different! You are researching a topic. When you need to research a topic, you go to the library for books and journals on the topic. You are gathering data from these sources. Finally, you are analyzing the data and putting it together to meet whatever needs you have. It might be a class presentation or a paper.

# How Can SQ3R *Help You Own* What You Read?

Even with all the time and energy you spend reading textbook chapters, there's no guarantee you'll understand and remember what you read. The SQ3R study method will help you grasp ideas quickly, remember more, and review effectively for tests. SQ3R stands for *survey, question, read, recite,* and *review*—all steps in the studying process. Developed about 60 years ago by Francis Robinson, the technique is still used today because it works.[6]

Moving through the stages of SQ3R requires that you know how to skim and scan. **Skimming** involves the rapid reading of chapter elements, including introductions, conclusions, and summaries; the first and last lines of paragraphs; boldfaced or italicized terms; and pictures, charts, and diagrams. The goal of skimming is a quick construction of the main ideas. In contrast, **scanning** involves the careful search for specific ideas and facts. You might use scanning during the review phase of SQ3R to locate particular information (such as a chemistry formula).

SQ3R is a studying framework, not a rigid system. You can follow the steps exactly as they are described or adjust them according to your preferences. You may decide, for example, to survey chapter elements in a different order than your classmates or to write different questions or favor different review strategies. Explore the strategies, evaluate what works, and then make the system your own. Although SQ3R will help you as you study almost every subject, it is not suited for literature.

**SKIMMING**

Rapid, superficial reading of material that involves glancing through to determine central ideas and main elements.

**SCANNING**

Reading material in an investigative way to search for specific information.

## Survey

*Surveying* involves previewing, or prereading, material before you actually study it. Compare it to looking at a map before a trip; taking a few minutes to analyze the route may save hours when you are on the road. You are combining your analytical and practical thinking skills to assess the material as quickly as possible.

When you survey, pay attention to the following textwide and chapter-by-chapter elements:

### Front Matter

Before you even get to page 1, most textbooks have a table of contents, a preface, and other materials. The table of contents tells you about coverage, topic order, and features. The preface, in particular, can point out the book's unique approach. For example, the preface for the American history text *Out of Many* states that it highlights "the experiences of diverse communities of Americans in the unfolding story of our country."[7] In other words, cultural diversity is a central theme.

### Chapter Elements

Chapters generally include devices that help you learn material. Among these are:

- Chapter title, which establishes the topic and perhaps the author's perspective on the topic
- Chapter introduction, outline, list of objectives, or list of key topics
- Headings, tables and figures, quotes, marginal notes, and photographs, which help you understand the structure and identify important concepts within the chapter
- Special chapter features, often presented in boxes set off from the main text, that point to textwide themes

- Particular styles or arrangements of type (boldface, italics, underline, larger fonts, bullet points, boxed text) that call attention to important words and concepts
- Chapter summary, which reviews the concepts that were presented
- Review questions and exercises, which help you review and think critically about the material

Skimming these elements before reading the chapter will lead you to identify what is important.

### Back Matter

Some texts include a glossary at the back of the book, an index to help you locate topics, and a bibliography that lists additional readings.

Figure 6.4 shows the many devices that texts employ. Think about how many of these devices you already use and which you will start using to boost comprehension.

## Question

Your next step in the SQ3R process is to examine the chapter headings and, on a separate page or in the book margins, to *write questions* linked to them. If your reading material has no headings, develop questions as you read. These questions help you build comprehension and relate new ideas

**FIGURE 6.4**  Survey with text and chapter previewing devices

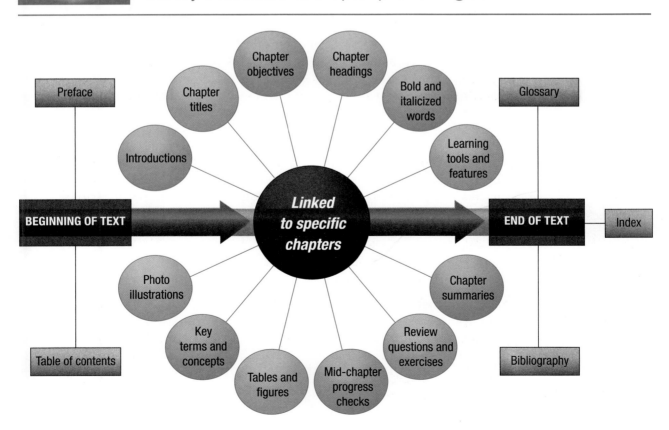

FIGURE 6.5   Use headings to form questions

| | |
|---|---|
| The Meaning of Freedom | What did freedom mean for both slaves and citizens in the United States? |
| Moving About | Where did African Americans go after they were freed from slavery? |
| The African American Family | How did freedom change the structure of the African American family? |
| African American Churches and Schools | What effect did freedom have on the formation of African American churches and schools? |
| Land and Labor After Slavery | How was land farmed and maintained after slaves were freed? |
| The Origins of African American Politics | How did the end of slavery bring about the beginning of African American political life? |

to what you already know. You can take questions from the textbook or from your lecture notes, or come up with them when you survey, based on the ideas you think are most important.

Figure 6.5 shows how this works. The column on the left contains primary- and secondary-level headings from a section of *Out of Many*. The column on the right rephrases these headings in question form.

There is no "correct" set of questions. In fact, given the same headings, you could write many different questions. As you develop the type of probing questions discussed in Chapter 4—questions that delve into the material and help you learn—you are engaging your creative and analytical abilities.

# Read

Your questions give you a starting point for *reading*, the first R in SQ3R. Learning from textbooks requires that you read actively. Active reading means engaging with the material through questioning, writing, note taking, and other activities. As you can see in Figure 6.6, the activities of SQ3R promote active reading. Following are some analytical, creative, and practical strategies that encourage active involvement.

## Focus on your Q-Stage Questions

Read the material with the purpose of answering each question. As you discover ideas and examples that relate to your question, write them down or note them in the text.

## Take Notes on Important Concepts

As you read, record keywords, phrases, and concepts in your notebook. Some students divide the notebook page into two columns, writing

**FIGURE 6.6**   Use SQ3R to become an active reader

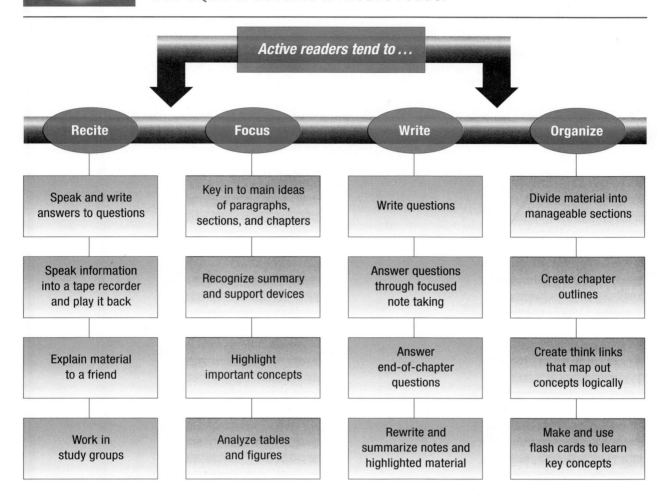

questions on the left and answers on the right. This method is called the Cornell note-taking system (see Chapter 7).

## Mark Up Your Textbook

Writing notes in the text margins and circling or highlighting key ideas will help you make sense of the material. Figure 6.7 shows effective highlighting and marginal notes on the page of a marketing text. Owning your own texts and marking them up is an invaluable learning tool.

Selective highlighting may help you pinpoint material to review before an exam, although excessive highlighting may actually interfere with comprehension. Here are tips on striking a balance:

- **Mark the text after you read the material once through.** If you do it on the first reading, you may mark less important passages.

- **Highlight key terms and concepts.** Mark the examples that explain and support important ideas.

- **Avoid overmarking.** A phrase or two in any paragraph is usually enough because too much underlining may overwhelm your eyes. Set off long passages with brackets rather than marking every line.

*(continued)*

**FIGURE 6.7** Effective highlighting and marginal notes aid memory

# Markets

The term *market* has acquired many meanings over the years. In its original meaning, a market is a physical place where buyers and sellers gather to exchange goods and services. Medieval towns had market squares where sellers brought their goods and buyers shopped for goods. In today's cities, buying and selling occur in shopping areas rather than markets. To an economist, a market describes all the buyers and sellers who transact over some good or service. Thus, the soft-drink market consists of sellers such as Coca-Cola and PepsiCo, and of all the consumers who buy soft drinks. To a marketer, a market is the set of all actual and potential buyers of a product or service.

O rganizations that sell to consumer and business markets recognize that they cannot appeal to all buyers in those markets, or at least not to all buyers in the same way. Buyers are too numerous, too widely scattered, and too varied in their needs and buying practices. And different companies vary widely in their abilities to serve different segments of the market. Rather than trying to compete in an entire market, sometimes against superior competitors, each company must identify the parts of the market that it can serve best.

*Definition of a market*

*Companies can't appeal to everyone*

Sellers have not always practiced this philosophy. Their thinking has passed through three stages:

*One-size-fits-all approach*

- *Mass marketing.* In mass marketing, the seller mass produces, mass distributes, and mass promotes one product to all buyers. At one time, Coca-Cola produced only one drink for the whole market, hoping it would appeal to everyone. The argument for mass marketing is that it should lead to the lowest costs and prices and create the largest potential market.

*Offer variety to buyers*

- *Product-variety marketing.* Here, the seller produces two or more products that have different features, styles, quality, sizes, and so on. Later, Coca-Cola produced several soft drinks packaged in different sizes and containers that were designed to offer variety to buyers rather than to appeal to different market segments. The argument for product-variety marketing is that consumers have different tastes that change over time. Consumers seek variety and change.

*A tailored approach to specific market segments*

- *Target marketing.* Here, the seller identifies market segments, selects one or more of them, and develops products and marketing mixes tailored to each. For example, Coca-Cola now produces soft drinks for the sugared-cola segment (Coca-Cola Classic and Cherry Coke), the diet segment (Diet Coke and Tab), the no-caffeine segment (Caffeine-Free Coke), and the noncola segment (Minute Maid sodas).

*Current approach is usually TARGET MARKETING*

Today's companies are moving away from mass marketing and product-variety marketing toward target marketing. Target marketing can better help sellers find their marketing opportunities. Sellers can develop the right product for each target market and adjust their prices, distribution channels, and advertising to reach the target market efficiently. Instead of scattering their marketing efforts (the "shotgun" approach), they can focus on the buyers who have greater purchase interest (the "rifle" approach).

87

*Source: Marketing: An Introduction*, 4th ed., by Kotler/Armstrong, © 1997. Reprinted with permission of Pearson Education, Inc., Upper Saddle River, NJ.

- **Don't confuse highlighting for learning.** You will not learn what you highlight unless you interact with it through careful review—questioning, writing, and reciting.

## Divide Your Reading into Digestible Segments

If you are losing the thread of the ideas, try smaller segments or take a break. Try to avoid reading according to the clock—such as, "I'll read for 30 minutes and then quit"—or you may short-circuit your understanding by stopping in the middle of a key explanation.

## Find the Main Idea

A crucial analytical skill in textbook reading is the ability to find the main idea: the thoughts that are at the heart of the writing, the ideas that create its essential meaning. Comprehension depends on your ability to recognize main ideas and to link the author's other thoughts to them. Here are places you are likely to find these core ideas:

- In a topic sentence at the beginning of the paragraph, stating the topic of the paragraph and what about that topic the author wants to communicate, followed by sentences adding support.
- At the end of the paragraph, following supporting details that lead up to it.
- Buried in the middle of the paragraph, sandwiched between supporting details.
- In a compilation of ideas from various sentences, each of which contains a critical element. It is up to the reader to piece these elements together to create the essence of meaning.
- Never explicitly stated, but implied by the information presented in the paragraph.

How, then, do you decide just what is the main idea? Ophelia H. Hancock, a specialist in improving reading skills for college students, suggests a three-step approach:[8]

1. *Search for the topic of the paragraph.* The topic of the paragraph is not the same thing as the main idea. Rather, it is the broad subject being discussed—for example, former President John F. Kennedy, hate crimes on campus, or the Internet.

2. *Identify the aspect of the topic that is the paragraph's focus.* If the general topic is former President John F. Kennedy, the writer may choose to focus on any of thousands of aspects of that topic, such as his health problems, his civil rights policies, or his effectiveness as a public speaker.

3. *Find what the author wants you to know about the specific aspect being discussed, which is the main idea.* The main idea of a paragraph dealing with President Kennedy as a public speaker may be this: *President Kennedy was a gifted, charismatic speaker who used his humor, charm, and intelligence to make the presidency accessible to all Americans during regularly televised presidential news conferences.*

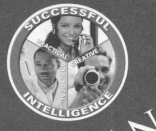

# Find the Main Idea

*Develop your ability to analyze the parts of a paragraph.*

Use the three-step approach described on page 191 to find the main idea of the following paragraph:

*Tone relates not so much to what you say as to how you say it. The tone of your writing has a major impact on what you are trying to communicate to your audience. Tone involves your choice of words interacting with your message. Have you ever reacted to someone's understanding of what you wrote with "That's not what I meant to say"? Your tone can be what has thrown your readers off track, although you can only be misunderstood if your writing is unclear or imprecise.*[9]

- What is the topic of this paragraph?
- What aspect of tone is being discussed?
- What main idea is being communicated?

Now choose a meaty paragraph from one of the texts you are currently studying, and use the same questions to find the paragraph's main idea. How do these questions help you focus on the paragraph's most important points?

## Recite

Once you finish reading a topic, stop and answer the questions you raised in the Q stage of SQ3R. Engage your practical thinking skills to choose the best way to do this. You may decide to *recite* each answer aloud, silently speak the answers to yourself, tell or teach the answers to another person, or write your ideas and answers in brief notes. Writing is often the most effective way to solidify what you have read because writing from memory checks your understanding.

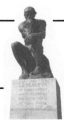

*Knowledge is power* they say. Knowledge is not only power, it is good fun.

E. M. FORSTER

Keep your learning styles in mind when you explore different strategies (see Chapter 3). For example, an intrapersonal learner may prefer writing, whereas an interpersonal learner might want to recite answers aloud to a classmate. A logical-mathematical learner may benefit from organizing material into detailed outlines, whereas a musical learner might want to chant information aloud to a rhythm.

After you finish one section, read the next. *Repeat the question-read-recite cycle until you complete the entire chapter.* If you find yourself fumbling for thoughts, you may not yet own the ideas. Reread the section that's giving you trouble until you master its contents. Understanding each section as you go is crucial because the material in one section often forms a foundation for the next.

## Review

*Review* soon after you finish a chapter. Reviewing immediately and periodically in the days and weeks after you read solidifies understanding. Chances are good that if you close the book after you read, you will forget most of the material. Here are reviewing techniques that engage all three components of successful intelligence. Try many, and use what works best for you.

- Skim and reread your notes. Then try summarizing them from memory.
- Answer the text's end-of-chapter review, discussion, and application questions.
- Quiz yourself, using the questions you raised in the Q stage. If you can't answer any of your own or the text's questions, scan the text for answers.
- Create a chapter outline in standard outline or think link form.
- Reread the preface, headings, tables, and **summary**.
- Recite important concepts to yourself, or record important information on a recorder/digital recorder/MP3 player and play it in your car or on a portable player.
- Make flash cards that have an idea or word on one side and examples, a definition, or other related information on the other. Test yourself.
- Review and summarize in writing the material you have highlighted or bracketed. Your goal is to create a summary that focuses on the central ideas, setting the stage for critical thinking.
- Think critically: Break ideas down into examples, consider similar or different concepts, recall important terms, evaluate ideas, and explore causes and effects.
- Discuss the concepts with a classmate or in a study group. Trying to teach study partners what you learned will pinpoint the material you know and what still needs work.

SUMMARY
A concise restatement of the material, that covers the main points.

If a concept is still unclear, ask your instructor for help. Pinpoint the material you wish to discuss, schedule a meeting during office hours, and bring a list of questions.

Refreshing your knowledge is easier and faster than learning it the first time. Set up regular review sessions—for example, once a week. Reviewing in different ways increases the likelihood of retention.

# How Can You *Respond Critically* to What You Read?

The fundamental purpose of all college reading is understanding. Think of your reading process as an archaeological dig. The first step is to excavate a site and uncover the artifacts: That's your initial survey and reading of the material. As important as the excavation is, the process is incomplete if you stop there. The second step is to investigate each item, evaluate what they all mean, and derive knowledge from what you discover. Critical reading allows you to complete that crucial second step.

Like critical thinking, critical reading is a part of analytical thinking (see Chapter 4). Instead of simply accepting what you read, seek understanding by questioning the material as you move from idea to idea. The best critical readers question every statement for accuracy, relevance, and logic. They also extend critical analysis to all media.

## Use Knowledge of Fact and Opinion to Evaluate Arguments

Critical readers evaluate arguments to determine whether they are accurate and logical. In this context, *argument* refers to a persuasive case—a set of connected ideas supported by examples—that a writer makes to prove or disprove a point.

It's easy—and common—to accept or reject an argument outright, according to whether it fits with your point of view. If you ask questions, however, you can determine the argument's validity and understand it in greater depth. Evaluating an argument involves

- Evaluating the quality of the evidence.
- Evaluating whether support fits the concept.
- Evaluating the logical connections.

When quality evidence combines with appropriate support and tight logic, the argument is solid.

### What Is the Quality of the Evidence?

Ask the following questions to evaluate the evidence:

- What is the source?
- Is the source reliable and free of bias?
- Who wrote this and with what intent?
- What assumptions underlie this material?
- Is the argument based on opinion?
- How does the evidence compare with evidence from other sources?

### How Well Does the Evidence Support the Idea?

Ask these questions to determine whether the evidence fits the concept:

- Is there enough evidence to support the central idea?
- Do examples and ideas logically connect to one another?

- Is the evidence convincing? Do the examples build a strong case?
- What different and perhaps opposing arguments seem just as valid?

Approach every argument with healthy skepticism. Have an open mind to assess whether you are convinced or have serious questions. Use critical thinking to make an informed decision.

If, for example, you read an article with this premise: "The dissolution of the traditional family unit (working father, stay-at-home mother, dependent children) is contributing to society's problems," you might examine the facts and examples the writer uses to support this statement, looking carefully at the cause-and-effect structure of the argument. You might question the writer's sources. You might think of examples that support the statement. You might find examples that disprove this argument, such as statistics that show strong job numbers and college degree completion in areas where nontraditional family units are common. Finally, you might think of opposing arguments, including the ideas and examples to support those arguments.

## Media Literacy

Use your analytical thinking skills to analyze the information you receive through the **media**, including television, radio, film, the Internet, newspapers, magazines, and books. By improving your *media literacy*, you will approach every media message with a healthy skepticism that leads you to ask questions, look for evidence, recognize perspectives, and challenge assumptions. This approach will help you decide which information you can trust and use.

MEDIA
The agencies of mass communication—television, film, journalism (magazines and newspapers), books, and the Internet.

The Center for Media Literacy explains "Five Core Concepts of Media Literacy":[10]

1. *All media are constructions.* All media are carefully constructed presentations designed for particular effect—to encourage you to feel certain emotions, to develop particular opinions, or to buy advertised products.

2. *Media use unique "languages."* Creators of media carefully choose wording, music, colors, timing, and other factors to produce a desired effect.

3. *Different audiences understand the same media message differently.* Individuals understand media in the context of their unique experiences. Someone who has climbed a mountain, for example, will experience a Mount Everest documentary differently than someone who has not.

4. *Media have commercial interests.* Creators of media are driven by the intent to sell products, services, or ideas. Advertising is chosen to appeal to the most likely audience (for example, beer and automobile ads, directed at 20- to 30-year-old men, often appear during sporting events).

5. *Media have embedded values and points of view.* Any media product reflects the values and biases of the people who created it.

Critical reading of texts and the media takes time and focus. You can learn from others by working in pairs or groups whenever you can.

# Why and How Should You *Study with Others*?

Tap your practical thinking skills to set up or find a study partner or group. When you study with others, you benefit from shared knowledge, solidified knowledge, increased motivation, and increased teamwork ability.

- **Shared knowledge.** It takes less time for study group members to pass on their knowledge to each other than for each member to learn all the material alone.

- **Solidified knowledge.** When you discuss concepts or teach them to others, you reinforce what you know and strengthen your critical thinking. Part of the benefit comes from repeating information aloud, and part comes from how you think through information before you pass it on to someone else.

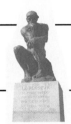

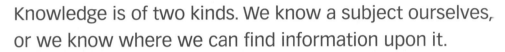

Knowledge is of two kinds. We know a subject ourselves, or we know where we can find information upon it.

SAMUEL JOHNSON

- **Increased motivation.** When you study by yourself, you are accountable to yourself alone. In a study group, however, others see your level of preparation, which may increase your motivation.

- **Increased teamwork ability.** The more experience you have with group dynamics, the more effective your teamwork will be.

A group of students taking the same course may get together once or twice a week or right before exams. Instructors sometimes initiate study groups for their students. Known as peer-assisted study sessions or supplemental instruction, these groups are common in math and science courses.

Roommates sometimes become study partners. When Lucila Crena, a freshman at Emory University and a native of Argentina, met her roommate Jolyn Taylor, she was fortunate enough to also find a partner who helped her focus. "I'm very easily distracted— she's definitely the more committed one," said Lucila. "With another student, I don't know that I would learn less, but it might be harder for me to actually do the work." The arrangement also benefited Jolyn, who turned to Lucila for help with Spanish.[11]

Group study can make a real difference if group members are dedicated. Choosing a leader, meeting at regular times, and setting goals all help groups accomplish their work.

## Leaders and Participants

Study groups and other teams rely on both leaders and participants to accomplish goals. Becoming aware of the roles each plays will increase your effectiveness.[12] Keep in mind that participants sometimes perform leadership tasks and vice versa. In addition, some teams shift leadership frequently during a project.

# Form a Study Group

*Form a study group for one of your courses.*

Get a group together and use this form to decide on and record the details.

- Course name:
- Study group members (names, phone numbers, e-mail addresses):

  Member #1

  Member #2

  Member #3

  Member #4

  Member #5

- Regular meeting time(s):
- Regular meeting place(s):
- Three strategies you plan to use to make the most of group time:

  Strategy #1:

  Strategy #2:

  Strategy #3:

## Being an Effective Participant

Some people are most comfortable when participating in a group that someone else leads. Participants are "part owners" of the team process with a responsibility for, and a stake in, the outcome. The following strategies will help you become more effective in this role.

- **Get involved.** Let people know your views on decisions.
- **Be organized.** The more focused your ideas, the more others will take them seriously.
- **Be willing to discuss.** Be open to different opinions. Always be respectful.
- **Keep your word.** Carry out whatever tasks you promise to do.

## Being an Effective Leader

Some people prefer to initiate the action, make decisions, and control how things proceed. Leaders often have a "big-picture" perspective that allows them to envision and plan group projects. The following strategies help a leader succeed.

- **Define and limit projects.** The leader should define the group's purpose (Is it to brainstorm, to make decisions, or to collaborate on a project?) and limit tasks so the effort remains focused.
- **Assign work and set a schedule.** A group functions best when everyone has an assigned task and when deadlines are clear.
- **Set meeting and project agendas.** The leader should, with advice from other members, establish and communicate goals and define how the work will proceed.
- **Focus progress.** It is the leader's job to keep everyone headed in the right direction.
- **Set the tone.** If the leader is fair, respectful, encouraging, and hardworking, group members are likely to follow the example.
- **Evaluate results.** The leader should determine whether the team is accomplishing its goals on schedule. If the team is not moving ahead, the leader should make changes.

## Strategies for Study Group Success

Every study group is unique. The way a group operates may depend on members' personalities, the subject being studied, and the group's size. No matter the particulars, the following general strategies will foster success.

- **Choose a leader for each meeting.** Rotating the leadership helps all members take ownership of the group.
- **Set long-term and short-term goals.** At your first meeting, determine what the group wants to accomplish over the semester. At the beginning of each meeting, have one person compile a list of questions to address.
- **Adjust to different personalities.** The art of getting along will serve you well no matter what you do.
- **Share the work.** The most important factor is a willingness to work, not a particular level of knowledge.
- **Set a regular meeting schedule.** Try every week, every two weeks, or whatever the group can manage.
- **Create study materials for one another.** Give each group member the task of finding a piece of information to compile, photocopy or e-mail, and review for other group members.
- **Help each other learn.** Have group members teach pieces of information, make up quizzes for each other, or go through flash cards together.
- **Pool your note-taking resources.** Compare notes with your group members and fill in any information you don't have. Try different note-taking styles (see Chapter 7 for more on note taking).
- **Be aware of cultural differences.** When members of a study group come from different countries, cultural values may impact how easily members get along. For example, whereas a student from a high-context culture such as Greece may want to begin every meeting with social talk, Americans and others from low-context cultures are likely to want to focus on assignments right away. Or students from a high-context

culture like Japan may be uncomfortable talking about personal accomplishments in the way Americans do and, instead, want to emphasize what the group does together.

Addressing the communication issues that result from these and other cultural differences requires group members to talk openly about what they observe and to work to accommodate each other's style. Making such adjustments will prepare you well for the twenty-first-century workplace. (For more on high-context and low-context cultures, see Chapter 2.)

Think of the vast amounts of information your mind processes as you read and study your textbooks. Challenge yourself to raise the bar of achievement by reading often and using the strategies suggested in this chapter. You will understand more, remember more, and have more to use as you work toward goals in school and beyond.

# читать

People who read Russian, Japanese, Greek, Arabic, or other languages process the symbols of their alphabets as easily as you process the letters on this page. If you read Russian, for example, you know that the word preceding this paragraph means "read." The brain's ability to process and group letters to form words, phrases, and sentences is the basis for reading and studying.

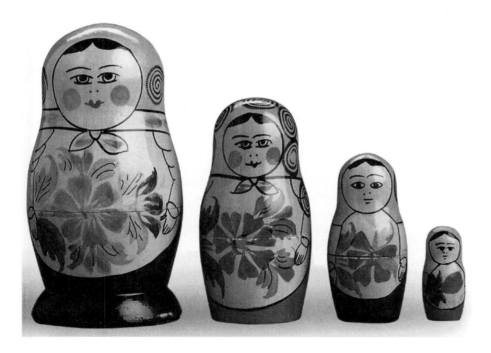

## Create Your Future

# DEVELOPING SUCCESSFUL INTELLIGENCE
## *Putting It All Together*

**Studying a Text Page.** The following excerpt is from "Evaluation and Exercise Prescription," Fardy and Yanowitz, *Cardiac Rehabilitation, Adult Fitness, and Exercise Testing,* 3rd edition. Read the material using the study techniques in this chapter, and complete the questions that follow.

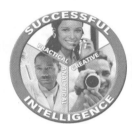

### Exercise Prescription

The exercise prescription represents the carefully regulated dosage of physical activity of a long-term training program. The dosage consists of a coalescence of intensity, duration, and frequency of effort that is undertaken in an exercise mode to achieve specific program objectives. The prescription should be developed in a manner similar to that of prescribing medication, that is, administered in specified amounts based on individual needs. When designed for cardiac rehabilitation and adult fitness, the exercise modes are usually selected for the purpose of enhancing cardiovascular function and lessening the risk of coronary heart disease. Other training objectives such as strength and flexibility have very different prescriptions and are addressed briefly in this chapter, although the reader is referred elsewhere for more in-depth information. The purposes of this chapter are to present the rationale for an exercise prescription that promotes cardiovascular function; to present the physiologic basis and design of the prescription, the factors that affect the prescription; and to apply the prescription formula to an exercise training program.

### Physiologic Basis of the Exercise Prescription

The physiologic basis of the exercise prescription is the overload principle and the relationship between training stimuli (dosage) and adaptation (response).

#### Overload Principle

Overload by definition means that the training stimulus must surpass normal daily physical exertion to be beneficial. The training stimulus, however, should not provoke undue fatigue, musculoskeletal strain, or mental or emotional burnout. Optimal benefit necessitates regular updating of the overload threshold.

### Dose Response

Adaptation is related to the amount of physical exertion, although the relationship is not consistently linear. Dose-response curves depicted in Figure A-1 represent a relationship illustrating that adaptation does not occur until some minimal effort is expended, that is, overload. The curves do not represent physiologic measures, but rather represent a conceptual comparison of effort versus gain under different circumstances. Training adaptation is modest or nonexistent for most persons until effort approximates 50 to 60% of maximum intensity. Thereafter, gains are rapid until they plateau at the top of the curves, between 85 and 90% of maximal effort, indicating that exercise is too intense or that there is insufficient time for recovery, or both. The dose-response curves shift to the right as physical condition improves. The rate of adaptation varies among individuals, although improvements are generally similar at different ages and for males and females.

## Components of the Prescription

The prescription dosage consists of intensity, duration, frequency, and mode of exercise.

### Intensity

The single most important factor of the exercise prescription is intensity of effort, usually expressed as a percentage of functional aerobic capacity or maximal heart rate (MHR). There is a strong and consistent correlation between oxygen uptake and heart rate as a percentage of maximum regardless of the level of physical condition, gender, or muscle groups being compared.

Several approaches may be used to prescribe training intensity. In any case maximal exercise testing is recommended for best results. The ACSM Guidelines provide clear recommendations for testing. Heart rate prescriptions based on submaximal testing or age-estimated maximal heart rates have the potential for considerable error and, as a result, may be too strenuous and pose the risk of injury or too easy and, hence, ineffective.

The target heart rate (THR) is ordinarily established between 70 and 90% MHR, approximately 60 to 80% VO2max. Those who are poorly conditioned as well as patients with cardiopulmonary disease can benefit from training at heart rates less than 70% MHR, while competitive athletes may require greater than 90% MHR for training adaptation.

**FIGURE A-1**  Improvement anticipated from effort expended

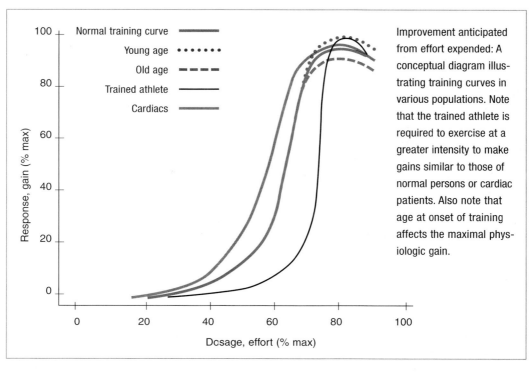

Improvement anticipated from effort expended: A conceptual diagram illustrating training curves in various populations. Note that the trained athlete is required to exercise at a greater intensity to make gains similar to those of normal persons or cardiac patients. Also note that age at onset of training affects the maximal physiologic gain.

*Source:* P. S. Fardy and F. G. Yanowitz, *Cardiac Rehabilitation, Adult Fitness, and Exercise Testing*, 3rd ed. © Williams & Wilkins, Baltimore, MD, 1995, pp. 246–247. Used with permission.

1. Identify the headings of the excerpt and the relationship among them. Which headings are primary-level headings; which are secondary; which are tertiary (third-level heads)? Which heading serves as an umbrella for the rest?

   _____

   _____

   _____

   _____

2. What do the headings tell you about the content of the excerpt?

   _____

   _____

   _____

   _____

3. Identify the terms with abbreviations after them. What does this tell you about these words? How is the graph in Figure A-1 useful?

   _____

   _____

   _____

   _____

4. After reading the chapter headings, write three study questions:

   _____

   _____

   _____

5. Using a marker pen, highlight key phrases and sentences. Write short marginal notes to help you review the material at a later point.

6. After reading this article, list three key concepts that you will need to study:

   a. _____

   b. _____

   c. _____

**Focusing on Your Purpose for Reading.** Read the material on the following page on kinetic and potential energy and the first law of thermodynamics taken from *Life on Earth* by Teresa Audesirk and Gerald Audesirk. When you have finished, answer the questions following the selection.

Among the fundamental characteristics of all living organisms is the ability to guide chemical reactions within their bodies along certain pathways. The chemical reactions serve many functions, depending on the nature of the organism: to synthesize the molecules that make up the organism's body, to reproduce, to move, even to think. Chemical reactions either require or release energy, which can be defined simply as *the capacity to do work*, including synthesizing molecules, moving things around, and generating heat and light. In this chapter we discuss the physical laws that govern energy flow in the universe, how energy flow in turn governs chemical reactions, and how the chemical reactions within living cells are controlled by the molecules of the cell itself. Chapters 7 and 8 focus on photosynthesis, the chief "port of entry" for energy into the biosphere, and glycolysis and cellular respiration, the most important sequences of chemical reactions that release energy.

## ENERGY AND THE ABILITY TO DO WORK

As you learned in Chapter 2, there are two types of energy: **kinetic energy** and **potential energy**. Both types of energy may exist in many different forms. Kinetic energy, or *energy of movement*, includes light (movement of photons), heat (movement of molecules), electricity (movement of electrically charged particles), and movement of large objects. Potential energy, or *stored energy*, includes chemical energy stored in the bonds that hold atoms together in molecules, electrical energy stored in a battery, and positional energy stored in a diver poised to spring (Fig. 4-1). Under the right conditions, kinetic energy can be transformed into potential energy, and vice versa. For example, the diver converted kinetic energy of movement into potential energy of position when she climbed the ladder up to the platform; when she jumps off, the potential energy will be converted back into kinetic energy.

To understand how energy flow governs interactions among pieces of matter, we need to know two things: (1) the quantity of available energy and (2) the usefulness of the energy. These are the subjects of the laws of thermodynamics, which we will now examine.

## The Laws of Thermodynamics Describe the Basic Properties of Energy

All interactions among pieces of matter are governed by the two **laws of thermodynamics**, physi-cal principles that define the basic properties and behavior of energy. The laws of thermodynamics deal with "isolated systems," which are any parts of the universe that cannot exchange either matter or energy with any other parts. Probably no part of the universe is completely isolated from all possible exchange with every other part, but the concept of an isolated system is useful in thinking about energy flow.

## The First Law of Thermodynamics States That Energy Can Be Neither Created nor Destroyed

The **first law of thermodynamics** states that within any isolated system, energy can be neither created nor destroyed, although it can be changed in form (for example, from chemical energy to heat energy). In other words, within an isolated system *the total quantity of energy remains constant.* The first law is therefore often called the law of conservation of energy. To use a familiar example, let's see how the first law applies to driving your car (Fig. 4-2). We can consider that your car (with a full tank of gas), the road, and the surrounding air roughly constitute an isolated system. When you drive your car, you convert the potential chemical energy of gasoline into kinetic energy of movement and heat energy. The total amount of energy that was in the gasoline before it was burned is the same as the total amount of this kinetic energy and heat.

An important rule of energy conversions is this: Energy always flows "downhill," from places with a high concentration of energy to places with a low concentration of energy. This is the principle behind engines. As we described in Chapter 2, temperature is a measure of how fast molecules move. The burning gasoline in your car's engine consists of molecules moving at extremely high speeds: a high concentration of energy. The cooler air outside the engine consists of molecules moving at much lower speeds: a low concentration of energy. The molecules in the engine hit the piston harder than the air molecules outside the engine do, so the piston moves upward, driving the gears that move the car. Work is done. When the engine is turned off, it cools down as heat is transferred from the warm engine to its cooler surroundings. The molecules on both sides of the piston move at the same speed, so the piston stays still. No work is done.

*Source:* T. Audesirk and G. Audesirk, *Life on Earth* (Upper Saddle River, NJ: Prentice Hall, 1997). Reprinted by permission of Prentice Hall.

1. *Reading for critical evaluation.* Evaluate the material by answering these questions:

   Were the ideas clearly supported by examples? If you feel one or more were not supported, give an example.

   _____

   _____

   _____

   _____

   Did the author make any assumptions that weren't examined? If so, name one or more.

   _____

   _____

   _____

   _____

   Do you disagree with any part of the material? If so, which part, and why?

   _____

   _____

   _____

   _____

   Do you have any suggestions for how the material could have been presented more effectively?

   _____

   _____

   _____

   _____

2. *Reading for practical application.* Imagine you have to give a presentation on this material the next time the class meets. On a separate sheet of paper, create an outline or think link that maps out the key elements you would discuss.

3. *Reading for comprehension.* Answer the following questions to determine the level of your comprehension.

   What are the two types of energy?

   _____

   _____

   Which one "stores" energy?

   _____

   _____

   Can kinetic energy be turned into potential energy?

   _____

   _____

What is the term for the physical principles that describe the basic properties and behaviors of energy?

_____

_____

Mark the following statements as true (T) or false (F).

_____ Within any isolated system, energy can be neither created nor destroyed.

_____ Energy always flows downhill, from high concentration levels to low.

_____ All interactions among pieces of matter are governed by two laws of thermodynamics.

_____ Some parts of the universe are isolated from other parts.

# TEAM BUILDING

## *Collaborative Solutions*

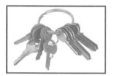

**Organizing a Study Group.** Organize a study group with three or four members of your class. At the group's first meeting:

- **Set a specific goal for the group.** For example, to prepare for an upcoming test or project, create a weekly schedule. Write everything down and make sure everyone has a copy.

- **Talk about the specific ways you will work together.** Discuss which of the following methods you want to try in the group: pooling your notes; teaching each other difficult concepts; making up, administering, and grading quizzes for each other; creating study flash cards; using SQ3R to review required readings. Set specific guidelines for how group members will be held accountable.

As an initial group exercise, try the following:

- **Review the study questions that you wrote for number 3 on page 204.** Each person should select one question to focus on while reading (no two people should have the same question). Group members should then reread the excerpt individually, thinking about their questions as they read and answering them in writing.

- **When you finish reading critically, gather as a group.** Each person should take a turn presenting the question, the response or answer that was derived through critical reading, and any other ideas that came up while reading. The other members of the group may then present any other ideas to add to the discussion. Continue until all group members have had a chance to present their concepts.

Over several weeks, try the group study methods you have chosen. Then evaluate the methods as a group, singling out the methods that most effectively helped group members master the course material. Finally, revise the group's methods if necessary, to focus on those most useful methods.

# WRITING

## Discovery Through Journaling

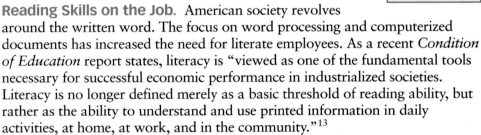

*Record your thoughts on a separate piece of paper or in a journal.*

**Reading Challenges.** What course this semester presents your most difficult reading challenge? What makes it tough—the type of material you have to read, the amount, the level of difficulty? Thinking about the strategies in this chapter, create and describe a plan that addresses this challenge. What techniques might help, and how will you use them? What positive effects do you think they'll have?

# CAREER PORTFOLIO

## Plan for Success

*Complete the following in your electronic portfolio or on separate sheets of paper.*

**Reading Skills on the Job.** American society revolves around the written word. The focus on word processing and computerized documents has increased the need for literate employees. As a recent *Condition of Education* report states, literacy is "viewed as one of the fundamental tools necessary for successful economic performance in industrialized societies. Literacy is no longer defined merely as a basic threshold of reading ability, but rather as the ability to understand and use printed information in daily activities, at home, at work, and in the community."[13]

For each of the following skill areas listed, indicate all of the ways in which you use that skill on the job or know you will need to use it in your future career. Then, also for each skill, rate your ability on a scale from 1 to 10, with 10 being the highest. Finally, on the same document or sheet of paper, highlight or circle the two skills that you think will be most important for your career as well as for your success as a learner in college.

- Ability to define your reading purpose
- Reading speed
- Reading comprehension
- Vocabulary building
- Identification and use of text-surveying devices
- Using analytical thinking skills when reading
- Evaluating reading material with others
- Ability to understand and use visual aids

For the two skill areas in which you rated yourself lowest, think about how you can improve your abilities. Make a problem-solving plan for each (you may want to use a flowchart like the one on page 166). Check your progress in one month and at the end of the semester.[14]

*Source: Sociology,* 6th ed. by John J. Macionis, © 1977. Reprinted by permission of Pearson Education, Inc., Upper Saddle River, NJ.

# Suggested Readings

Armstrong, William H., and M. Willard Lampe II. *Barron's Pocket Guide to Study Tips: How to Study Effectively and Get Better Grades*. New York: Barron's Educational Series, 2004.

Chesla, Elizabeth. *Reading Comprehension Success: In 20 Minutes a Day*, 2nd ed. Florence, KY: Thomson Delmar Learning, 2002.

Frank, Steven. *The Everything Study Book*. Holbrook, MA: Adams Media, 1997.

Labunski, Richard E. *The Educated Student: Getting the Most Out of Your College Years*. Versailles, KY: Marley and Beck, 2003.

Luckie, William R., Wood Smethurst, and Sarah Beth Huntley. *Study Power Workbook: Exercises in Study Skills to Improve Your Learning and Your Grades*. Cambridge, MA: Brookline Books, 1999.

Silver, Theodore. *The Princeton Review Study Smart: Hands-on, Nuts and Bolts Techniques for Earning Higher Grades*. New York: Villard Books, 1996.

# Internet Resources

Academictips.org (study tips and links):
**www.academictips.org**

How to Study (study advice with valuable links):
**www.howtostudy.com**

Prentice Hall Student Success Supersite Study Skills:
**www.prenhall.com/success**

# Endnotes

[1] Richard J. Light, *Making the Most of College: Students Speak Their Minds* (Cambridge, MA: Harvard University Press, 2001), pp. 23–24.

[2] Sherwood Harris, *The New York Public Library Book of How and Where to Look It Up* (Englewood Cliffs, NJ: Prentice Hall, 1991), p. 13.

[3] Roxanne Ruzic, CAST, "Lessons for Everyone: How Students with Reading-Related Learning Disabilities Survive and Excel in College Courses with Heavy Reading Requirements." Paper presented at the Annual Meeting of the American Educational Research Association (April 13, 2001). Retrieved February 2004, from: www.cast.org/udl/index.cfm?i=1540.

[4] Steve Moidel, *Speed Reading* (Hauppauge, NY: Barron's Educational Series, 1994), p. 18.

[5] Ibid.

[6] Francis P. Robinson, *Effective Behavior* (New York: Harper & Row), 1941.

[7] John Mack Faragher et al., *Out of Many*, 3rd ed. (Upper Saddle River, NJ: Prentice Hall), p. xxxvii.

[8] Ophelia H. Hancock, *Reading Skills for College Students*, 5th ed. (Upper Saddle River, NJ: Prentice Hall, 2001), pp. 54–59.

[9] Excerpted from Lynn Quitman Troyka, *Simon & Schuster Handbook for Writers*, 5th ed. (Upper Saddle River, NJ: Prentice Hall, 1999), p. 12.

[10] Center for Media Literacy, 1998.

[11] Eric Hoover, "Peer Factor: Do Smart Students Improve the Performance of Others?" *The Chronicle of Higher Education* (February 7, 2003). Retrieved March 2004, from: http://chronicle.com/weekly/v49/i22/22a02901.htm.

[12] Louis E. Boone, David L. Kurtz, and Judy R. Block, *Contemporary Business Communication* (Englewood Cliffs, NJ: Prentice Hall, 1994), pp. 489–499.

[13] U.S. Department of Education, National Center for Education Statistics, *The Condition of Education, 1996*, NCES 96–304, by Thomas M. Smith (Washington, DC: U.S. Government Printing Office, 1996), p. 84.

[14] John J. Macionis, *Sociology*, 6th ed. (Upper Saddle River, NJ: Prentice Hall, 1997), p. 174.

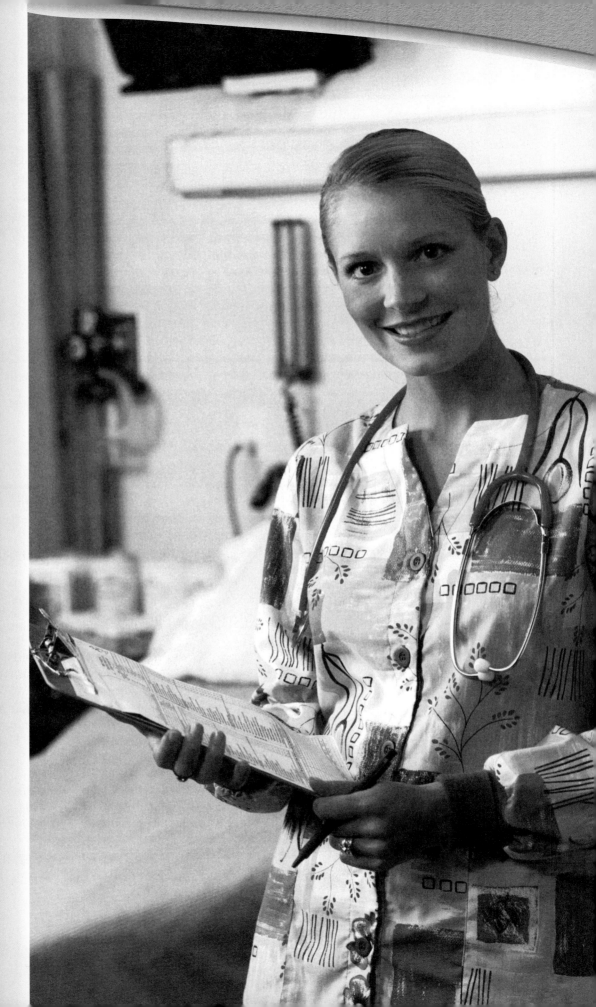

**EXPRESS: LISTENING, NOTE TAKING, AND MEMORY**

*TAKING IN, RECORDING, AND REMEMBERING INFORMATION*

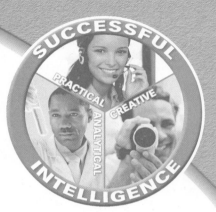

**C**ollege exposes you daily to all kinds of information, and your job as a student is to take it in, sort through it, and keep what is important. This chapter shows you how to do just that by building your listening (taking in information), note taking (recording what's important), and memory skills (remembering information).

Compare these skills to using a camera: You start by locating an image through the viewfinder, then you carefully focus the lens (listening), record the image on film or a digital card (note taking), and produce a print (remembering). The whole process engages your analytical, creative, and practical abilities and helps you build knowledge you can use.

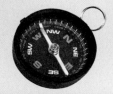

# Q & A BLUE SKY QUESTIONS DOWN-TO-EARTH ANSWERS

### How can I balance time restrictions, along with other nursing responsibilities and still provide quality patient care?

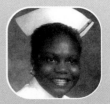

Lillan A. Kanda
*Lewis University*
*Romeoville, Ilinois*

I have a two-year associate degree in nursing, and I'm now enrolled in a bachelor's program. Writing was not emphasized much in the two-year nursing program. Students only had to take a minimum basic college English course, but this doesn't provide what you need in the real world. I work at a hospital, and I'm realizing that I need to improve my writing skills. With charting it's important to be accurate. I've tried following older nurses as my role models, but I've found that I still must adapt to my own way of charting. In the hospital, mistakes do happen. When I have to make an incident report stating what happened I wish my writing skills were better. The four-year degree involves more about writing and research, and it's giving me a chance to polish my writing skills.

One of my required courses is called "Concepts of Professional Nursing," My first paper for that class was about collaboration, in which I described teamwork among my coworkers. I was ready to quit the class, but the teacher was patient and I completed the course. The hardest part was doing the citations. One of the rules, of course, is that you can't use someone else's words, and I found it hard to paraphrase. If I can write about something that I'm very familiar with, the writing comes easier for me. For example, I wrote a paper about my growing up in Ghana, West Africa. That was one of my favorite writing assignments.

In some ways I think computers spoil nurses in regard to writing. Technology makes nursing easier, but it doesn't encourage nurses to write more. In school we are taught to write in narrative form, but with charting you usually have to abbreviate, so grammar is often disregarded. We do some narrative charting, but at the hospital I used to work for, we used only computer checklists for charting. Sometimes when we have new in-service programs for the computer it's so scary to me because I'm not used to anything that advanced. In spite of my apprehensions, I see the value of writing on many levels. For example, following a charting system helps me focus on the patient and anticipate problems that I might have overlooked had I not taken the time to write out my observations. Information that might not have initially seemed important may be vital to another health care professional, especially if the patient's condition changes. The reflective aspect of writing helps me look at the patient holistically.

Last semester I had a patient with a skin integrity problem, and I noticed how writing down my interpretation of the issues facing this patient helped me coordinate an effective plan. This brings me to the heart of my concern. During clinicals, I only take care of one patient at a time. What about when I must juggle five or more patients all at once? I know the nursing profession is demanding. But without writing to stimulate my thinking, I'm concerned that I won't be able to provide the kind of care that I envision. It feels like I'm cheating myself and the patient.

## Experience and learning will help you.

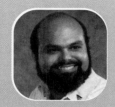

Ray Salva Jr.
*Registered Nurse, Gottlieb Memorial Hospital, Melrose Park, Illinois*

Providing quality patient care can feel like a tug-of-war game. As a nurse, you will be pulled in many directions all at once, but with experience you can manage your patient load so that each person receives the best care possible.

One of the keys to providing quality care is organizational skills. Knowing which patients need the most care can help you set priorities during your particular shift. The severity of each patient's physical condition determines, at least in part, how much care you can and should give to them. Some patients require a lot more individual attention because of the seriousness of their condition. Remembering the basic ABCs—airway, breathing, and circulation—has helped me makes this determination.

It might also help to be aware that day shifts are busier than evening shifts. Most hospital procedures, such as X-rays, are scheduled during the day, and that's also when doctors and families make their visits. Since you've found it gratifying to focus on one patient at a time, you may prefer to specialize in ICU or CCU, because these patients frequently require one-on-one nursing care.

Another key or quality patient care is knowing what resources are available at your hospital. For example, knowing whom to contact. If a patient is having respiratory distress or needs psychiatric care can make a difference. When you begin your first nursing position, you should receive a policy and procedures manual that lists these resources. For the sake of your patients, read through this so that you are aware of the options for them.

As you probably know, not every hospital uses SOAP notes, and most hospitals are now computerized. You may find that you don't have time to do much writing and charting until near the end of your shift, after the necessary and urgent tasks are completed. At my hospital, every patient has his or her own computer checklist and other prompts that nurses are expected to fill out. At the bottom there is a narrative section where I can be creative and make note of something important concerning the patient.

Since writing is a crucial learning tool for you, perhaps you could write about nursing in your free time. You could keep a journal and after the close of certain shifts, you could write down your observations and insights, and use these note as a reminder of what worked for you that day and what didn't work.

Keep in mind that written care plans are only one part of the puzzle in providing quality care. Your training, your instinct, and even your individual personality all comprise the other pieces that help you become an excellent nurse. When I started my nursing career seven yours ago I was a nervous wreck because I wanted to be the "perfect" nurse. Over time a more relaxed style began to emerge, and I brought "me" into the job. Once that happened I found nursing to be the kind of rewarding profession I always knew it could be.

# How Can You Become a *Better Listener?*

The act of hearing isn't the same as the act of **listening**. Hearing refers to sensing spoken messages from their source. Listening, however, involves a complex process of communication. Successful listening occurs when the listener understands the speaker's intended message. The good news is that

LISTENING
*A process that involves sensing, interpreting, evaluating, and reacting to spoken messages.*

listening is a teachable—and learnable—skill that engages analytical and practical abilities.

## Know the Stages of Listening

Listening is made up of four stages that happen instantaneously and build on one another: sensing, interpreting, evaluating, and reacting. You move through these stages without being aware as they take the message from the speaker to the listener and back to the speaker (see Figure 7.1).

During the *sensation* stage, your ears pick up sound waves and transmit them to the brain. For example, you are sitting in class and hear your instructor say, "The only opportunity to make up last week's test is Tuesday at 5 P.M."

In the *interpretation* stage, listeners attach meaning to a message. This involves understanding what is being said and relating it to what you already know. You relate this message to your knowledge of the test, whether you need to make it up, and what you are doing on Tuesday at 5 P.M.

In the *evaluation* stage, you decide how you feel about the message, whether, for example, you like it or agree with it and how it relates to your needs and values. If the message goes against your values or does not fulfill your needs, you may reject it, stop listening, or argue in your mind with the speaker. In this example, if you do need to make up the test but have to work on Tuesday at 5 P.M., you may evaluate the message as less than satisfactory.

The final stage of listening is a *reaction* to the message in the form of direct feedback. In a classroom, direct feedback comes in the form of questions and comments. Your reaction, in this case, may be to ask the instructor if she can schedule another test time.

**FIGURE 7.1**  Understand the stages of listening

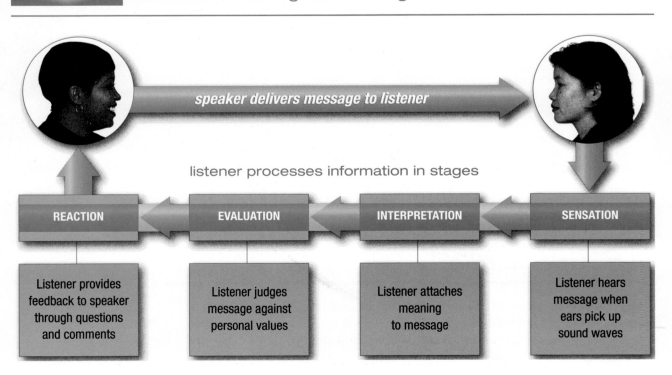

Improving your listening skills involves two primary goals: managing listening challenges (maximizing the sensation stage) and becoming an active listener (maximizing the interpretation and evaluation stages).

## Manage Listening Challenges

Classic studies have shown that immediately after listening, students are likely to recall only half of what was said. This is partly due to such listening challenges as divided attention and distractions, the tendency to shut out the message, the inclination to rush to judgment, and partial hearing loss or learning disabilities.[1] Fortunately, you can minimize these challenges. Here are some ways to do it.

### Divided Attention and Distractions

Internal and external distractions often divide your attention. *Internal distractions* include anything from hunger to headache to personal worries. Something the speaker says may also trigger a reaction that causes your mind to drift. In contrast, *external distractions* include anything from noises (whispering, police sirens) to excessive heat or cold to a wobbly seat. It is hard to listen when you are sweating, uncomfortable, or distracted by talkers.

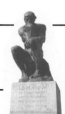

Opportunities are often missed because we are broadcasting when we should be listening.

AUTHOR UNKNOWN

Use practical strategies to reduce distractions so you can concentrate on what you're hearing. Sitting near the front of the room will help, as will moving away from chatting classmates. Work to concentrate when you're in class and save worrying about personal problems for later. Get enough sleep to stay alert, eat enough to avoid hunger, and dress comfortably.

### Shutting Out the Message

If students perceive that a subject is difficult or uninteresting, they may tune out and miss material that forms the foundation for what comes next. To avoid this kind of listening lapse, remind yourself that instructors often use their lectures to supplement the text and then include that material on tests. If you pay attention to the entire lecture, you will be able to read over your notes later, compare your notes to the textbook, and use your analytical thinking skills to figure out how everything fits together.

If you experience a listening lapse, refocus your concentration quickly, instead of worrying about what you missed. Later, connect with a classmate to fill in the gaps in your notes.

### The Rush to Judgment

It is common for people to stop listening when they hear something they don't like. Their focus turns to their personal reactions and away from the message. Students who disagree during a lecture often spend valuable class time figuring out how to word a question or comment in response.

Judgments may also involve reactions to the speakers themselves. If you do not like your instructors or if you have preconceived notions about their ideas or background, you may decide you don't value what they have to say. Anyone whose words have ever been ignored because of race, ethnicity, gender, physical characteristics, or disability understands how prejudice can interfere with listening. Although it is human nature to stop listening, at times, in reaction to a speaker or message, this tendency can get in the way of your education.

### Partial Hearing Loss and Learning Disabilities

If you have a hearing loss, seek out special services, including tutoring and equipment that can help you listen in class. For example, listening to a taped lecture at a higher-than-normal volume can help you hear things you missed in the classroom. Meeting with your instructor outside of class to clarify your notes may also help. It is also smart to sit near the front of the room.

Other disabilities, such as attention deficit disorder (ADD) or a problem with processing spoken language, can add to listening difficulties. People with these problems may have trouble paying attention or understanding what they hear. If you have a disability that creates a listening challenge, seek help through the counseling or student health center, an adviser, or an instructor.

## Become an Active Listener

On the surface, listening seems like a passive activity: you sit back and take in information as someone else speaks. Effective listening, however, is an active process that involves setting a listening purpose, asking questions, paying attention to verbal signposts, and expecting the unexpected.

### Set Purposes for Listening

Begin by establishing what you want to achieve, such as understanding the material better or mastering a specific task. Many instructors state their purpose at the beginning of the class. Writing it down will help you focus on the message.

### Ask Questions

A willingness to ask questions shows a desire to learn and is the mark of an active, analytical thinker and listener. Among the most important types of questions you will ask are *clarifying questions*, which state your understanding of what you heard and ask whether that understanding is correct.

Although questions and comments turn you into an active, analytical participant, they may sometimes distract you from the speaker. One practical way to avoid this is to jot down your questions quickly and come back to them during a discussion period. This strategy helps you relax and continue to listen.

Students from different cultures may take different approaches to questioning. American students are more likely to actively question instructors than students from Japan and other high-context cultures who tend to avoid confronting someone in authority. In addition, because students from high-context cultures are accustomed to hearing vague, indirect language designed to move them to form their own conclusions, they may be less likely to ask for clarification. (For more on high-context and low-context cultures, see Chapter 2.)

VERBAL
SIGNPOSTS
Spoken words or phrases that call attention to the information that follows.

## Pay Attention to Verbal Signposts

Speakers' choice of words may tell you a lot about the information they consider important and help you predict test questions. For example, an idea described as "new and exciting" or "classic" is more likely to be on a test than one described as "interesting." **Verbal signposts** often involve transition words and phrases that help organize information, connect ideas, and indicate what is important and what is not. Listen for phrases like those in Figure 7.2 and pay attention to the material that follows.

## Expect the Unexpected

Active listening requires opening your mind to diverse points of view and to the heated classroom debates that may result. When the literature students in the following example listened actively, they were surprised where the discussion led:

> The professor said she had attended a symposium where the author Ward Just said: "In my books, I always make sure readers know by about page 35 how each of the key characters earns their living. I just think this is critical to help each reader put all the characters in my writing in a context."
>
> My instructor then assigned two books for us to read. One was by Ward Just, and it was organized exactly as promised. The other was by a different writer, who . . . obviously couldn't care less whether readers ever learned how characters earned their living. Each of us was asked to come prepared to either agree or disagree with Mr. Just's idea. . . . It was clear the professor was hoping for some disagreement.

| **FIGURE 7.2** | Verbal signposts point out important information |
|---|---|

| SIGNALS POINTING TO KEY CONCEPTS | SIGNALS OF SUPPORT |
|---|---|
| There are two reasons for this . . . | For example, . . . |
| A critical point in the process involves . . . | Specifically, . . . |
| Most important, . . . | For instance, . . . |
| The result is . . . | Similarly, . . . |

| SIGNALS POINTING TO DIFFERENCES | SIGNALS THAT SUMMARIZE |
|---|---|
| On the contrary, . . . | Finally, . . . |
| On the other hand, . . . | Recapping this idea, . . . |
| In contrast, . . . | In conclusion, . . . |
| However, . . . | As a result, . . . |

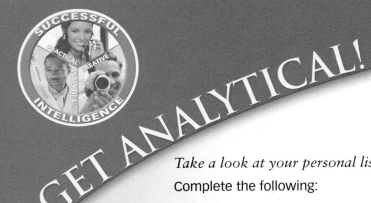
*Take a look at your personal listening habits.*

Complete the following:

- Analyze how present you are as a listener. Are you easily distracted, or can you focus well? Do you prefer to listen, or do you tend to talk?
- When you are listening, what tends to distract you?
- What happens to your listening skills when you become confused?
- How do you react when you strongly disagree with something your instructor says—when you are convinced that you are "right" and your instructor is "wrong"?
- Thinking about your answers and about your listening challenges, list two strategies from the chapter that can help you focus and improve your listening skills.

1.

2.

Well, she got it. Three of us took the same position as Mr. Just. The other five strongly disagreed. And about a half-hour into the discussion, which was as spirited as we had all semester, one of the women said she couldn't help noticing that the three who shared Mr. Just's view just happened to be the three men in the class, while the five who disagreed happened to be the five women. "Does that imply anything?" she wondered. Which, as you can easily imagine, quickly led to an even more spirited discussion about how gender of both author and reader might influence the way we think about the structure of writing.[2]

Effective listening skills prepare you to take effective notes—a necessary and powerful study tool.

# How Can You Make the Most of *Note Taking?*

By encouraging you to decide what is worth remembering, the act of note taking gets you thinking analytically and practically. Note taking involves you in the learning process in many important ways:

- Having notes to read after class can help you process and learn information for tests.

- When you take notes, you listen better and become more involved in class.

- Notes help you think critically and organize ideas.

- When a lecture includes information not found in your text, you will have no way to study it without writing it down.

- Note taking is a lifetime skill that you will use at work and in your personal life.

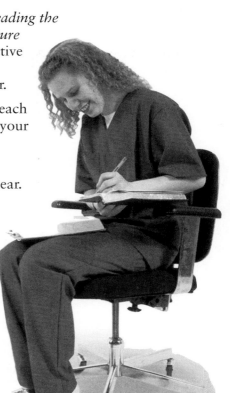

He listens well who takes notes.

DANTE ALIGHIERI

# Record Information in Class

Taking useful notes involves effort before class (preparation), during class (focus and note-taking strategies), and after class (reviewing and revising notes).

## Preparing to Take Class Notes

There are a number of ways to prepare for note-taking sessions:

**Preview your reading material.** *More than anything else you do, reading the assigned materials before class prepares you to understand the lecture and class discussion.* It also gives you the background to take effective notes. The class syllabus should tell you when specific reading assignments are due. If you have any questions, ask your instructor.

**Gather your supplies.** Use separate pieces of notebook paper for each class. Punch holes in handouts and insert them immediately into your binder following your notes for that day. If you take notes on a laptop, open the file containing your class notes right away.

**Location, location, location.** Find a seat where you can see and hear. Sitting near the front will minimize distractions. Be ready to write when the instructor begins speaking.

**Choose the best note-taking system.** Later in the chapter, you will learn about different note-taking systems. Take the following factors into account when choosing an appropriate system for any situation:

- **The instructor's style** (you'll be able to identify it after a few classes). Whereas one instructor may deliver organized lectures at a normal speaking rate, another may jump from topic to topic or talk very quickly.

- **The course material.** You may decide that an informal outline works best for a highly structured philosophy course, but that a think link is better for a looser sociology course. Try a note-taking system for a few classes; then make adjustments.

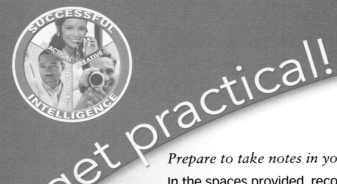

# Face a Note-Taking Challenge

*Prepare to take notes in your toughest class.*

In the spaces provided, record the specific steps you will take to prepare to take notes in what you consider to be your most challenging course.

_____

_____

- Course name and date of class:
- List all the reading you must complete before your next class (include pages from text and supplemental sources):
- Where will you sit in class to focus your attention and minimize distractions?
- Which note-taking system is best suited for the class, and why?
- Write the names and e-mail addresses of two classmates whose notes you can borrow if you miss a class:

- **Your learning style.** Choose strategies that make the most of your strong points and help boost weaker areas. A visual–spatial learner might prefer think links or the Cornell system; a thinker type might stick to outlines; an interpersonal learner might use the Cornell system and fill in the cue column in a study group setting (see Chapter 3 for a complete discussion of learning styles). You might even find that one system is best in class and another works best for review sessions.

**Gather support.** Set up a support system with two students in each class. Then, when you are absent, you can ask either one for the notes you missed.

## Record Information Effectively During Class

Because no one has time to write everything down, the following practical strategies will help you record what you consider important for later study. This is not a list of "musts." Rather, it is a list of ideas to try as you work to find the right note-taking strategy for you.

- Date and identify each page. When you take several pages of notes, add an identifying letter or number to the date on each page: 11/27A, 11/27B, 11/27C, for example, or 11/27—1 of 3, 11/27—2 of 3, 11/27—3 of 3. This will help you keep track of page order. Add the specific lecture topic at the top of the page so you can gather all your notes on that topic.
- If your instructor jumps from topic to topic during a single class, it may help to start a new page for each new topic.

**FIGURE 7.3**   How to pick up on instructor cues

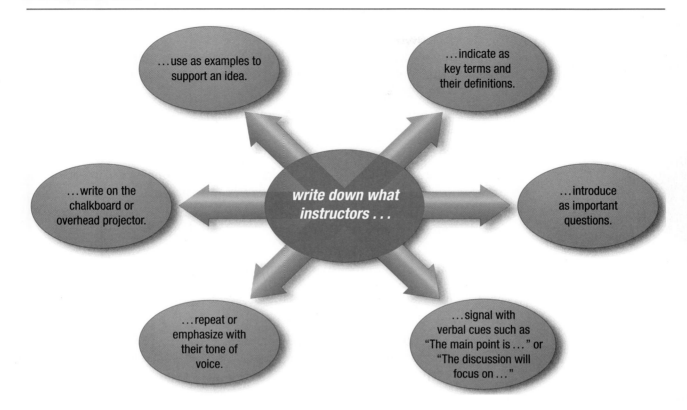

- Record whatever an instructor emphasizes—key terms, definitions, ideas, and examples. (Figure 7.3 shows methods an instructor might use to call attention to information.)

- Write down all questions raised by the instructor; these questions may appear on a test.

- Leave one or more blank spaces between points. This "white space" will help you review your notes, which will be in segments. (This suggestion does not apply to a think link.)

- Draw pictures and diagrams to illustrate ideas.

- Write quickly but legibly, perhaps using a form of personal shorthand. (See the section on shorthand on p. 227.) Remember that you can always make improvements and additions later.

- Mark important material with a star, underlining, a highlighter pen, a different color pen, or capital letters.

- If you don't understand a concept, leave a space and place a question mark in the margin. Then take advantage of your resources—ask the instructor to explain it after class, discuss it with a classmate, or consult your text—and fill in the blank when the idea is clear.

- Try to use the same system to indicate importance—such as indenting, spacing, or underlining—on each page. This will allow you to perceive key information with a minimum of effort.

## Taking Notes During Class Discussions

During discussion periods, one student may say something, then another, and finally the instructor may summarize the comments or link them together to make a point. Frequently, class discussion periods have tremendous value, but just as frequently information is presented in a disorganized, sometimes chaotic way. Here are suggestions for recording what you need to know during these discussions:

- Listen carefully to everyone. Jot down relevant points and ignore points that seem irrelevant.
- Listen for idea threads that weave through comments.
- Listen for ideas the instructor picks up on and emphasizes and for encouraging comments to students, such as "You make a great point," "I like your idea," and so on.
- Take notes when the instructor rephrases and clarifies a student's point.
- Try using a think link as your note-taking system, because discussions often take the form of brainstorming sessions. A think link will help you connect ideas that come at you from different perspectives and in different voices.
- Finally, if you are unsure, ask the instructor (during the discussion or in office hours) whether a student's statement is important.

## Review and Revise Your Notes

Reviewing your notes helps solidify information in memory. Review also helps you link new information to information you already know, which is a key step in building new ideas. The review-and-revision stage of note taking should include time for planning, critical thinking, adding information from other sources, summarizing, and working with a study group.

### Plan a Review Schedule

**Review within a day of the lecture.** You don't have to spend hours memorizing every word. Just set some time aside to reread your notes and perhaps write questions and comments on them. An hour between classes, for example, would be an ideal time for a quick review.

**Review regularly.** Try to schedule times during the week for reviewing notes from that week's class meetings. For example, if you know you are free from 2 P.M. to 5 P.M. every Tuesday and Thursday, plan to review notes from two courses on Tuesday and from two others on Thursday. Having a routine helps assure that you will look at material regularly.

**Review with an eye toward tests.** Step up your efforts before a test. Schedule longer review sessions, call a study group meeting, and review more frequently. Shorter sessions of intense review work interspersed with breaks may get more results than long hours of continuous studying. Some students find that recopying their notes, before an exam or earlier in the study process, helps them remember key concepts.

## Revise Using Other Sources and Critical Thinking

Adding text material, other required course readings, and Internet material to your notes is one of the best ways to link and apply new information to what you already know. Try using the following analytical, creative, and practical strategies to build understanding as you revise:

- Brainstorm and record examples from other sources that illustrate ideas in your notes.
- Pay attention to similarities between your text materials and class notes (ideas that appear in both are probably important to remember).
- Think of material from the readings that supports and clarifies ideas in your notes.
- Consider what in your class notes differs from your readings and why.
- Write down new ideas that occur to you as you review.
- Extend and apply the concepts from your notes and other sources to new situations.

When you use your notes to inspire successfully intelligent thinking, your grades may reflect your efforts. The student in the following example learned this lesson after doing poorly on some tests. He explains,

> All four of us in my rooming group are taking Economics. I would say we are all about equally smart. . . . Yet they are getting A's and I kept getting C's. I just couldn't figure out why.
>
> Finally, it was driving me nuts, so I went for help. My resident advisor asked if she could see my notes from that class. She looked them over carefully, and then asked me a few questions based on those notes. She helped me realize that I was great on "giving back the facts," but not so good at all at extending those facts to new situations. Yet here at college, all the questions on exams are about new situations. . . .
>
> It took someone here to help me refocus how I study. . . . I still am not getting A's, but at least solid B+'s. I don't know what would have happened if I hadn't asked for help and had just continued using that old high school style.[3]

## Summarize

Summarizing your notes involves critically evaluating which ideas and examples are most important and then rewriting the material in a shortened form. You may prefer to summarize as you review, with the notes in front of you. If you are using the Cornell system (see page 223), you would summarize in space at the bottom of the page.

Some students summarize from memory after review, to see how much they have retained. Others summarize as they read, then summarize from memory, and compare the two.

## Work with Study Groups

When you work with a study group, you have the opportunity to review both your personal notes and those of your classmates. This can be an enormous help if, for example, you lost concentration during part of a lecture and your notes don't make sense. You and another student may even have notes that have radically different information. When this happens, try to reconstruct what the instructor said and, if necessary, bring in a third person to clear up the confusion. See Chapter 5 for more on effective studying in groups.

# Which *Note-Taking System* Should You Use?

The most common note-taking systems include outlines, the Cornell system, and think links. Consider two factors when choosing which to use—what feels comfortable to you and what works best with course content. For example, someone who prefers the Cornell system might use it for European history but switches to a think link for French.

## Take Notes in Outline Form

When a reading assignment or lecture seems well organized, you may choose to take notes in outline form. Outlining means constructing a line-by-line representation, with certain phrases set off by varying indentations, showing how concepts, facts, and examples are related.

*Formal outlines* indicate ideas and examples with Roman numerals, uppercase and lowercase letters, and numbers. In contrast, *informal outlines* show the same associations but replace the formality with a system of consistent indenting and dashes. Figure 7.4 shows the difference between the two outline forms. Many students find informal outlines easier for in-class

**FIGURE 7.4**   Choose between different outline structures

| FORMAL OUTLINE | INFORMAL OUTLINE |
|---|---|
| Topic | Topic |
| I. First Main Idea | First Main Idea |
| A. Major supporting fact | —Major supporting fact |
| B. Major supporting fact | —Major supporting fact |
| 1. First reason or example | —First reason or example |
| 2. Second reason or example | —Second reason or example |
| a. First supporting fact | —First supporting fact |
| b. Second supporting fact | —Second supporting fact |
| II. Second Main Idea | Second Main Idea |
| A. Major supporting fact | —Major supporting fact |
| 1. First reason or example | —First reason or example |
| 2. Second reason or example | —Second reason or example |
| B. Major supporting fact | —Major supporting fact |

note taking. Figure 7.5 shows how a student has used the structure of a formal outline to write notes on the topic of civil rights legislation.

From time to time, an instructor may give you a guide, usually in outline form, to help you take notes in class. This outline may be on the board, on an overhead projector, or on a handout that you receive at the beginning of class. Because these *guided notes* are usually general and sketchy, they require that you fill in the details.

## Use the Cornell Note-Taking System

The Cornell note-taking system, also known as the T-note system, developed by Walter Pauk at Cornell University, consists of three sections on ordinary notepaper.[4]

**FIGURE 7.5**  Use a formal outline to organize your notes

CIVIL RIGHTS LEGISLATION: 1860–1968

I. Post–Civil War Era
   A. Fourteenth Amendment, 1868: equal protection of the law for all citizens
   B. Fifteenth Amendment, 1870: constitutional rights of citizens regardless of race, color, or previous servitude
II. Civil Rights Movement of the 1960s
   A. National Association for the Advancement of Colored People (NAACP)
      1. Established in 1910 by W.E.B. DuBois and others
      2. Legal Defense and Education fund fought school segregation
   B. Martin Luther King Jr., champion of nonviolent civil rights action
      1. Led bus boycott: 1955–1956
      2. Marched on Washington, D.C.: 1963
      3. Awarded NOBEL PEACE PRIZE: 1964
      4. Led voter registration drive in Selma, Alabama: 1965
   C. Civil Rights Act of 1964: prohibited discrimination in voting, education, employment, and public facilities
   D. Voting Rights Act of 1965: gave the government power to enforce desegregation
   E. Civil Rights Act of 1968: prohibited discrimination in the sale or rental of housing

- Section 1, the largest section on the right, is the *note-taking column*. Record your notes here in whatever form is most comfortable for you.

- Section 2, to the left of your notes, is the *cue column*. Leave it blank while you read or listen, then fill it in later as you review. You might fill it with comments that highlight main ideas, clarify meaning, suggest examples, or link ideas and examples. You can even draw diagrams. Many students use this column to raise questions that they will ask themselves when they study. By placing specific questions in the cue column, you can help yourself focus on critical details.

- Section 3, at the bottom of the page, is known as the *summary area*. Here you briefly summarize the notes on the page. Use this section during the review process to reinforce concepts and provide an overview of what the notes say.

Create this note-taking structure before class begins. Picture an upside-down letter T as you follow these directions:

- Start with a sheet of standard loose-leaf paper. Label it with the date and title of the lecture.

- To create the cue column, draw a vertical line about 2.5 inches from the left side of the paper. End the line about 2 inches from the bottom of the sheet.

- To create the summary area, start at the point where the vertical line ends (about 2 inches from the bottom of the page) and draw a horizontal line that spans the entire paper.

Figure 7.6 shows how a student used the Cornell system to take notes in a business course.

## Create a Think Link

A *think link*, also known as a *mind map* or *word web*, is a visual form of note taking. When you draw a think link, you diagram ideas by using shapes and lines that link ideas and supporting details and examples. The visual design makes the connections easy to see, and the use of shapes and pictures extends the material beyond just words. Many learners respond well to the power of **visualization**. You can also use think links to brainstorm ideas for paper topics.

To create a think link, start by circling or boxing your topic in the middle of a sheet of paper. Next, draw a line from the topic and write the name of one major idea at the end of the line. Circle that idea also. Then, jot down specific facts related to the idea, linking them to the idea with lines. Continue the process, connecting thoughts to one another by using circles, lines, and words. Figure 7.7 shows how a student used this particular think link structure to map out the sociology concept of social stratification. Other think link designs include stair steps showing connected ideas that build toward a conclusion or a tree shape with roots as causes and branches as effects.

A think link may be difficult to construct in class, especially if your instructor talks quickly. In this case, use another note-taking system during class. Then, create a think link as part of the review process.

VISUALIZATION
The interpretation of verbal ideas through the use of visual images.

**FIGURE 7.6**

## The Cornell system adds note-taking flexibility

October 3, 2008, p. 1

UNDERSTANDING EMPLOYEE MOTIVATION

| | |
|---|---|
| Why do some workers have a better attitude toward their work than others? | Purpose of motivational theories<br>— To explain role of human relations in motivating employee performance<br>— Theories translate into how managers actually treat workers |
| Some managers view workers as lazy; others view them as motivated and productive. | 2 specific theories<br>— Human resources model, developed by Douglas McGregor, shows that managers have radically different beliefs about motivation.<br>— Theory X holds that people are naturally irresponsible and uncooperative<br>— Theory Y holds that people are naturally responsible and self-motivated |
| Maslow's Hierarchy<br><br>self-actualization needs (challenging job)<br>esteem needs (job title)<br>social needs (friends at work)<br>security needs (health plan)<br>physiological needs (pay) | — Maslow's Hierarchy of Needs says that people have needs in 5 different areas, which they attempt to satisfy in their work.<br>— Physiological need: need for survival, including food and shelter<br>— Security need: need for stability and protection<br>— Social need: need for friendship and companionship<br>— Esteem need: need for status and recognition<br>— Self-actualization need: need for self-fulfillment<br>Needs at lower levels must be met before a person tries to satisfy needs at higher levels.<br>— Developed by psychologist Abraham Maslow |

Two motivational theories try to explain worker motivation. The human resources model includes Theory X and Theory Y. Maslow's Hierarchy of Needs suggests that people have needs in 5 different areas: physiological, security, social, esteem, and self-actualization.

## Use Other Visual Note-Taking Strategies

Several other note-taking strategies will help you organize information and are especially useful to visual learners. These strategies may be too involved to complete during class, so you may want to use them when taking notes on a text chapter or when rewriting your notes for review.

### Timelines

A timeline can help you organize information—such as dates in the French Revolution—into chronological order. Draw a vertical or horizontal line on the page and connect each item to the line, in order, noting the dates.

**FIGURE 7.7**   Think links provide a visual approach to note taking

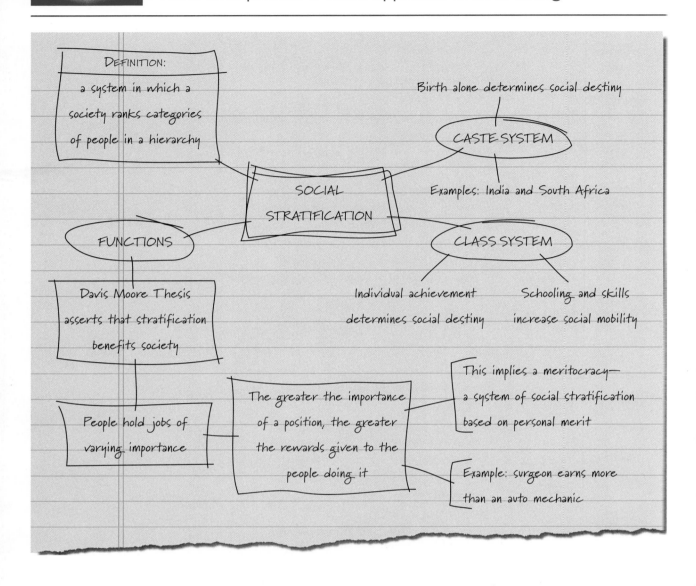

DEFINITION:
a system in which a society ranks categories of people in a hierarchy

Birth alone determines social destiny

CASTE SYSTEM

SOCIAL STRATIFICATION

Examples: India and South Africa

FUNCTIONS

CLASS SYSTEM

Davis Moore Thesis asserts that stratification benefits society

Individual achievement determines social destiny

Schooling and skills increase social mobility

People hold jobs of varying importance

The greater the importance of a position, the greater the rewards given to the people doing it

This implies a meritocracy—a system of social stratification based on personal merit

Example: surgeon earns more than an auto mechanic

## Tables

Tables throughout this text display information in vertical or horizontal columns. Use tables to arrange information according to categories.

## Hierarchy Charts

HIERARCHY
A graded or ranked series.

Charts showing the **hierarchy** of information can help you visualize how each piece fits into the hierarchy. A hierarchy chart could show levels of government, for example, or levels of scientific classification of animals and plants.

No matter what note-taking system you choose, your success will depend on how well you use it. Mastering the practical skill of personal shorthand will help you make the most of your choice.

# How Can You *Write Faster* When Taking Notes?

Using some form of personal **shorthand**, you can push your pen faster. Because you alone are the intended reader, you can misspell and abbreviate words in ways that only you understand.

To avoid forgetting what shorthand notations mean, review your notes while they are fresh in your mind. If anything confuses you, spell out words as you review.

Here are some suggestions that will help you master this important practical skill:

SHORTHAND

A system of rapid handwriting that employs symbols, abbreviations, and shortened words to represent words and phrases.

1. Use standard abbreviations in place of complete words.

| | | | |
|---|---|---|---|
| w/ | with | cf | compare, in comparison to |
| w/o | without | ff | following |
| → | means; resulting in | Q | question |
| ← | as a result of | p. | page |
| ↑ | increasing | * | most important |
| ↓ | decreasing | < | less than |
| ∴ | therefore | > | more than |
| Θ or b/c | because | = | equals |
| ≈ | approximately | % | percent |
| + or & | and | Δ | change |
| − | minus; negative | 2 | to; two; too |
| no. or # | number | vs | versus; against |
| i.e. | that is, | eg | for example |
| etc. | and so forth | c/o | care of |
| ng | no good | lb | pound |

2. Shorten words by removing vowels from the middle of words.

| | | |
|---|---|---|
| prps | = | purpose |
| lwyr | = | lawyer |
| cmptr | = | computer |

3. Substitute word beginnings for entire words.

| | | |
|---|---|---|
| assoc | = | associate; association |
| info | = | information |
| subj | = | subject |

4. Form plurals by adding *s* to shortened words.

| | | |
|---|---|---|
| prblms | = | problems |
| drctrys | = | directories |
| prntrs | = | printers |

5. Make up your own symbols and use them consistently.

| b/4 | = | before |
| 4tn | = | fortune |
| 2thake | = | toothache |

6. Use standard or informal abbreviations for proper nouns such as places, people, companies, scientific substances, events, and so on.

| DC | = | Washington, D.C. |
| $H_2O$ | = | water |
| Moz. | = | Wolfgang Amadeus Mozart |

7. If you are repeatedly writing a word or phrase throughout a class, write it out once and then create an abbreviation. For example, if you are taking notes on Argentina's former first lady Eva Perón, you might start by writing *Eva Perón (EP)* and then use *EP* through the rest of your notes for that class.

Finally, throughout your note taking, remember that the primary goal is to generate materials that help you learn and remember information. No matter how sensible any note-taking strategy might be, it won't do you any good if it doesn't help you reach that goal. Keep a close eye on what works for you and stick to it.

If you find that your notes aren't comprehensible, legible, or focused, analyze the problem. Can't read your notes? You might have been sleepy. Confusing gaps in information? You might be distracted in class, have an instructor who jumps around in the lecture, or lack an understanding of the course material. Put your problem-solving skills to work and brainstorm solutions from the variety of strategies in this chapter. With effort, your notes will become a helpful learning tool in school and beyond.

Learning listening skills and finding a system for taking effective notes prepare you for one of the most important challenges you face in school: developing your memory so you can remember what you hear in class, study in your texts, and record in your notes.

# How Does *Memory* Work?

Your accounting instructor is giving a test tomorrow on the double-entry accounting system. You feel confident because you spent hours last week memorizing your notes. Unfortunately, by the time you take the test, you remember very little. This is not surprising because most forgetting occurs within minutes after memorization.

In a classic study conducted in 1885, researcher Herman Ebbinghaus memorized a list of meaningless three-letter words such as CEF and LAZ. He then examined how quickly he forgot them. Within one hour he forgot more than 50% of what he had learned; after two days, he knew fewer than 30% of the material. Although Ebbinghaus's recall of the nonsense syllables remained fairly stable after that, his experiment shows how fragile memory can be, even when you take the time and expend the energy to memorize information.[5]

# How Your Brain Remembers: Short-Term and Long-Term Memory

Memories are stored in three different "storage banks" in your brain. The first, called *sensory memory*, is an exact copy of what you see and hear and lasts for a second or less. Certain information is then selected from sensory memory and moved into *short-term memory*, a temporary information storehouse that lasts no more than 10 to 20 seconds. You are consciously aware of material in short-term memory. Unimportant information is quickly dumped. Important information is transferred to *long-term memory*, the mind's more permanent storehouse.

Although all three stages are important, targeting long-term memory will solidify learning the most. "Short-term—or working—memory is useful when we want to remember a phone number until we can dial," says biologist James Zull. "We use short-term memory for these momentary challenges, all the time, every day, but it is limited in capacity, tenacity, and time."[6] Zull explains that short-term memory can hold only small amounts of information for brief periods. In addition, it is unstable—a distraction can easily dislodge information.

## Retaining Information in Long-Term Memory

To retain information in long-term memory, your brain moves through a four-stage process, which relates directly to the stages of the listening process described on pages 212–213. Figure 7.8 illustrates the process.

**FIGURE 7.8**     Long-term memory involves four stages

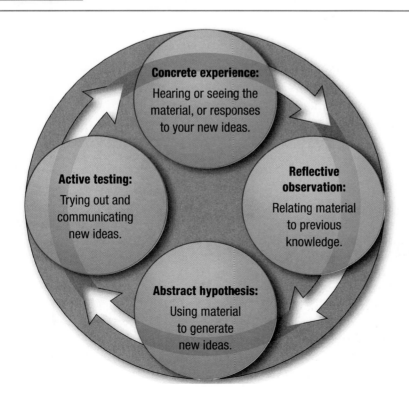

Concrete experience:
Hearing or seeing the material, or responses to your new ideas.

Reflective observation:
Relating material to previous knowledge.

Abstract hypothesis:
Using material to generate new ideas.

Active testing:
Trying out and communicating new ideas.

1. *Experiencing the material* (concrete experience). Your brain takes in the information through one or more of your senses.

2. *Relating the material to what you already know* (reflexive observation). You reflect on the new information and connect it to previous knowledge.

3. *Forming new ideas* (abstract hypothesis). You come up with new insights from the combination of what you knew before and what you are learning now.

4. *Trying out and communicating new ideas* (active testing). You explore your ideas to see if they make sense and work.

Here's an example to illustrate the process.

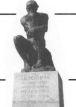

We rarely forget that which has made a deep impression on our minds.

TRYON EDWARDS

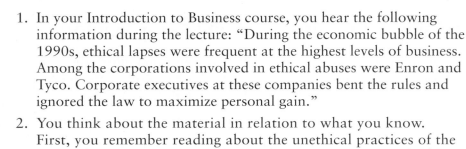

1. In your Introduction to Business course, you hear the following information during the lecture: "During the economic bubble of the 1990s, ethical lapses were frequent at the highest levels of business. Among the corporations involved in ethical abuses were Enron and Tyco. Corporate executives at these companies bent the rules and ignored the law to maximize personal gain."

2. You think about the material in relation to what you know. First, you remember reading about the unethical practices of the billionaires of the 1930s, including J. P. Morgan and Andrew Carnegie, who built corporate empires—and amassed personal fortunes—through unethical business practices. Second, you think about ethical and unethical behavior you have seen in people you know personally.

3. You form a new idea: Government regulations are necessary to curb the all-too-human tendency to bend rules for personal gain.

4. You try out your idea by talking to classmates and thinking further.

*Result*: Information about business ethics is solidly anchored in long-term memory.

## What *Memory Strategies* Can Improve Recall?

If forgetting is so common, why do some people have better memories than others? Some may have an inborn talent for remembering. More often, though, they succeed because they have practiced and mastered analytical, creative, and practical techniques for improving recall.

# Develop Helpful Strategies

The following practical and analytical strategies will help improve your recall.

## Have Purpose and Intention

Why can you remember the lyrics to dozens of popular songs but not the functions of the pancreas? Perhaps this is because you want to remember the lyrics or you have an emotional tie to them. To strengthen your intention to remember academic information, focus on why the information is important and how you can use it.

## Understand What You Memorize

The best way to guarantee that concepts become part of your long-term memory is to use your analytical ability to understand them inside and out. With a depth of learning comes the framework on which to place related concepts. Thus, if you are having trouble remembering something new, think about how the idea fits into what you already know. A simple example: If a new vocabulary word puzzles you, try to identify the word's root, prefix, or suffix. Knowing that the root *bellum* means "war" and the prefix *ante* means "before" will help you recognize and remember that *antebellum* means "before the war."

## Recite, Rehearse, and Write

When you *recite* material, you repeat key concepts aloud, in your own words, to help you memorize them. *Rehearsing* is similar to reciting but is done silently. It is the process of mentally repeating, summarizing, and associating information with other information. *Writing* is reciting on paper. Organizational tools, such as an outline or a think link, will help you record material in ways that show the logical connections within its structure.

## Study During Short, Frequent Sessions

Research has shown that you can improve your chances of remembering material if you learn it more than once. To get the most out of study sessions, spread them over time and rest in between. You may feel as though you accomplish a lot by studying for an hour without a break; however, you'll probably remember more from three 20-minute sessions.

Sleep can actually aid memory because it reduces interference from new information. Because you can't always go to sleep immediately after studying for an exam, try postponing the study of other subjects until your exam is over. When studying for several tests at once, avoid studying two similar subjects back to back. Your memory is likely to be more accurate when you study history right after biology rather than, for example, chemistry after biology.

## Limit and Organize Material

This involves two key activities:

- **Separate main points from unimportant details** Ask yourself: What is the most important information? Highlight only the key points in your texts, and write notes in the margins about central ideas. See the example in Figure 7.7 on page 226.
- **Divide material into manageable sections** Generally, when material is short and easy to understand, studying it from start to finish improves

recall. With longer material, however, you may benefit from dividing it into logical sections, mastering each section, putting all the sections together, and then testing your memory of all the material. Actors take this approach when learning the lines of a play, and it can work just as well for students trying to learn new concepts.

## Practice the Middle

When you are trying to learn something, you usually study some material first, attack other material in the middle of the session, and approach still other topics at the end. The weak link in your recall is likely to be the material you study midway. It pays to give this material special attention.

## Create Groupings

When items do not have to be remembered in any particular order, the act of grouping can help you recall them better. Say, for example, that you have to memorize these four 10-digit numbers:

9806875087 9876535703 7636983561 6724472879

It may look impossible. If you group the numbers to look like telephone numbers, however, the job may become more manageable:

(980) 687–5087    (987) 653–5703    (763) 698–3561    (672) 447–2879

In general, try to limit groups to 10 items or fewer. It's hard to memorize more at one time.

## Use Flash Cards

Flash cards are a great visual memory tool. They give you short, repeated review sessions that provide immediate feedback, and they are portable, which gives you the flexibility to use them wherever you go. Use the front of a 3 × 5 index card to write a word, idea, or phrase you want to remember. Use the back for a definition, an explanation, and other key facts. Figure 7.9 shows two flash cards used to study for a psychology exam.

Here are some suggestions for making the most of your flash cards:

- Carry the cards with you and review them frequently.
- Shuffle the cards and learn the information in various orders.

**FIGURE 7.9**    Flash cards help you memorize important facts

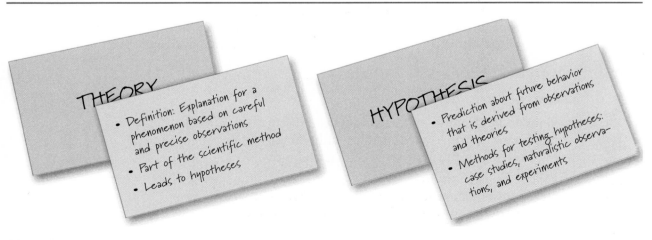

THEORY
- Definition: Explanation for a phenomenon based on careful and precise observations
- Part of the scientific method
- Leads to hypotheses

HYPOTHESIS
- Prediction about future behavior that is derived from observations and theories
- Methods for testing hypotheses: case studies, naturalistic observations, and experiments

- Test yourself in both directions. First, look at the terms and provide the definitions or explanations. Then turn the cards over and reverse the process.

## Use a Tape Recorder

Use a tape recorder as an immediate feedback "audio flash card." Record short-answer study questions on tape, leave 10 to 15 seconds between questions to answer out loud, then record the correct answer after each pause. For example, a question for a writing class might be, "What are the three elements of effective writing? . . . (10–15 second pause) . . . topic, audience, and purpose."

# Use Mnemonic Devices

Certain performers entertain their audiences by remembering the names of 100 strangers or flawlessly repeating 30 ten-digit phone numbers. Although these performers probably have superior memories, they also rely on memory techniques, known as **mnemonic devices** (pronounced neh-MAHN-ick), for assistance.

MNEMONIC DEVICES
Memory techniques that involve associating new information with information you already know.

Mnemonic devices depend on vivid associations (relating new information to other information). Instead of learning new facts by rote (repetitive practice), associations give you a hook on which to hang these facts and retrieve them later. Mnemonic devices make information familiar and meaningful through unusual, unforgettable mental associations and visual pictures. Forming mnemonics depends on activating your creative ability.

There are different kinds of mnemonic devices, including visual images and associations, acronyms, and songs and rhymes. Study how these devices work, and then use your creative thinking skills to apply them to your own memory challenges.

## Create Visual Images and Associations

You are more likely to remember a piece of information if you link it to a visual image. The best mental images often involve bright colors, three dimensions, action scenes, inanimate objects with human traits, ridiculousness, and humor.

Turning information into mental pictures helps improve memory, especially for visual learners. To remember that the Spanish artist Picasso painted *The Three Women*, you might imagine the women in a circle dancing to a Spanish song with a pig and a donkey (pig-asso). The more outlandish the image the better, because these images are the most memorable.

> Memory is the stepping-stone to thinking because without remembering facts, you cannot think, conceptualize, reason, make decisions, create, or contribute.

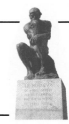

HARRY LORAYNE

## Use the Mental Walk Strategy to Remember Items in a List

Using the mental walk strategy, you imagine that you store new ideas in familiar locations. Say, for example, that for biology you have to remember the major endocrine glands. To do this, you can think of the route you take to the library. You pass the college theater, the science center, the bookstore, the cafeteria, the athletic center, and the social science building before reaching the library. At each spot along the route, you place the idea or concept you wish to learn. You then link the concept with a similar-sounding word that brings to mind a vivid image:

- At the campus theater, you imagine bumping into the actor Brad Pitt, who is holding two terriers (pituitary gland).
- At the science center, you visualize Mr. Universe with bulging thighs. When you are introduced, you learn that his name is Roy (thyroid gland).
- At the campus bookstore, you envision a second Mr. Universe with his thighs covered in mustard (thymus gland).
- In the cafeteria, you see an ad for Dean Al for president (adrenal gland).
- At the athletic center, you visualize a student throwing a ball into a pan and creatures applauding from the bleachers (pancreas).
- At the social science building, you imagine receiving a standing ovation (ovaries).
- And at the library, you visualize sitting at a table taking a test that is easy (testes).

## Create Acronyms

**ACRONYM**
*A word formed from the first letters of a series of words, created in order to help you remember the series.*

Another helpful association method involves the use of **acronyms**. In history class, you can remember the World War II Allies—Britain, America, and Russia—with the acronym BAR. This is an example of a word acronym because the first letters of the items you wish to remember spell a word. The word (or words) spelled don't necessarily have to be real words. As you see in Figure 7.10, the acronym Roy G. Biv will help you remember the colors of the spectrum.

Other acronyms take the form of an entire sentence in which the first letter of each word in each sentence stands for the first letter of the memorized term. This is called a *list order acronym*. For example, when science students want to remember the list of planets in order of their distance from the sun (Mercury, Venus, Earth, Mars, Jupiter, Saturn, Uranus, and Neptune), they can learn the sentence:

My very elegant mother just served us noodles.

**FIGURE 7.10**  An acronym will help you recall the colors of the spectrum

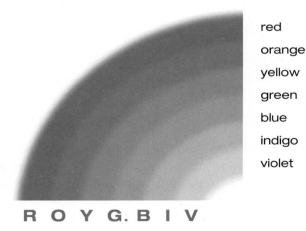

red
orange
yellow
green
blue
indigo
violet

R O Y G . B I V

# Craft Your Own Mnemonic

## get creative!

*Make a mnemonic device to help you remember something important to you.*

- As you study your texts in the next few weeks, identify a group of connected facts that you have to memorize—for example, for a political science course, the names of every presidential candidate after World War II; for an English literature course, the names of all the characters in Shakespeare's *Romeo and Juliet*. Indicate your choice here:

- Now create a mnemonic that will help you memorize the group. Use any of the mnemonic devices presented in this chapter including visual images and associations, acronyms, and songs and rhymes. Write the mnemonic here (use additional paper if necessary).

## Use Songs or Rhymes

Some of the classic mnemonic devices are rhyming poems that tend to stick in your mind. One you may have heard is the rule about the order of "i" and "e" in spelling:

> I before E, except after C, or when sounded like "A" as in "neighbor" and "weigh." Four exceptions if you please: either, neither, seizure, seize.

Make up your own poems or songs, linking tunes or rhymes that are familiar to you with information you want to remember. When Susan W. Fisher teaches introductory biology at Ohio State University, she uses this "biorap," performed by class members, to help everyone remember part of DNA replication (the rap includes references to the football coach and student-government president):

> *A pairs with T and G pairs with C*
>
> *It works 'cause the code's complementary*
>
> *It lets you be you and me be me*
>
> *From Coach Tressel to Eddie Pauline.*

The chorus "*DNA makes protein*" is then repeated four times. Said junior David S. Waterman of this musical mnemonic, "Because the performances are entertaining, students are more apt to pay attention and remember what we see or hear."[7]

Improving your memory requires energy, time, and work. In school, it also helps to master SQ3R, the textbook study technique introduced in Chapter 7.5. By going through the steps in SQ3R and using the specific memory techniques described in this chapter, you will be able to learn more in less time—and remember what you learn long after exams are over.

# PERSONAL TRIUMPH CASE STUDY

## CAROL COMLISH
### Graduate of the University of Alabama, Tuscaloosa, Alabama

*Life's twists and turns can put stubborn roadblocks in your path. With perseverance, and with a focus on hard work and memory that kept her coming back to school over a span of 29 years, Carol Comlish kept clearing the road that led to her goal of a college degree. Read the account; then use a separate piece of paper to answer the questions on page 237.*

The author Jack London once said, "You can't wait for inspiration. You have to go after it with a club." After pursuing my bachelor's degree for 29 years, London's statement keeps reminding me that, indeed, there were many times I had to flog myself for inspiration to persevere.

When I was in high school, I chose a business curriculum because I knew I had no means to attend college. My mother, a single parent of six, was left ill-equipped to provide the encouragement or the funds to help steer me toward a college education. After high school, I worked as a government secretary in Washington, D.C., and later as a flight attendant. Every penny I earned paid for much-needed dental work and for shoes and clothing my mother was unable to provide. There was no money left for schooling.

During those years, I married and had four children. I had much of what I had always wanted, but I still felt the drive to get an education. So, when my youngest child was two years old, I enrolled in my first college course—15 years after high school. I had not taken college prep courses to prepare me, and it was tough. Soon another baby appeared on the scene, and I quit school. Two years later, I had yet another baby. School and studying were out of the question. I could barely hold my head above water.

Then, when my youngest child began kindergarten, I tried school again. But it was so difficult to maintain a balance between the constant demands of the family and the demands of schoolwork that, after a couple of years of that grueling routine, I dropped out again.

Over the next 10 years, my desire for learning was exceptionally intense. Everything interested me. I learned to speak French, I read Shakespeare, and I devoured history. I was fairly self-educated but wanted the satisfaction of a formal education.

When my sixth child was in junior high, I began working to help pay for college expenses for my brood. But, in time, my personal desire to get a degree led me to the University of Alabama External Degree program. The program was difficult because it required that I complete assignments without the benefit of classroom lectures and the help of professors. For six years I toiled in the program while working full time and trying to maintain equilibrium in a household with two remaining children whose needs still had to be met.

The most difficult aspect of the program was cramming assignments into every single weekend. There was no time for leisure—not if I wanted to achieve my goal. However, with all my other responsibilities, I have to admit that I was not always as motivated as I might have been. I would burn out periodically and not open a book for months.

When the end was finally in sight, I was unable to continue my studies due to a particularly discouraging experience with one of my courses. I was ready to quit for good. But I soon realized that, since so much was invested, I had to go on. I pushed harder than ever. At last, on May 19, 2001, at the University of Alabama in Tuscaloosa, I received my B.A. degree in humanities, with high honors.

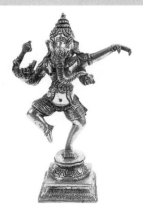

ཤེམས་མ་ཡེངད་ཞིག

In Sanskrit, the classical written language of India and other Hindu countries, these characters—pronounced as *sem ma yeng chik*—mean "do not be distracted." Think of this concept as you strive to improve your concentration for listening, note taking, and remembering. Focus on the ideas at hand. Try not to be distracted by other thoughts, other people's notions of what is "correct," or negativity as you take in and record information and commit it to memory. Be present in the moment so you can apply your skills to learning as much as you can.

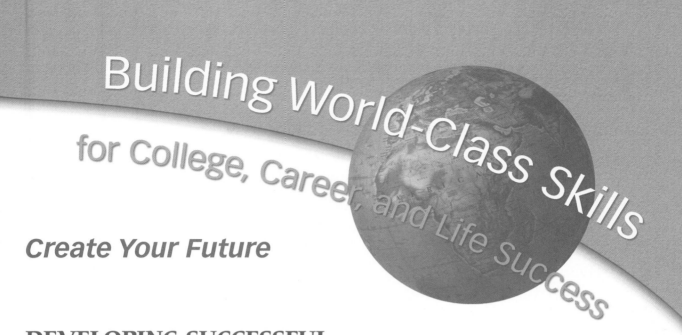

# Building World-Class Skills

## for College, Career, and Life Success

## *Create Your Future*

## DEVELOPING SUCCESSFUL INTELLIGENCE

### *Putting It All Together*

**Learn from the Experiences of Others.** Look back to Carol Comlish's Personal Triumph on p. 236. After you've read her story, relate her experience to your own life by completing the following:

**Step 1. Think it through:** *Analyze your experience and compare it to Carol's.* What academic goal are you trying to reach now that will take you a long time, and how does this relate to Carol's experience? Why is this goal important to you? From your memory of reaching other important goals, what strategies will help you achieve it?

**Step 2. Think out of the box:** *Let others inspire ideas.* Choose two people whom you respect. Put your listening skills to work: Spend a few minutes talking with each of them about your goal. Ask them about similar experiences they have had, and listen to the ideas that they used. From what you've heard, begin brainstorming ideas about how you will achieve your goal.

**Step 3. Make it happen:** *Put a practical plan together.* Map out how you will achieve your goal. Create a mnemonic device that will help you remember your plan. Envision your success as you put your plan into action.

## TEAM BUILDING

### *Collaborative Solutions*

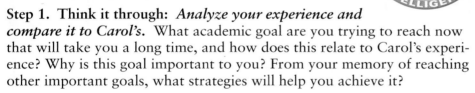

**Create a Note-Taking Team.** Although students often focus much more on taking notes in class than on taking notes while reading, reading notes are just as important to your understanding of the course material. In your most demanding course, form a study group with two other people and choose a reading assignment—a text chapter, an article, or any other assigned reading—to work on together. Agree to read it and take notes independently before your next meeting. Each student should make photocopies of his or her notes for the other group members.

When you meet again, compare your notes, focusing on the following characteristics:

- Legibility (Can everyone read what is written?)
- Completeness (Did you all record the same information? If not, why not?)
- Organizational effectiveness (Does everyone get an idea of how ideas flow?)
- Value of the notes as a study aid (Will this help everyone remember the material?)

Based on what you've discussed with your group, come up with specific ways to improve your personal note-taking skills. You can also work with your study group to compare notes taken in a particular class period and work on improving in-class note-taking techniques.

# WRITING
## *Discovery Through Journaling*

*Record your thoughts on a separate piece of paper or in a journal.*

**How People Retain Information.** How do you react to the following statement? "We retain 10% of what we read, 20% of what we hear, 30% of what we see, 50% of what we hear and see, 70% of what we say, 90% of what we say and do." How can you use this insight to improve your ability to retain information? What will you do differently as a result of this insight?

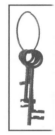

# CAREER PORTFOLIO
## *Plan for Success*

**Matching Career to Curriculum.** Your success in most career areas depends in part on your academic preparation. Some careers, such as medicine, require very specific curriculum choices (for example, specific biology and chemistry courses are required for medical school). Some careers require certain courses that teach basic competencies; for example, to be an accountant, you have to take accounting and bookkeeping. Other career areas, such as many business careers, don't have specific requirements, but employers often look for certain curriculum choices that indicate the mastery of particular skills and knowledge.

Put your listening and note-taking skills to work as you investigate your options. Choose a career area that interests you. Interview two people in that area—one from an academic setting (such as an instructor in a related subject area or an academic adviser) and one from the working world (such as a person working in that career or a career planning and placement office counselor). Choose a setting where you can listen well and take effective notes.

Ask your interviewees two questions: First, ask them about curriculum: What courses are required for this area, and what courses are beneficial but not required? Then ask them how you can stretch yourself outside of class in ways that will help you stand out—extracurricular activities, internships, leadership roles, part-time work, and any other helpful pursuits.

When you have completed your interviews, create two lists—one of recommended courses, marking the required ones with a star, and one of activities, internships, and any other recommendations.

## Suggested Readings

Burley-Allen, Madelyn. *Listening: The Forgotten Skill: A Self-Teaching Guide*. New York: Wiley, 1995.

DePorter, Bobbi, and Mike Hernacki. *Quantum Notes: Whole-Brain Approaches to Note-Taking*. Chicago: Learning Forum, 2000.

Dunkel, Patricia A., Frank Pialorsi, and Joane Kozyrez. *Advanced Listening Comprehension: Developing Aural & Note-Taking Skills*, 3rd ed. Boston: Heinle & Heinle, 2004.

Higbee, Kenneth L. *Your Memory: How It Works and How to Improve It*. New York: Marlowe, 2001.

Lebauer, R. Susan. *Learn to Listen, Listen to Learn: Academic Listening and Note-Taking*. Upper Saddle River, NJ: Prentice Hall, 2000.

Levin, Leonard. *Easy Script Express: Unique Speed Writing Methods to Take Fast Notes and Dictation*. Chicago: Legend Publishing, 2000.

Lorayne, Harry. *Super Memory—Super Student: How to Raise Your Grades in 30 Days*. Boston: Little, Brown, 1990.

Lorayne, Harry. *The Memory Book: The Classic Guide to Improving Your Memory at Work, at School, and at Play*. New York: Ballantine Books, 1996.

Robbins, Harvey A. *How to Speak and Listen Effectively*. New York: AMACOM, 1992.

Roberts, Billy. *Working Memory: Improving Your Memory for the Workplace*. London: Bridge Trade, 1999.

Roberts, Billy. *Educate Your Memory: Improvement Techniques for Students of All Ages*. London: Allison & Busby, 2000.

## Internet Resources

ForgetKnot: A Source for Mnemonic Devices: **http://members.tripod.com/~ForgetKnot/**

Prentice Hall Student Success Supersite—Study Skills: **www.prenhall.com/success/StudySkl/index.html**

Helpful advice on listening from the Kishwaukee College Learning Skills Center: **kish.cc.il.us/lsc/ssh/listening.shtml**

## Endnotes

[1]Ralph G. Nichols, "Do We Know How to Listen? Practical Helps in a Modern Age," *Speech Teacher* (March 1961): 118–24.

[2]Richard J. Light, *Making the Most of College: Students Speak Their Minds* (Cambridge, MA: Harvard University Press, 2001), pp. 48–49.

[3]Ibid., p. 38.

[4]Walter Pauk, *How to Study in College*, 7th ed (Boston: Houghton Mifflin, 2001), pp. 236–41.

[5]Herman Ebbinghaus, *Memory: A Contribution to Experimental Psychology*, trans. H. A. Ruger and C. E. Bussenius (New York: New York Teacher's College, Columbia University, 1885).

[6]James Zull, *The Art of Changing the Brain: Enriching Teaching by Exploring the Biology of Learning* (Sterling, VA: Stylus Publishing, 2002).

[7]Vyacheslav Kandyba, "Professor Uses Music to Bring Biology to Life," *The Chronicle of Higher Education* (March 30, 2003). Retrieved March 2004, from: http://chronicle.com/weekly/v49/i38/38a01002.htm.

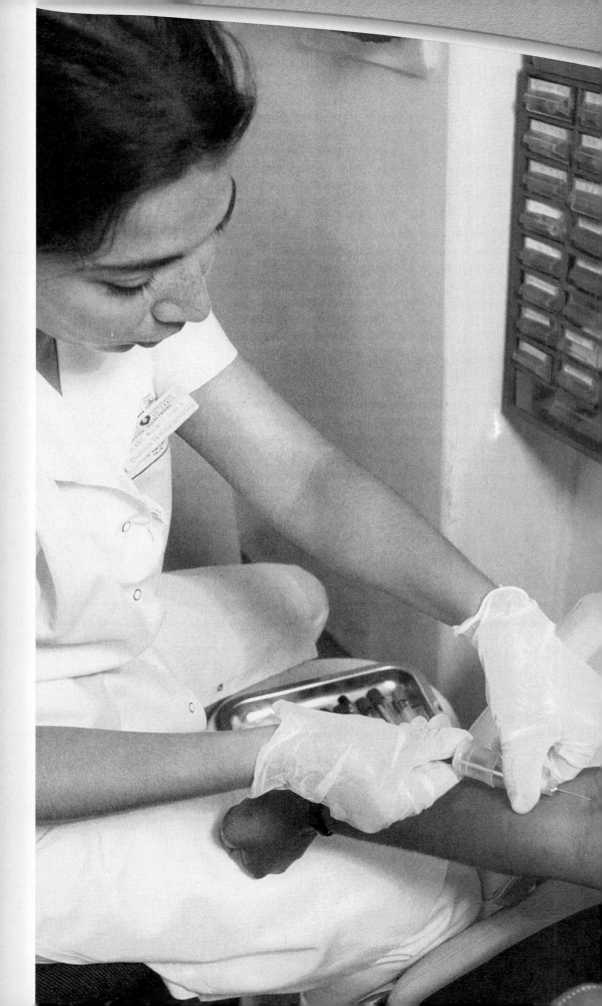

# ASSESS: TEST TAKING
## SHOWING WHAT YOU KNOW

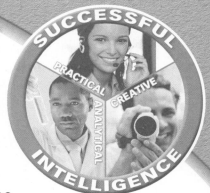

# 8

For a runner, a race is equivalent to a test because it measures ability at a given moment. Doing well in a race requires training similar to the studying you do for exams. The best runners—and test takers—understand that they train not just for the race or test, but to achieve a level of competence that they will use elsewhere.

When you show what you know successfully on tests, you achieve educational goals and develop confidence that you can perform well again and again. Exams also help you gauge your progress and, if necessary, improve your efforts. Most important, smart test preparation results in real learning that you take with you from course to course and into your career and life.

As you will see in this chapter, test taking is about preparation, persistence, and strategy—all of which tap into your analytical, creative, and practical abilities. It is also about conquering fears, paying attention to details, and learning from mistakes.

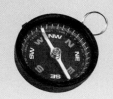

# Q & A BLUE SKY QUESTIONS DOWN-TO-EARTH ANSWERS

## How can I combat test anxiety?

I am a Yu'pik Eskimo from a village on the Yukon River. Before attending college, I worked for six years as a clerk at the Native Corporation, a gas station and general store. When the manager passed away, the business offered to make me a manager. Even though I knew how to do much of the work, I didn't feel I was ready, so I decided to go to school for more training.

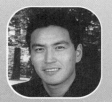

Peter Changsak
Sheldon Jackson College,
Sitka, Alaska

College life is different from what I am accustomed to. The hardest part has been taking tests. I study hard, but then when I get in class and the test begins, my mind goes blank. When I read, I understand what I'm reading, but as soon as I close the book, I can't remember what I just read. My favorite class is Biology Lab—probably because we can walk around.

I love mechanics and construction. When I worked at the Native Corporation, we built a new building. I felt like I was a success at work, but I don't feel successful as a student. Sometimes I feel like quitting, but I also think it can help me have more choices if I stick with it. I'm learning how to be a serious student, but it isn't easy. Can you give suggestions about how I can get over my test anxiety?

# PRACTICAL ANSWERS

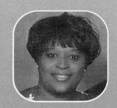

Tonjua Williams, M.Ed.
Associate Provost,
Health Programs,
St. Petersburg College

## Focus on preparation and work to change your attitude toward tests

Many students experience test anxiety, especially students who are new to the educational setting. Often, anxiety is a result of feeling uncomfortable or distressed when charting unfamiliar waters. The first test administered in a class can bring about a great deal of anxiety.

*First, it is important to prepare adequately for class exams:*

- Attend class regularly.
- Pay attention in class and take *good notes*.
- Join a *study group* with fellow classmates.
- Spend three hours outside of the classroom studying for every hour you spend in class. Start studying early (don't wait until the week of the exam to study).
- Communicate with your instructor to make sure you understand course expectations, lecture information, and special projects that are due.
- Before the exam, get plenty of rest and eat a light breakfast or snack.

*Second, when taking an exam:*

- Close your eyes, take a deep breath, then review the test.
- Begin by responding to the questions you are most comfortable/familiar with.
- Continue reviewing the test to look for clues to answer those questions that you are not sure about.

*Third, after taking the exam:*

- After each test/exam, review your test/exam to learn about the areas you need to improve.
- Continue studying the information from the last exam along with new course information.

Finally, remember not all anxiety is bad—test anxiety, believe it or not, can encourage us to rise to an occasion. The stress of an upcoming test can help you work very hard and be prepared for the exam. Once the preparation is done, it is important for you to remind yourself that an exam is your opportunity to show off your knowledge. Changing your attitude toward the exam and looking forward to the opportunity to share your knowledge will help you think more positively about tests.

# How Can Preparation Improve *Test Performance?*

You prepare for exams every day of the semester. By attending class, staying on top of assignments, completing readings and projects, and participating in class discussions, you are actively learning and retaining what you need to know to do well on exams. This knowledge is the most important test-preparation tool you have.

The following additional measures will help you to be as prepared as possible for exam day because they will help you put your analytical, creative, and practical thinking skills into action.

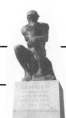

Ninety percent of life is just showing up.

WOODY ALLEN

## Identify Test Type and Material Covered

Before you begin studying, find out as much as you can about the test, including:

- **Topics that will be covered.** Will it cover everything since the semester began or will it be limited to a narrow topic?
- **Types of questions.** Objective (multiple choice, true/false, sentence completion), subjective (essay), or a combination?
- **Material you will be tested on.** Will the test cover only what you learned in class and in the text, or will it also cover outside readings?

Your instructors may answer many of these questions. They may tell you the question format and the topics that will be on the test. Some instructors may even drop hints about possible questions, either directly ("I might ask a question on this subject on your next exam") or more subtly ("One of my favorite theories is . . .").

Here are other practical strategies for predicting what may be on a test.

### Use SQ3R to Identify What's Important

Often, the questions you write and ask yourself when you read assigned materials may be part of the test. Textbook study questions are also good candidates.

# Write Your Own Test

## get creative!

*Prepare for an upcoming exam using a pretest you create yourself.*

Use the tips in this chapter to predict the material that will be covered, the types of questions that will be asked (multiple choice, essay, etc.), and the nature of the questions (a broad overview of the material or specific details).

Then be creative. Your goal is to write questions that your instructor is likely to ask—interesting questions that tap what you have learned and make you think about the material in different ways. Go through the following steps:

1. Write the questions you come up with on a separate sheet of paper.

2. Use what you created as a pretest. Set up test-like conditions—a quiet, timed environment—and see how well you do. Avoid looking at your text or notes unless the test is open book.

3. Evaluate your pretest answers against your notes and the text. How did you do?

4. Finally, after you take your instructor's exam, evaluate whether you think this exercise improved your performance on the actual exam. Would you use this technique again when you study for another exam? Why or why not?

## Talk to People Who Already Took the Course

Try to get a sense of test difficulty, whether tests focus primarily on assigned readings or class notes, what materials are usually covered, and what types of questions are asked. Also ask about instructors' preferences. If you learn that the instructor pays close attention to specific facts, for example, use flash cards to drill yourself on details. If the instructor emphasizes a global overview, focus on concepts.

## Examine Old Tests, If the Instructor Makes Them Available

You may find old tests in class, online, or on reserve in the library. Make sure you have the instructor's permission to consult them. Old tests will help you answer questions like these:

- Do tests focus on examples and details, general ideas and themes, or a combination?

- Are the questions straightforward or confusing and sometimes tricky?

- Will you be asked to integrate facts from different areas in order to draw conclusions?

After taking the first exam in the course, you will have a better idea of what to expect.

## Create a Study Plan and Schedule

Use the guidelines presented on page 170 to create a study plan and schedule. Make copies of the checklist on page 171 and complete it for every exam. It is an invaluable tool for organizing your pre-exam studying.

Studying for final exams, which usually take place the last week of the semester, is a big commitment that requires careful time management. Your college may schedule study days, sometimes known as "reading period" or "dead days," between the end of classes and the beginning of finals. Lasting from a day or two to several weeks, these days give you uninterrupted hours to prepare for exams and finish papers.

End-of-year studying often requires flexibility. For example, instead of working at the library during this period, students at the University of Texas at Austin are often seen at Barton Springs, a spring-fed pool near campus. Anna Leeker and Jillian Adams chose this site to study biology because of the beautiful surroundings—and because they had little choice. "We heard that the libraries are packed, and that students are waiting in line for tables," said Jillian. Both realize that they have to be vigilant about maintaining their focus, no matter where they study.[1]

## Prepare Through Careful Review

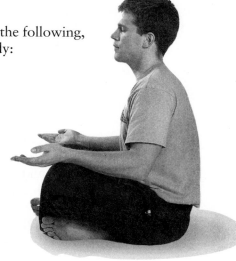

A thorough review, using analytical and practical strategies like the following, will give you the best shot at remembering the material you study:

### Use SQ3R

The reading method you studied in Chapter 8.5 provides an excellent structure for reviewing your reading materials.

- *Surveying* gives you an overview of topics.
- *Questioning* helps you focus on important ideas and determine the meaning.
- *Reading* (or, in this case, rereading) reminds you of concepts and supporting information.
- *Reciting* helps to anchor the concepts in your head.
- *Reviewing*, such as quizzing yourself on the Q-stage questions, summarizing highlighted sections, making key-concept flash cards, and outlining chapters, helps solidify learning.

### Review Your Notes

Use the following techniques to review your notes before an exam:

- **Time your reviews carefully.** Review notes for the first time within a day of the lecture, if you can, and then review again closer to the test day.
- **Mark up.** Reread your notes, filling in missing information, clarifying points, writing out abbreviations, and highlighting key ideas.

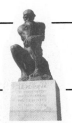

> Learning is what most adults will do for a living in the 21st century.

BOB PERELMAN

- **Organize.** Consider adding headings and subheadings to your notes to clarify the structure of the information. Rewrite your notes using a different organizing structure—for example, an outline if you originally used a think link.

- **Summarize.** Evaluate which ideas and examples are most important; then rewrite your notes in shortened form. Summarize your notes in writing or with a summary think link. Try summarizing from memory as a self-test.

## Take a Pretest

Use end-of-chapter text questions to create your own pretest. If your course doesn't have an assigned text, develop questions from your notes and assigned outside readings. Old homework problems will also help target areas you need to work on. Choose questions that are likely to be covered. Then answer them under test-like conditions—in a quiet place, with no books or notes to help you (unless the exam is open book), and with a clock to tell you when to quit.

The same test-preparation skills you learn in college will help you do well on standardized tests for graduate school. Sharon Smith describes how students in her preparatory program used practice tests and other techniques to help boost their scores on the Medical College Admission Test (MCAT). They 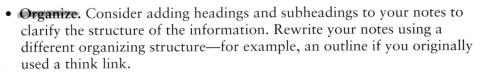 "started with un-timed practices in order to work on accuracy, and timed practices were incorporated as the semester progressed. Everyone tried to finish the tests/passages in the allotted time, and, at the end of each practice session, go over answer choices to understand why they are correct or incorrect." During spring semester they were "given mock exams, and it was important to treat the mock MCAT as if it were the real exam. This gave the best assessment of performance on test day."[2]

## Prepare Physically

Most tests ask you to work at your best under pressure. A good night's sleep will leave you rested and alert and improve your ability to remember the material you studied the night before. Eating a light, well-balanced meal is also important. When time is short, grab a quick-energy snack such as a banana, orange juice, or a granola bar. For more ideas on getting adequate sleep and eating a balanced diet, look ahead to the chapter on personal wellness (Chapter 10).

## Make the Most of Last-Minute Studying

*Cramming*—studying intensively and around the clock right before an exam—often results in information going into your head and popping right back out shortly after the exam is over. If learning is your goal, cramming is not a good idea. The reality, however, is that nearly every student crams during college, especially during midterms and finals. Use these hints to make the most of this intensive study time:

- **Review your flash cards.** If you use flash cards, review them one last time.
- **Focus on crucial concepts.** Resist reviewing notes or texts page by page.
- **Create a last-minute study sheet.** On a single sheet of paper, write down key facts, definitions, formulas, and so on. If you prefer visual notes, use think links to map out ideas and supporting examples.
- **Arrive early.** Study the sheet or your flash cards until you are asked to clear your desk.

After your exam, evaluate how cramming affected your recall. Within a few days, you will probably remember very little, a reality that will work against you in advanced courses that build on this knowledge and in careers that require it. Think ahead about how you can start studying earlier to prepare for your next exam.

Whether you cram or not, you may experience anxiety on test day. Many students do. Following are some ideas for how to handle test anxiety when it strikes.

# How Can You Work Through *Test Anxiety?*

A certain amount of stress can be a good thing. Your body is alert, and your energy motivates you to do your best. Some students, however, experience incapacitating stress before and during exams, especially midterms and finals.

**Test anxiety** can cause sweating, nausea, dizziness, headaches, and fatigue. It can reduce your ability to concentrate, make you feel overwhelmed, and cause you to blank out. As a result, test anxiety often results in lower grades that may not reflect what you really know. Take two steps to minimize your anxiety: Prepare thoroughly and build a positive attitude.

TEST ANXIETY
A bad case of nerves that can make it hard to think or to remember.

## Preparation

The more confident you feel about the material, the better you will perform on test day. In this sense, consider all the preparation and study information in *Keys to Success* as test-anxiety assistance. Also, finding out what to expect on the exam will help you feel more in control. Seek out information about the material that will be covered, the question format, the length of the exam, and the points assigned to each question.

Creating a detailed study plan builds your knowledge as it combats anxiety. Divide the plan into small tasks. As you finish each, you gain an increased sense of accomplishment, confidence, and control.

# Attitude

Here are ways to maintain an attitude that will help you succeed.

- **See the test as an opportunity to learn.** Instead of thinking of tests as contests that you either win or lose, think of them as signposts along the way to mastering the material. Learning is far more important than "winning."

- **Understand that tests measure performance, not personal value.** Your grade does not reflect your ability to succeed. Whether you get an A or an F, you are the same person.

- **Appreciate your instructor's purpose.** Your instructors want to help you succeed. Don't hesitate to visit them during office hours and send e-mail questions to clarify material.

- **Seek study partners who challenge you.** Find study partners who can inspire you to do your best. Try to avoid people who are also anxious because you both may pick up on each other's fears and negativity. (For more on study groups, see Chapter 6.)

- **Set yourself up for success.** Expect progress and success—not failure. Take responsibility for creating success through your work and attitude.

- **Practice relaxation.** When you feel test anxiety mounting, breathe deeply, close your eyes, and visualize positive mental images such as getting a good grade and finishing with time to spare. Try to ease muscle tension—stretch your neck; tighten and then release your muscles.

- **Practice positive self-talk.** Tell yourself that you can do well and it is normal to feel anxious, particularly before an important exam. As you walk into the testing room, give yourself a pep talk that builds confidence—something like, "I know this stuff, and I'm going to show everyone what I know." Also, slay your perfection monster by telling yourself, "I don't have to get a perfect score."

Students from other cultures may not experience test anxiety in the same way as Americans. Because of cultural differences, U.S. students may experience more anxiety than students from countries, such as England, where group achievement tends to be emphasized more than individual achievement.

Math exams are a special problem for many students. Dealing with the anxieties associated with these exams will be examined on pages 298–99, where you will find stress-management, studying, and exam-taking techniques.

## Test Anxiety and the Returning Student

If you're returning to school after years away, you may wonder how well you will handle exams. To deal with these feelings, focus on what you have learned through life experience, including the ability to handle work and family pressures. Without even knowing it, you have developed the time-management, planning, and communication skills necessary for college success.

In addition, your life experiences will give real meaning to abstract classroom ideas. For example, workplace relationships may help you understand social psychology concepts, and refinancing your home mortgage may help you grasp the importance of interest-rate swings, a key concept in economics.

Parents who have to juggle child care with study time can find the challenge especially difficult before a test. Here are some suggestions that might help:

- **Find help.** This is especially important with younger children.
- **Plan activities.** If you have younger children, have a supply of games, books, and videos on hand to use while you study.
- **Explain the time frame.** Tell school-age children your study schedule and the test date. Plan a reward after your test.

Preparing for an exam sets the stage for taking the exam. You are now ready to focus on methods to help you succeed when the test begins.

# What *General Strategies* Can Help You Succeed on Tests?

Even though every test is different, there are general strategies that will help you handle almost all tests, including short-answer and essay exams.

## Write Down Key Facts

Before you even look at the test, write down key information—including formulas, rules, and definitions—that you studied recently and you don't want to forget. Use the back of the question sheet or some scrap paper for your notes. (Be sure your instructor knows that you made these notes after the test began.)

## Begin with an Overview

Although exam time is precious, spend a few minutes at the start of the test gathering information about the questions— how many there are in each section, what types, and their point values. Then, analyze the situation and think practically to schedule your time. For example, if a two-hour test is divided into two sections of equal point value—an essay section with four questions and a short-answer section with 60 questions—you might spend an hour on the essays (15 minutes per question) and an hour on the short answers (one minute per question).

You may need to take level of difficulty into account as you come up with options for how to parcel out your time. For example, if you think you can get through the short-answer questions in 45 minutes and sense that you'll have a tougher time with the writing section, you can budget an hour and a quarter for the essays.

# Read Test Directions

Reading test directions carefully can save you trouble. For example, although a history test of 100 true/false questions and one essay may look straightforward, the directions may tell you to answer 80 of the 100 questions or that the essay is optional. If the directions indicate you are penalized for incorrect answers—meaning you lose points instead of simply not gaining points—avoid guessing unless you're fairly certain.

When you read the directions, you may learn that some questions or sections are weighted more heavily than others. For example, the short-answer questions may be worth 30 points, whereas the essays are worth 70. In this case, it's smart to spend more time on the essays than the short answers. To stay aware of the specifics of the directions, use the practical strategy of circling or underlining key information.

# Mark Up the Questions

Highlight instructions and keywords to avoid careless errors. As you read each question, circle qualifiers such as *always, never, all, none,* and *every,* verbs that communicate specific test instructions, and concepts that are tricky or need special attention.

# Take Special Care on Machine-Scored Tests

Use the correct pencil (usually a number 2) on machine-scored tests, and mark your answer in the proper space, filling the space completely. Periodically, use your practical thinking skills to check the answer number against the question number to make sure they match. If you mark the answer to question 4 in the space for question 5, not only will your response to question 4 be wrong, but your responses to all subsequent questions will be off by a line. To avoid this problem, put a small dot next to any number you skip and plan to return to later.

Neatness counts on these tests because the computer can misread stray pencil marks or partially erased answers. If you mark two answers to a question and partially erase one, the computer will read both responses and charge you with a wrong answer.

# Work from Easy to Hard

Begin with the easiest questions, and answer them as quickly as you can without sacrificing accuracy. This will boost your confidence and leave more time for questions that require more focus and effort. Mark tough questions as you reach them, and return to them after answering the questions you know.

# Watch the Clock

Keep track of how much time is left and how you are progressing. Some students are so concerned about time that they rush through the test and have time left over. If this happens to you, spend the remaining time refining and checking your work instead of leaving early. You may be able to correct mistakes, change answers, or add more information to an essay.

## Master the Art of Intelligent Guessing

When you are unsure of an answer on a short-answer test, you can leave it blank or guess. As long as you are not penalized for incorrect answers, guessing helps you. "Intelligent guessing," writes Steven Frank, an authority on student studying and test taking, "means taking advantage of what you do know in order to try to figure out what you don't. If you guess intelligently, you have a decent shot at getting the answer right."[3]

When you check your work at the end of the test, use your analytical ability to decide whether you would make the same guesses again. Chances are that you will leave your answers alone, but you may notice something that changes your mind: a qualifier that affects meaning, a miscalculation in a math problem. Or you may recall information that you drew a blank on the first time around.

## Maintain Academic Integrity

Cheating as a strategy to pass a test or get a better grade robs you of the opportunity to learn the material, which, ultimately, is your loss. Cheating also jeopardizes your future if you are caught. You may be seriously reprimanded—or even expelled—if you violate your school's code of academic integrity.

Now that you have explored these general strategies, you can use what you've learned to address specific types of test questions.

# How Can You Master *Different Types* of Test Questions?

Every type of test question has a different way of finding out how much you know about a subject. For **objective questions**, you choose or write a short answer, often making a selection from a limited number of choices. Multiple-choice, fill-in-the-blank, matching, and true/false questions fall into this category. **Subjective questions** require you to plan, organize, draft, and refine a response. All essay questions are subjective. In general, subjective questions tap your creative abilities more than short-answer questions do.

Figure 8.1 shows samples of real test questions from Western civilization, macroeconomics, Spanish, and biology college texts published by Pearson Education. Included are multiple-choice, true/false, fill-in-the-blank, matching, and essay questions, including a short-answer essay. Seeing these questions firsthand will help you feel more comfortable with testing formats and question types when you take your first exams.

OBJECTIVE QUESTIONS

Short-answer questions that test your ability to recall, compare, and contrast information and to choose the right answer from a limited number of choices.

SUBJECTIVE QUESTIONS

Essay questions that require you to express your answer in terms of your own personal knowledge and perspective.

FIGURE 8.1 Real test questions from real college texts

## From Chapter 29, "The End of Imperialism," in *Western Civilization: A Social and Cultural History,* 2nd edition.

■ **MULTIPLE-CHOICE QUESTION**

India's first leader after independence was:

A. Gandhi      B. Bose      C. Nehru      D. Sukharno      *(answer: C)*

■ **FILL-IN-THE-BLANK QUESTION**

East Pakistan became the country of _____ in 1971.

A. Burma      B. East India      C. Sukharno      D. Bangladesh      *(answer: D)*

■ **TRUE/FALSE QUESTION**

The United States initially supported Vietnamese independence.    T    F      *(answer: false)*

■ **ESSAY QUESTION**

Answer one of the following:

1. What led to Irish independence? What conflicts continued to exist after independence?
2. How did Gandhi work to rid India of British control? What methods did he use?

## From Chapter 6, "Unemployment and Inflation," in *Macroeconomics: Principles and Tools,* 3rd edition.

■ **MULTIPLE-CHOICE QUESTION**

If the labor force is 250,000 and the total population 16 years of age or older is 300,000, the labor-force participation rate is

A. 79.5%      B. 83.3%      C. 75.6%      D. 80.9%      *(answer: B)*

■ **FILL-IN-THE-BLANK QUESTION**

Mike has just graduated from college and is now looking for a job, but has not yet found one. This causes the employment rate to _____ and the labor-force participation rate to _____.

A. increase; decrease      C. stay the same; stay the same

B. increase; increase      D. increase; stay the same      *(answer: C)*

■ **TRUE/FALSE QUESTION**

The Consumer Price Index somewhat overstates changes in the cost of living because it does not allow for substitutions that consumers might make in response to price changes.    T    F    *(answer: true)*

■ **SHORT-ANSWER ESSAY QUESTION**

During a press conference, the Secretary of Employment notes that the unemployment rate is 7.0%. As a political opponent, how might you criticize this figure as an underestimate? In rebuttal, how might the Secretary argue that the reported rate is an overestimate of unemployment?

*(Possible answer: The unemployment rate given by the secretary might be considered an underestimate because discouraged workers, who have given up the job search in frustration, are not counted as unemployed. In addition, full-time workers may have been forced to work part-time. In rebuttal, the secretary might note that a portion of the unemployed have voluntarily left their jobs. Most workers are unemployed only briefly and leave the ranks of the unemployed by gaining better jobs than they had previously held.)*

**FIGURE 8.1**    Continued

---

**From *Mosaicos: Spanish as a World Language,* 3rd edition.**

■ **MATCHING QUESTION**

You are learning new words and your teacher asks you to think of an object similar to or related to the words he says. His words are listed below. Next to each word, write a related word from the list below.

| el reloj | el cuaderno | el pupitre | una computadora |
| el televisor | la tiza | el lápis | la mochila |

1. el escritorio _____       4. la pizarra _____

2. el bolígrafo _____       5. el libro _____

3. la videocasetera _____

*(answers: 1. el pupitre; 2. el lápis; 3. el televisor; 4. la tiza; 5. el cuaderno)*

■ **ESSAY QUESTION**

Your mother always worries about you and wants to know what you are doing with your time in Granada. Write a short letter to her describing your experience in Spain. In your letter, you should address the following points:

1. What classes you take

2. When and where you study

3. How long you study every day

4. What you do with your time (mention three activities)

5. Where you go during your free time (mention two places)

---

**From Chapter 13, "DNA Structure and Replication," in *Biology: A Guide to the Natural World,* 2nd edition.**

■ **MULTIPLE-CHOICE QUESTION**

What units are bonded together to make a strand of DNA?

A. chromatids      B. cells      C. enzymes      D. nucleotides      E. proteins      *(answer: D)*

■ **TRUE/FALSE QUESTION**

Errors never occur in DNA replication, because the DNA polymerases edit out mistakes.      T      F

*(answer: false)*

■ **FILL-IN-THE-BLANK QUESTION**

In a normal DNA molecule, adenine always pairs with _____ and cytosine always pairs with _____.

*(answers: thymine; guanine)*

■ **MATCHING QUESTION**

Match the scientist and the approximate time frames (decades of their work) with their achievements.

| Column 1 | Column 2 |
|---|---|
| _____ 1. Modeled the molecular structure of DNA | A. George Beadle and Edward Tatum, 1930s and 1940s |
| _____ 2. Generated X-ray crystallography images of DNA | B. James Watson and Francis Crick, 1950s |
| _____ 3. Correlated the production of one enzyme with one gene | C. Rosalind Franklin and Maurice Wilkins, 1950s |

*(answers: 1–B; 2–C; 3–A)*

# Multiple-Choice Questions

Multiple-choice questions are the most popular type of question on standardized tests. The following analytical and practical strategies can help you answer them:

## Carefully Read the Directions

Directions can be tricky. For example, whereas most test items ask for a single correct answer, some give you the option of marking several choices that are correct. For some tests, you might be required to answer only a certain number of questions.

## Read Each Question Thoroughly

Then look at the choices, and try to choose an answer. This strategy makes it less likely that you'll get confused.

## Underline Keywords and Phrases

If the question is complicated, try to break it down into small sections that are easy to understand.

## Pay Attention to Words That Could Throw You Off

For example, it is easy to overlook negatives in a question ("Which of the following is not . . .").

## If You Don't Know the Answer, Eliminate Answers That You Know or Suspect Are Wrong

If you can leave yourself with two possible answers, you will have a 50–50 chance of making the right choice. To narrow down, ask questions about each of the choices:

- **Is the choice accurate on its own terms?** If there's an error in the choice—for example, a term that is incorrectly defined—the answer is wrong.

- **Is the choice relevant?** An answer may be accurate, but unrelated to the question.

- **Are there any qualifiers?** Absolute qualifiers, like *always, never, all, none,* or *every,* often signal an exception that makes a choice incorrect. For example, the statement "Normal children always begin talking before the age of 2" is untrue (most normal children begin talking before age 2, but some start later). Analysis has shown that choices containing conservative qualifiers like *often, most, rarely,* or *may sometimes be* are often correct.

- **Do the choices give clues?** Does a puzzling word remind you of a word you know? Does any part of an unfamiliar word—its prefix, suffix, or root—ring a bell?

## Make an Educated Guess by Looking for Patterns

Certain patterns tend to appear in multiple-choice questions and may help you make smart guesses. Although these patterns may not apply to the specific test questions you encounter, they're important to keep in mind.

Experts advise you to:

- Consider the possibility that a choice that is *more general* than the others is the right answer.
- Consider the possibility that a choice that is *longer* than the others is the right answer.
- Look for a choice that has a *middle value in a range* (the range can be from small to large or from old to recent). It is likely to be the right answer.
- Look for two choices that have *similar meanings*. One of these answers is probably correct.
- Look for answers that *agree grammatically* with the question. For example, a fill-in-the-blank question that has an *a* or *an* before the blank gives you a clue to the correct answer.

### Make Sure You Read Every Word of Every Answer

Instructors have been known to include answers that are almost right, except for a single word. Focus especially on qualifying words such as *always, never, tend to, most, often,* and *frequently.*

### When Questions Are Linked to a Reading Passage, Read the Questions First

This will help you focus on the information you need to answer the questions.

## True/False Questions

Read true/false questions carefully to evaluate what they are asking. If you're stumped, guess (unless you're penalized for wrong answers).

Look for qualifiers in true/false questions—such as *all, only,* and *always* (the absolutes that often make a statement false) and *generally, often, usually,* and *sometimes* (the conservatives that often make a statement true)— that can turn a statement that would otherwise be true into one that is false or vice versa. For example, "The grammar rule 'I before E except after C' is *always* true" is false, whereas "The grammar rule 'I before E except after C' is *usually* true" is true. The qualifier makes the difference.

## Matching Questions

Matching questions ask you to match the terms in one list with the terms in another list, according to the directions. For example, the directions may tell you to match a communicable disease with the germ that usually causes it. The following practical strategies will help you handle these questions.

### Make Sure You Understand the Directions

The directions tell you whether each answer can be used only once or more than once.

### Work from the Column with the Longest Entries

The left-hand column usually contains terms to be defined or questions to be answered, whereas the right-hand column contains definitions or answers. As a result, entries in the right-hand column are usually longer than those on the left. Reading the items on the right only once each will save time as you work to match them with the shorter phrases on the left.

## Start with the Matches You Know

On your first run-through, mark these matches with a penciled line, waiting to finalize your choices after you've completed all the items. Keep in mind that if you can use an answer only once, you may have to change answers if you reconsider any of your original choices.

## Finally, Tackle the Matches You're Not Sure Of

On your next run-through, focus on the more difficult matches. Look for clues and relationships you might not have considered.

If one or more phrases seem to have no correct answer, look back at your easy matches to be sure you did not jump too quickly. Consider the possibility that one of your sure-thing answers is wrong.

# Fill-in-the-Blank Questions

Fill-in-the-blank questions, also known as sentence completion questions, ask you to supply one or more words or phrases with missing information that completes the sentence. These strategies will help you make successful choices.

## Be Logical

Insert your answer; then reread the sentence from beginning to end to be sure it is factually and grammatically correct and makes sense.

## Note the Length and Number of the Blanks

These are important clues but not absolute guideposts. If two blanks appear right after one another, the instructor is probably looking for a two-word answer. If a blank is longer than usual, the correct response may require additional space. However, if you are certain of an answer that doesn't seem to fit the blanks, trust your knowledge and instincts.

## Pay Attention to How Blanks Are Separated

If there is more than one blank in a sentence and the blanks are widely separated, treat each one separately. Answering each as if it were a separate sentence-completion question increases the likelihood that you will get at least one answer correct. Here is an example:

> When Toni Morrison was awarded the _____ Prize for Literature, she was a professor at _____ University.
>
> *(Answer: Morrison received the Nobel Prize and is a professor at Princeton University.)*

## Think Out of the Box

If you can think of more than one correct answer, put them both down. Your instructor may be impressed by your assertiveness and creativity.

## If You Are Uncertain of an Answer, Make an Educated Guess

Have faith that after hours of studying, the correct answer is somewhere in your subconscious mind and your guess is not completely random.

# Write to the Verb

*Hone your ability to read and follow essay instructions accurately.*

Focusing on the action verbs in essay test instructions can mean the difference between giving instructors what they want and answering off the mark.

- Start by choosing a topic you learned about in this text—for example, the concept of successful intelligence or internal and external barriers to listening. Write your topic here:

- Put yourself in the role of instructor. Write an essay question on this topic, using one of the action verbs in Figure 8.2 to frame the question. For example, "List the three aspects of successful intelligence," or "Analyze the classroom-based challenges associated with internal barriers to listening."

- Now choose three other action verbs from Figure 8.2. Use each one to rewrite your original question.

    1.

    2.

    3.

- Finally, analyze how each new verb changes the focus of the essay.

    1.

    2.

    3.

## Essay Questions

An essay question allows you to express your knowledge and views more extensively than a short-answer question. With this freedom comes the challenge to organize and express that knowledge clearly.

The following steps will help improve your responses to essay questions. The process is basically a less extensive version of the writing process: You plan, draft, revise, and edit your response (see Chapter 9). The primary differences here are that you are writing under time pressure and that you are working from memory.

1. *Start by reading the questions.* Decide which to tackle (if there's a choice). Use your analytical ability to focus on what each question is asking. Then engage practical strategies as you read the directions carefully and do everything asked.

Some essay questions may contain more than one part, so it is important to budget your time. For example, if you have one hour to answer three question sections, you might budget 20 minutes for each section, and

## FIGURE 8.2    Focus on action verbs on essay tests

| | |
|---|---|
| **Analyze**—Break into parts and discuss each part separately. | **Explain**—Make the meaning of something clear, often by making analogies or giving examples. |
| **Compare**—Explain similarities and differences. | **Illustrate**—Supply examples. |
| **Contrast**—Distinguish between items being compared by focusing on differences. | **Interpret**—Explain your personal view of facts and ideas and how they relate to one another. |
| **Criticize**—Evaluate the positive and negative effects of what is being discussed. | **Outline**—Organize and present the main examples of an idea or sub-ideas. |
| **Define**—State the essential quality or meaning. Give the common idea. | **Prove**—Use evidence and argument to show that something is true, usually by showing cause and effect or giving examples that fit the idea to be proven. |
| **Describe**—Visualize and give information that paints a complete picture. | **Review**—Provide an overview of ideas and establish their merits and features. |
| **Discuss**—Examine in a complete and detailed way, usually by connecting ideas to examples. | **State**—Explain clearly, simply, and concisely, being sure that each word gives the image you want. |
| **Enumerate/List/Identify**—Recall and specify items in the form of a list. | **Summarize**—Give the important ideas in brief. |
| **Evaluate**—Give your opinion about the value or worth of something, usually by weighing positive and negative effects, and justify your conclusion. | **Trace**—Present a history of the way something developed, often by showing cause and effect. |

break that down into writing stages (3 minutes for planning, 15 minutes for drafting, 2 minutes for revising and editing).

2. *Watch for action verbs.* Certain verbs can help you figure out how to think. Figure 8.2 explains some words commonly used in essay questions. Underline these words as you read and use them to guide your writing.

3. *Plan.* Use your creative thinking skills to brainstorm ideas and examples. Create an informal outline or a think link to map your ideas and list supporting examples.

4. *Draft.* Start with a thesis statement that states clearly what your essay will say. Then, devote one or more paragraphs to the main points in your outline. Back up the general statement that starts each paragraph with evidence in the form of examples, statistics, and so on. Use simple, clear language, and look back at your outline to make sure you cover everything. Wrap it up with a short, pointed conclusion. Because you probably won't have time for redrafting, try to be as complete and organized as possible.

5. *Revise.* Make sure you answer the question completely and include all of your points. Look for ideas you left out, general statements that need more support, paragraphs that don't hold together well, unnecessary

**FIGURE 8.3**   Create an informal outline during essay tests

Roles of BL in IC
1.  To contradict or reinforce words
    —e.g., friend says "I'm fine"
2.  To add shades of meaning
    —saying the same sentence in 3 diff. ways
3.  To make lasting 1st impression
    —impact of nv cues and voice tone greater than words
    —we assume things abt person based on posture, eye contact, etc.

material, and confusing sentences. Fix problems by adding new material in the margins and crossing out what you don't need. When adding material, you can indicate with an arrow where it fits or note that inserts can be found on separate pages. If you have more than one insert, label each to avoid confusion (e.g., Insert #1, Insert #2, etc.).

6. *Edit.* Check for mistakes in grammar, spelling, punctuation, and usage. No matter your topic, being technically correct in your writing makes your work more impressive.

Neatness is a crucial factor in essay writing. No matter how good your ideas are, if your instructor can't read them, your grade will suffer. If your handwriting is a problem, try printing your answers, skipping every other line, and writing on only one side of the paper. Students with illegible handwriting might ask to take the test on a laptop computer.

To answer the third essay question from the box below, one student created the planning outline shown in Figure 8.3. Notice how abbreviations and shorthand help the student write quickly. It is much faster to write "Role of BL in IC" than "Role of Body Language in Interpersonal Communication" (see Chapter 6 for shorthand strategies). Figure 8.4 shows the student's essay, including the word changes and inserts she made while revising the draft.

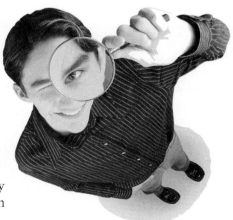

# How Can You Learn from *Test Mistakes?*

The purpose of a test is to see how much you know, not merely to get a grade. Use the following strategies to analyze and learn from your mistakes so that you avoid repeating them.

## FIGURE 8.4    Response to an essay question with revision marks

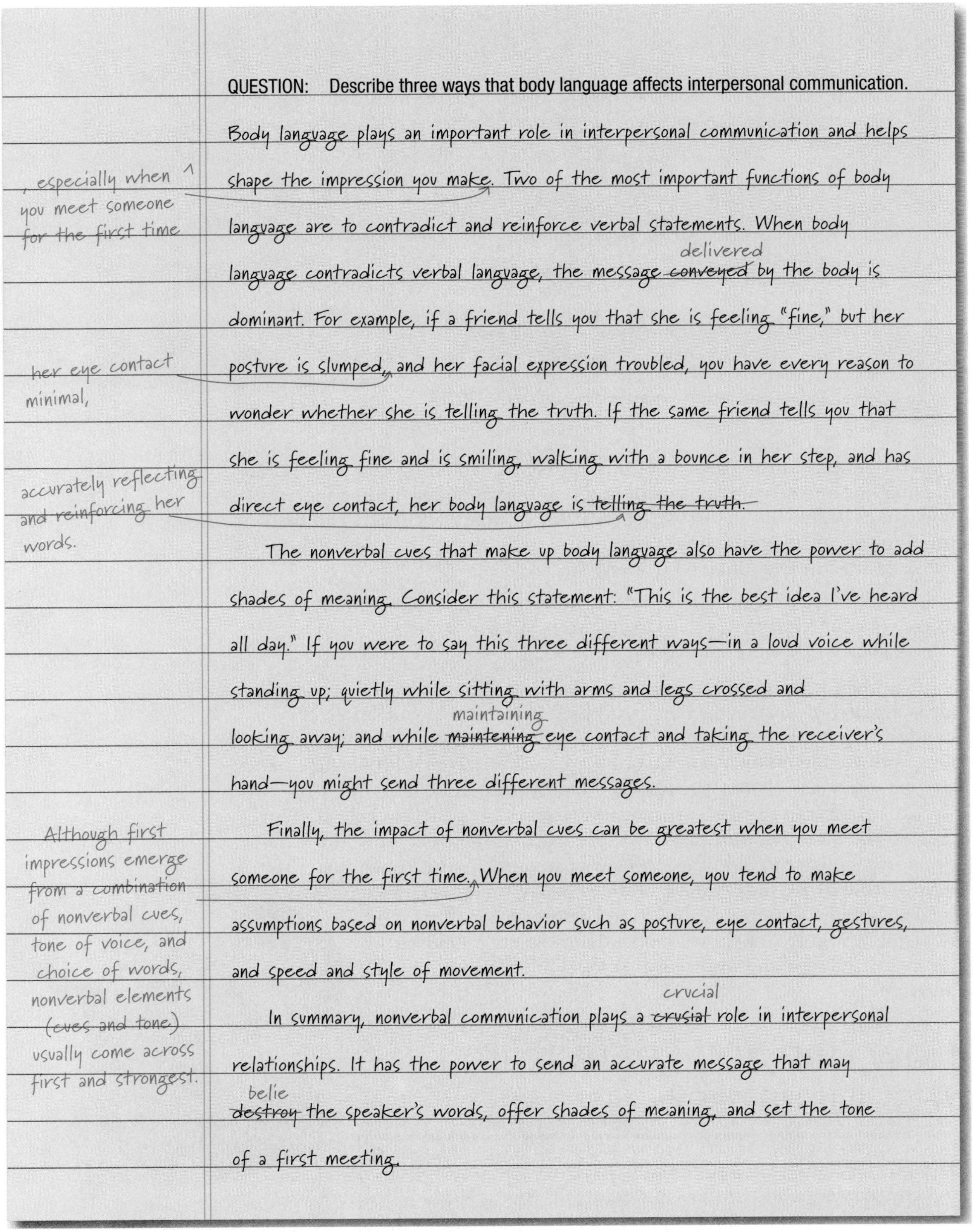

QUESTION:    Describe three ways that body language affects interpersonal communication.

Body language plays an important role in interpersonal communication and helps
shape the impression you make. Two of the most important functions of body
language are to contradict and reinforce verbal statements. When body

*, especially when
you meet someone
for the first time*

*delivered*

language contradicts verbal language, the message ~~conveyed~~ by the body is
dominant. For example, if a friend tells you that she is feeling "fine," but her

*her eye contact
minimal,*

posture is slumped, and her facial expression troubled, you have every reason to
wonder whether she is telling the truth. If the same friend tells you that
she is feeling fine and is smiling, walking with a bounce in her step, and has

*accurately reflecting
and reinforcing her
words.*

direct eye contact, her body language is ~~telling the truth.~~

The nonverbal cues that make up body language also have the power to add
shades of meaning. Consider this statement: "This is the best idea I've heard
all day." If you were to say this three different ways—in a loud voice while
standing up; quietly while sitting with arms and legs crossed and

*maintaining*

looking away; and while ~~maintaining~~ eye contact and taking the receiver's
hand—you might send three different messages.

*Although first
impressions emerge
from a combination
of nonverbal cues,
tone of voice, and
choice of words,
nonverbal elements
(cues and tone)
usually come across
first and strongest.*

Finally, the impact of nonverbal cues can be greatest when you meet
someone for the first time. When you meet someone, you tend to make
assumptions based on nonverbal behavior such as posture, eye contact, gestures,
and speed and style of movement.

*crucial*

In summary, nonverbal communication plays a ~~crucial~~ role in interpersonal
relationships. It has the power to send an accurate message that may

*belie*

~~destroy~~ the speaker's words, offer shades of meaning, and set the tone
of a first meeting.

## Try to Identify Patterns in Your Mistakes

Look for the following:

- **Careless errors.** In your rush to finish, did you misread the question or directions, blacken the wrong box on the answer sheet, skip a question, write illegibly?

- **Conceptual or factual errors.** Did you misunderstand a concept? Did you fail to master facts or concepts? Did you skip part of the text or miss classes in which ideas were covered?

## Rework the Questions You Got Wrong

Based on instructor feedback, try to rewrite an essay, recalculate a math problem from the original question, or redo questions following a reading selection. If you discover a pattern of careless errors, redouble your efforts to be more careful and save time to double-check your work.

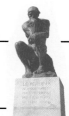

Our greatest glory is not in never falling, but in rising every time we fall.

CONFUCIUS

## After Reviewing Your Mistakes, Fill in Your Knowledge Gaps

If you made mistakes because of a lack of understanding, develop a plan to learn the material. Solidifying your knowledge can help you on future exams and in life situations that involve the subject you're studying.

## Talk to Your Instructors

Talk with your instructor about your specific mistakes on short-answer questions or about a weak essay. If you are not sure why you were marked down on an essay, ask what you could have done to improve your grade. Take advantage of this opportunity to determine how to do better on the next exam.

## If You Fail a Test, Don't Throw It Away

Use it as a way to review material that you had trouble with or didn't know as well as you should have. You might also want to keep it as a reminder that you can improve if you have the will to succeed. When you compare a failure to later successes, you'll see how far you've come.

The willingness to learn from test mistakes is critical for all students, including those with reading-related learning disabilities. When CAST researcher Roxanne Ruzic examined how students who are learning disabled prepare for tests, she found that successful students took advantage of instructor feedback; they applied what they learned from their mistakes on one test to their preparation for others. Students who dismissed this feedback did not excel.

Jack is a case in point, as Ruzic explains: "When Jack received his graded midterm exam [in his course Introduction to International Business], he discounted some of what the instructor wrote in his blue book, claiming she was wrong, rather than trying to figure out how to ensure that he knew the material

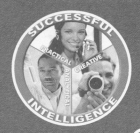

# Learn from Your Mistakes

*Examine what went wrong on a recent exam to build knowledge for next time.*

Look at an exam on which your performance fell short of expectations. If possible, choose one that contains different types of objective and subjective questions. With the test and answer sheet in hand, use your analytical and practical thinking skills to answer the following questions:

- Identify the types of questions on which you got the most correct answers (for example, matching, essay, multiple choice).

- Identify the types of questions on which you made the greatest number of errors.

- Analyze your errors to identify patterns: For example, did you misread test instructions or did you ignore qualifiers that changed the questions' meanings? What did you find?

- Finally, what are two practical actions you are committed to take during your next exam to avoid the same problems?

  Action 1:

  Action 2:

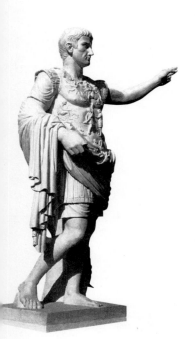

and she knew that he knew it. Although Jack did not do as well on the midterm as he would have liked, he used the same study techniques to prepare for the final exam as he had used for the midterm. Had Jack talked more to other people (including instructors) regularly to assess his understanding of content and expectations and worked in study groups, he would have been much more successful in his courses." Jack's final course grade was a C+—not where he could have been had he made the effort to learn from earlier setbacks.

# *Sine qua non*

Although Latin is no longer spoken and is considered a dead language, it plays an important role in modern English because many English words and phrases have Latin roots. The Latin phrase *sine qua non* (pronounced sihn-ay kwa nahn) means, literally, "without which not." In other words, a sine qua non is "an absolutely indispensable or essential thing."

Think of learning as the sine qua non of test taking. When you have worked hard to learn, review, and retain information, you will be well prepared for tests, no matter what form they take. Focus on knowledge to transform test taking from an intimidating challenge into an opportunity to demonstrate what you know.

# Building World-Class Skills
## for College, Career, and Life Success

*Create Your Future*

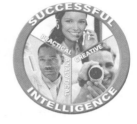

## DEVELOPING SUCCESSFUL INTELLIGENCE

### *Putting It All Together*

**Prepare Effectively for Tests.** Take a detailed look at your performance on and preparation for a recent test.

**Step 1. Think it through:** *Analyze how you did.* Were you pleased or disappointed with your performance and grade? Why?

Thinking about your performance, look at the potential problems listed here. Circle any that you feel were a factor in this exam. Fill in the empty spaces with any key problems not listed.

- Incomplete preparation
- Feeling rushed during the test
- Poor guessing techniques
- Test anxiety
- 

- Fatigue
- Shaky understanding of concepts
- Feeling confused about directions
- 
- 

If you circled any problems, think about why you made mistakes (if it was an objective exam) or why you didn't score well (if it was an essay exam).

**Step 2. Think out of the box:** *Be creative about test-preparation strategies.* If you had absolutely no restrictions on time or on access to materials, how would you have prepared for this test?

*Describe briefly what your plan would be and how it would minimize any problems you encountered.*

*Now think back to your actual preparation for this test. Describe techniques you used and note time spent.*

*How does what you would like to do differ from what you actually did?*

**Step 3. Make it happen:** *Improve preparation for the future.* Think about the practical actions you will take the next time you face a similar test.

*Actions I took this time but do not intend to take next time:*

*Actions I did not take this time but intend to take next time:*

# TEAM BUILDING
## Collaborative Solutions

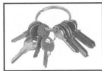

**Test Study Group.** Form a study group with two or three other students. When your instructor announces the next exam, ask each study group member to record everything he or she does to prepare for the exam, including:

- Learning what to expect on the test (topics and material that will be covered, types of questions that will be asked)
- Examining old tests
- Creating and following a study schedule and checklist
- Using SQ3R to review material
- Taking a pretest
- Getting a good night's sleep before the exam
- Doing last-minute cramming
- Mastering general test-taking strategies
- Mastering test-taking strategies for specific types of test questions (multiple choice, true/false, matching, fill in the blank, essay)

After the exam, come together to compare preparation strategies. What important differences can you identify in the routines followed by group members? How did learning styles play a role in those differences? How do you suspect that different routines affected test performance and outcome? On a separate piece of paper, for your own reference, write down what you learned from the test-preparation habits of your study mates that may help you as you prepare for upcoming exams.

# WRITING
## Discovery Through Journaling

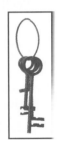

*Record your thoughts on a separate piece of paper or in a journal.*

**Test Anxiety.** Do you experience test anxiety? Describe how tests generally make you feel (you might include an example of a specific test situation and what happened). Identify your specific test-taking fears, and brainstorm ideas for how to overcome fears and self-defeating behaviors.

# CAREER PORTFOLIO
## Plan for Success

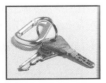

*Complete the following in your electronic portfolio or on separate sheets of paper.*

**On-the-Job Testing.** Depending on what careers you are considering, you may encounter one or more tests throughout your career. Some are for entry into the field (e.g., medical boards); some test your proficiency on particular equipment (e.g., a proficiency test on Microsoft Word); some move you to the next level of employment (e.g., a technical certification test to become a certified actuary). Choose one career you are thinking about and investigate what tests are involved as you advance through different stages of the field. Be sure to look for tests in any of the areas just described. Write down everything you find out about each test involved. For example:

- What it tests you on
- When, in the course of pursuing this career, you would need to take the test
- What preparation is necessary for the test (including course work)
- Whether the test needs to be retaken at any time (e.g., airline pilots usually need to be recertified every few years)

Finally, see if you can review any of the tests you will face if you pursue this career. For example, if your career choice requires proficiency on a specific computer program, your college's career or computer center may have the test available.

## Suggested Readings

Browning, William G., Ph.D. *Cliffs Memory Power for Exams* (Lincoln, NE: CliffsNotes Inc., 1990).

Frank, Steven. *Test Taking Secrets: Study Better, Test Smarter, and Get Great Grades* (Holbrook, MA: Adams Media Corporation, 1998).

Fry, Ron. *"Ace" Any Test*, 5th ed. (Florence, KY: Thomson Delmar Learning, 2004).

Hamilton, Dawn. *Passing Exams: A Guide for Maximum Success and Minimum Stress* (New York: Continuum International, 2003).

Kesselman-Turkel, Judy, and Franklynn Peterson. *Test Taking Strategies* (Madison: University of Wisconsin Press, 2004).

Luckie, William R., and Wood Smethurst. *Study Power: Study Skills to Improve Your Learning and Your Grades* (Cambridge, MA: Brookline Books, 1997).

Meyers, Judith N. *Secrets of Taking Any Test: Learn the Techniques Successful Test-Takers Know* (New York: Learning Express, July 2000).

## Internet Resources

Prentice Hall Student Success SuperSite (testing tips in study skills section): **www.prenhall.com/success**

Florida State University (list of sites offering information on test-taking skills): **http://osi.fsu.edu/hot/testtaking/skills.htm**

Test Taking Tips.com (test taking and study skills): **www.testtakingtips.com**

University of North Dakota (study strategies home page): **www.d.umn.edu/student/loon/acad/strat/**

## Endnotes

[1]Ben Gose, "Notes from Academe: Living It Up on the Dead Days," *The Chronicle of Higher Education* (June 7, 2002). Retrieved April 2004, from: http://chronicle.com/weekly/v48/i39/39a04801.htm.

[2]"Students Speak," MEDPREP: Medical/Dental Education Preparatory Program, Southern Illinois University School of Medicine. Retrieved March 2004, from: www.som.siu.edu/medprep/students_speak.html.

[3]Steven Frank, *The Everything Study Book* (Holbrook, MA: Adams Media Corporation, 1996), p. 208.

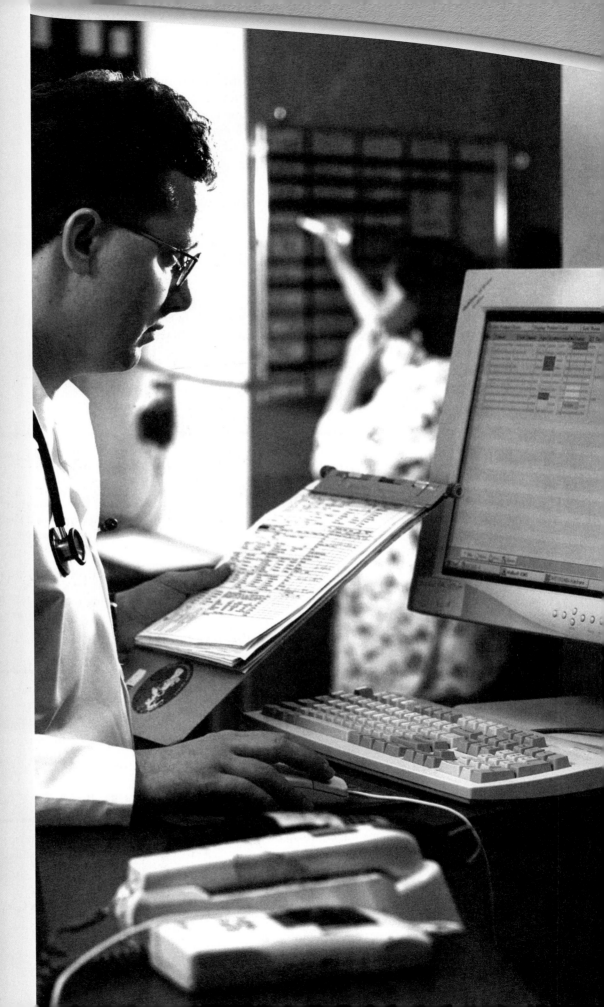

EMPOWER: RESEARCHING AND WRITING

*GATHERING AND COMMUNICATING IDEAS*

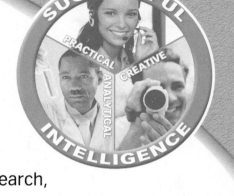

R esearch and writing, powerful tools that engage your successful intelligence, are at the heart of your education. In Chapter 5 we talked about the importance of evidence-based practice and research. In this chapter we are talking about research as gathering information. Through library and Internet research, you gather and analyze information from sources all over the world. Through writing, you analyze ideas, think creatively about what they mean, and communicate information and perspectives to others. Whether you write an essay in English class or a summary of a scientific study for your biology course, the writing process helps sharpen your thinking and your practical communication skills.

This chapter has two goals: to help you improve your skill in finding information at your college library and on the Internet, and to reinforce some of the writing basics that most students study in an English composition course. In school and in your career, researching and writing are essential to success to becoming a nurse.

### IN THIS CHAPTER ...

*you will explore answers to the following questions:*

- How can you make the most of your library? 269
- How can you do research on the Internet? 275
- What is the writing process? 278
- How can you do an effective presentation in any language? 290

# Q & A BLUE SKY QUESTIONS DOWN-TO-EARTH ANSWERS

## How can I become more confident about my writing?

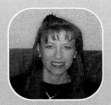

Beverly Andre
Triton College, Continuing
Education Program, River
Grove, Illinois

The best thing I ever wrote was in the sixth grade. My teacher let us pick a topic, and I chose to write about riding horses because I loved it and knew a lot about it. In high school, writing was okay because my teacher was helpful. College papers, however, have been a real challenge. I don't think my topic ideas are very original, and I feel that my vocabulary is not that advanced. If a professor assigns a topic I know nothing about, I usually don't have as much interest as with something familiar.

One of the reasons I don't like to write is because I don't like researching. Knowing how to begin gets confusing because there's so much to choose from. Once I do pull the information together, I can't seem to expand on an idea without being redundant. I also go off on all sorts of tangents. The bottom line is that I find it difficult to put my thoughts to paper. How can I become a better writer?

## PRACTICAL ANSWERS

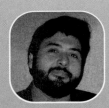

Raymond Montolvo Jr.
Writers' Program, University
of Southern California,
Los Angeles, California

### Concentrate on trying to improve your skills instead of worrying about getting a good grade.

No matter your writing goal, in most cases the person you are writing for, your instructor, wants you to improve. Keeping this in mind may help you concentrate on trying to improve your skills instead of worrying about getting a good grade.

I suggest a two-pronged approach to better writing. The first step is to read. Read novels, the newspaper, and nonfiction articles. Reading helps you learn to organize your thoughts, and it increases your vocabulary. If you want to focus on a specific area of study, read publications in that area. Create file folders for pieces of writing that you like. For example, make a copy of a business letter that you think is well written, and refer to it when you need to write a similar correspondence.

Second, bridge the gap between what you should know and what an instructor can tell you. Ask your instructor what he or she thinks you need to work on. Focus your energy on understanding the assignment and strengthening technical skills such as sentence structure and grammar. Another tip is to read what you've written, sentence by sentence, and think about how you could say it better.

If you don't know where to begin your research, start with what feels comfortable. If you are at ease with computers, use the Internet. If you prefer libraries, start by asking the reference librarian for assistance. The main point with research is to jump right in. Once you read something that relates to your topic, it will refer you to something else.

Finally, don't get frustrated by setbacks. Writing is a process that you learn as you would a type of exercise. Set goals you can attain. Finishing something builds confidence.

# How Can You *Make the Most* of Your Library?

A library is a home for information; consider it the brain of your college. Your practical thinking skills will help you to find what you need quickly and efficiently.

## Start with a Road Map

Make your life easier right away by learning how your library is organized:

### Circulation Desk

All publications are checked out at the circulation desk, which is usually near the library entrance.

### Reference Area

Here you'll find reference books, including encyclopedias, directories, dictionaries, almanacs, and atlases. You'll also find librarians and other library employees who can direct you to information. Computer terminals, containing the library's catalog of holdings as well as online bibliographic and full-text databases, are usually part of the reference area.

### Book Area

Books—and, in many libraries, magazines and journals in bound or boxed volumes—are stored in the stacks. A library with *open stacks* allows you to search for materials on your own. In a *closed-stack* system, a staff member retrieves materials for you.

### Periodicals Area

Here you'll find recent issues of popular and scholarly magazines, journals, and newspapers. Because you usually cannot check out unbound **periodicals**, you may find photocopy machines nearby where you can copy pages.

PERIODICALS
Magazines, journals, and newspapers that are published regularly throughout the year.

### Audiovisual Materials Areas

Many libraries have special areas for video, art and photography, and recorded music collections.

### Computer Areas

Computer terminals, linked to college databases and the Internet, may be scattered throughout the building or set off in particular areas. You may be able to access these databases and the Internet from computer labs and writing centers. Many college dorm rooms are also wired for computer access, enabling students to connect via personal computers.

## Microform Areas

Most libraries have microform reading areas. *Microforms* are materials printed in reduced size on film, either *microfilm* (a reel of film) or *microfiche* (a sheet or card of film), viewed through special machines.

Almost all college libraries offer orientation sessions on how to find what you need. In addition, library Web pages usually contain online catalogs from your college and associated colleges, online databases, and phone numbers and e-mail addresses for reference librarians. If you need help, take a real or virtual tour and sign up for training.

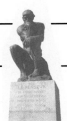

## My library was dukedom large enough.

WILLIAM SHAKESPEARE

## Learn How to Conduct an Information Search

The most successful and time-saving search for information involves a specific *search strategy*—a practical, step-by-step method that takes you from general to specific sources. Starting with general sources provides an overview of your topic and can lead to more specific information and sources.

For example, an encyclopedia article on the archaeological discovery of the Dead Sea Scrolls—manuscripts written between 250 B.C.E. and 68 C.E. that trace the roots of Judaism and Christianity—may mention that one of the most important books on the subject is *Understanding the Dead Sea Scrolls*, edited by Hershel Shanks. This book, in turn, leads you to 13 experts who wrote specialized text chapters.

It's important to narrow your topic because broad topics yield too much data. Instead of using the topic "Dead Sea Scrolls" in your search, for example, consider narrowing it to any of the following:

- How the Dead Sea Scrolls were discovered by Bedouin shepherds in 1947
- The historical origins of the scrolls
- The process archaeologists used to reconstruct scroll fragments

### Conducting a Keyword Search

To find materials related to your topic, conduct a *keyword search* of the library database, a method for locating sources through the use of topic-related words and phrases. To narrow your topic and reduce the number of hits, add more keywords. For example, instead of searching through the broad category *art*, focus on *nineteenth-century French impressionist art.*

Keyword searches use natural language, rather than specialized classification vocabulary. Figure 9.1 provides tips to help you use the keyword system.

As you search, keep in mind that

- Double quotes around a word or phrase will locate the exact term you entered ("financial aid").
- Using uppercase or lowercase does not affect the search (*Scholarships* will find *scholarships*).
- Singular terms will find the plural (*scholarship* will find *scholarships*).

**FIGURE 9.1** How to perform an effective keyword search

| IF YOU ARE SEARCHING FOR . . . | DO THIS | EXAMPLE |
|---|---|---|
| A word | Type the word normally | aid |
| A phrase | Type the phrase in its normal word order (use regular word spacing) or surround the phrase with double quotation marks | financial aid *or* "financial aid" |
| Two or more keywords without regard to word order | Type the words in any order, surrounding the words with quotation marks (use *and* to separate the words) | "financial aid" and "scholarships" |
| Topic A or topic B | Type the words in any order, surrounding the words with quotation marks (use *or* to separate the words) | "financial aid" or "scholarships" |
| Topic A but not topic B | Type topic A first within quotation marks, and then topic B within quotation marks (use *not* to separate the words) | "financial aid" not "scholarships" |

# Conduct Research Using a Search Strategy

Knowing where to look during each phase of your search helps you find information quickly and efficiently. A successful search strategy often begins with general references and moves to more specific references (see Figure 9.2).

## Use General Reference Works

Begin your research with general reference works. These works cover many different topics in a broad, nondetailed way. General reference guides are often available on-line or on **CD-ROM**. Works that fall into the general reference category include the following:

- Encyclopedias such as the multivolume *Encyclopedia Americana* and the single-volume *New Columbia Encyclopedia*
- Almanacs such as the *World Almanac* and *Book of Facts*
- Yearbooks such as the *McGraw-Hill Yearbook of Science and Technology* and the *Statistical Abstract of the United States*
- Dictionaries such as *Webster's New World College Dictionary*
- Biographical reference works such as the *New York Times Biographical Service*, *Webster's Biographical Dictionary*, and various editions of *Who's Who*
- Bibliographies such as *Books in Print* (especially the *Subject Guide to Books in Print*)

Scan these sources for an overview of your topic. Bibliographies at the end of encyclopedia articles may also lead to important sources.

## Search Specialized Reference Works

Turn next to specialized reference works for more specific facts. Specialized reference works include encyclopedias and dictionaries that focus on a narrow field. Although the entries in these volumes are short, they focus on critical ideas

*CD-ROM*
*A compact disc, containing words and images in electronic form, that can be read by a computer (CD-ROM stands for "compact disc read-only memory").*

**FIGURE 9.2** A library search strategy will help you find information

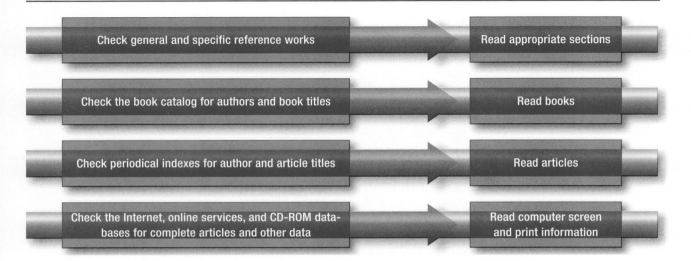

| Check general and specific reference works | → | Read appropriate sections |
| Check the book catalog for authors and book titles | → | Read books |
| Check periodical indexes for author and article titles | → | Read articles |
| Check the Internet, online services, and CD-ROM data-bases for complete articles and other data | → | Read computer screen and print information |

and on the keywords you need to conduct additional research. Bibliographies that accompany the articles point to the works of recognized experts. Examples of specialized reference works, organized by subject, include the following:

- History (*Encyclopedia of American History*)
- Science and technology (*Encyclopedia of Biological Sciences*)
- Social sciences (*Dictionary of Education*)
- Current affairs (*Social Issues Resources Series [SIRS]*)

## Browse Through Books on Your Subject

Use the computerized *library catalog* to find books and other materials on your topic. The catalog, searchable by author, title, and subject, tells you which publications the library owns. Each catalog listing refers to the library's classification system, which in turn tells you exactly where the publication can be found.

## Use Periodical Indexes to Search for Periodicals

Periodicals, a valuable source of current information, include journals, magazines, and newspapers. *Journals* are written for readers with specialized knowledge. Whereas *Newsweek* magazine may run a general-interest article on AIDS research, the *Journal of the American Medical Association* may print the original scientific study for an audience of scientists. Many libraries display periodicals that are up to a year or two old and convert older copies to microform. Many full-text articles are also available on computer databases and via the Internet.

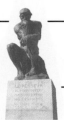

The outcome of any serious research can only be to make two questions grow where only one grew before.

THORSTEIN VEBLEN

# Discover Your College Library

*get practical!*

*Learn the nuts and bolts of your college's library system.*

Identify the following:

- Name and location of the college library. (If your college has more than one library, identify the branch you are most likely to use.)
- Hours of operation.
- Library website address.
- Important e-mail addresses and phone numbers, including those of the reference and circulation desks.
- Stack locations of the books and other publications you may need in this semester's courses.
- Names and URLs of computer databases you are likely to use.
- Location of a library nook or chair that is ideal for studying.

Periodical indexes lead you to specific articles. *The Reader's Guide to Periodical Literature*, available in print and on CD-ROM, indexes general information sources including articles in hundreds of general-interest publications. Look in the Infotrac family of databases (available online or on CD-ROM) for other periodical indexes such as *Health Reference Center* and *General Business File*.

Indexing information is listed in the *Standard Periodical Directory, Ulrich's International Periodicals Directory*, and *Magazines for Libraries*. Each database lists the magazines and periodicals it indexes. Because there is no all-inclusive index for technical, medical, and scholarly journal articles, you'll have to search indexes that specialize in narrow subject areas. Such indexes also include abstracts (article summaries). Among the available indexes are *ERIC (Educational Resources Information Center), The Humanities Index, Index Medicus*, and *Psychological Abstracts*. You'll also find separate newspaper indexes in print, in microform, on CD-ROM, or online.

Almost no library owns all of the publications listed in these and other specialized indexes. However, journals that are not part of your library's collection or are not available in full-text form online may be available through an interlibrary loan, which allows patrons to request materials from other libraries. The librarian will help you arrange the loan.

## Ask the Librarian

Librarians can assist you in solving research problems. They can help you locate sources, navigate catalogs and databases, and uncover research shortcuts. Say, for example, you are researching recent federal gun-control legislation, and you want to contact groups on both sides of the issue. Using Google to conduct a keyword Internet search, you come up with nearly 17,000 hits—and you have no way of knowing which organizational websites are the best. To help you make a decision, the librarian may lead you to the *Encyclopedia of Associations*, which lists the National Rifle Association, a pro-gun organization, and Handgun Control Inc., a gun-control group.

Librarians are not the only helpful people in the library. For simplicity's sake, this book uses the term *librarian* to refer to both librarians and other staff members who are trained to help. Here are some tips that will help you get the advice you are seeking from the librarian.

- **Be prepared and be specific.** Instead of asking for information on the American presidency, focus on the topic you expect to write about in your American history paper—for example, President Franklin D. Roosevelt's leadership during World War II.

- **Ask for help when you can't find a specific source.** For example, when a specific book is not on the shelf, the librarian may direct you to another source that works as well.

- **Ask for help with computers and other equipment.** Librarians are experts in using the computers and other equipment, so turn to them for help with technical problems.

Following are typical inquiries reference librarians received at Moraine Valley Community College in Illinois, along with where the information was found and how long each search took. The librarians successfully located information using analytical, creative, and practical thinking. Note that the Internet did not always yield the answer; librarians often used traditional reference works.[1]

- **"I want to find information about holistic medicine and nursing in nursing journals."** Search time: 9 minutes. The librarian introduced the student to a specialized health care database and showed her how to narrow the search range.

- **"We need movie advertising costs per week and box-office receipts to make a comparison of return on investment for a business class."** Search time: 45 minutes. The librarian and student scanned business and general databases and searched the Web. They found what they needed for some movies, but not others.

- **"I need literary criticism about the poetry of Adrienne Rich."** Search time: 15 minutes. The librarian used online databases and reference books to find several articles.

- **"What Cajun restaurant in Blue Island, Illinois, is supposed to be haunted?"** Search time: 45 minutes. A Web search was fruitless, so the librarian led the student to several books about haunted buildings in suburban Chicago.

The library is an indispensable tool in your efforts to gather information—the foundation of knowledge. Chad Clunie, a political science major at Indiana University's Southeast Campus, is driven to use the library by what he describes as the "quest for knowledge." As an officer in the local student branch of the American Civil Liberties Union, Chad uses library resources to formulate debates on current topics, such as same-sex marriage and the Patriot Act. "There's so much to learn," said Chad. "There's no way of knowing it all."[2]

Internet research supplements library research as it connects you almost instantaneously to billions of information sources. A miracle of technology, the Internet allows you to search for information at lightning speed.

# How Can You Do *Research* on the Internet?

The *Internet* is a computer network that links organizations and people around the world. To get what you need from it, you need to think analytically about what you want to know, conduct creative searches in which you explore topics from different perspectives, and use practical tools to locate information.

According to Bob Kieft, library director at Pennsylvania's Haverford College, students must "think critically and independently about the sources they use, be curious and imaginative about the projects they are working on, be open to the topic in ways that lead them to ask good questions, and bring their analytical powers to bear. . . . What students know about technology is less important than how they think about their work"[3] and the steps they take to find answers.

## The Basics

With a basic knowledge of the Internet, you can access facts and figures, read articles and reports, purchase products, download files, send messages electronically via e-mail, and even "talk" to people in real time. Following is some information you should know:

- **Access.** Users access the Internet through Internet Service Providers (ISPs). Some ISPs are commercial, such as America Online. Others are linked to companies, colleges, and other organizations.

- **Information locations.** Most information is displayed on *websites*, cyberspace locations developed by companies, government agencies, organizations, and individuals. Together, these sites make up the *World Wide Web*.

- **Finding locations.** The string of text and numbers that identifies an Internet site is called a *URL* (Universal Resource Locator). You can type in a URL to access a specific site. Many websites include *hyperlinks*—URLs, usually underlined and highlighted in color—that when clicked on will take you directly to another Web location.

## Use Search Directories and Search Engines

Commercial search engines and directories are your portal to the World Wide Web. Among the most powerful and popular search sites are Google (www.google.com), Yahoo! (www.yahoo.com), MSN Search (www.msnsearch.com), Overture (www.overture.com), Excite (www.excite.com),

Alta Vista (http://altavista.com), HotBot (www.hotbot.com), Ask (www. ask.com), and Lycos (www.lycos.com). Information is accessible through keyword searches.

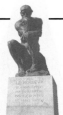

The flood of unedited information on Google demands that users sharpen critical thinking skills, to filter the results. Google forces us to ask, "What do we really want to know?"

ESTHER DYSON

The academic publications that you may need in higher level courses are generally inaccessible through Google and other popular search tools even though these publications are available online, free of charge, through university libraries. For example, although the University of Michigan includes the full texts of 22,000 scholarly volumes in its digital collection, these collections are all but invisible to search engines. This is changing as Google, Yahoo!, and other search engines are working with librarians and colleges to make digitized academic archives available to everyone.[4]

## Internet Search Strategy

The World Wide Web has been called "the world's greatest library, with all its books on the floor." *Your goal is to find enough information without being overwhelmed by too much information.* With no librarian in sight, engage successful intelligence to use this basic search strategy:

1. *Think carefully about what you want to locate.* Professor Eliot Soloway recommends phrasing your search in the form of a question. For example, *What vaccines are given to children before age five?* Then he advises identifying the important words in the question (*vaccines, children, before age five*) as well as other related words (*chicken pox, tetanus, polio, shot, pediatrics,* and so on). This will give you a collection of terms to use in different combinations as you search.[5]

2. *Use a search engine or directory to isolate sites under your desired topic or category.* Save the sites that look useful. Most Internet browsers have a "bookmark" or "favorites" feature for recording sites you want to find again.

3. *Explore these sites to get a general idea of what's out there.* If the search engine or directory takes you where you need to go, you're in luck. More often, in academic research, you will need to dig deeper. Use what you find to notice useful keywords and information locations.

4. *Use your keywords in a variety of ways to uncover different possibilities.* Make sure to spell keywords correctly.

- Vary word order if you are using more than one keyword (for example, search under "*education, college, statistics*" and "*statistics, education, college*").

- Use the words "and," "not," and "or" in ways that limit your search (see Figure 9.1 for tips for using keywords in library searches).

5. *Evaluate the list of links that appears.* If there are too many, narrow your search by using more keywords or more specific keywords (Broadway

# Google (Yes, It's a Verb)

*get creative!*

*Explore ways to use Google and other search engines effectively.*

Google accesses 6 billion documents and has the capacity to return 750,000 Internet links in a third of a second. Despite this, Leon Botstein, president of Bard College, warns of Google's pitfalls: "In general, Google overwhelms you with too much information, much of which is hopelessly unreliable or beside the point. It's like looking for a lost ring in a vacuum bag. What you end up with mostly are bagel crumbs and dirt."[6]

With this warning in mind, use your creativity and analysis to complete the following:

1. Choose a common topic—for example, apples, kitchen sinks, snowflakes. Google the topic to see how many websites you access. Write that number here. _____ Now spend 10 minutes scanning the Web listings. How many different topics did your search uncover other than the topic you intended?

2. Pick three of the off-the-topic links you found, and write a thesis statement to a paper that would require you to use these leads in your research. Be creative.

3. In all likelihood, your thesis statement makes little sense. What does this tell you about the need for critical thinking when using Google and other search directories and engines in your research?

4. Finally, open your mind to the creative possibilities your research uncovered. Did any of the websites spark ideas about your topic that you had never considered? Write down two ideas you never thought of before.

   a.

   b.

could become Broadway AND "fall season" AND 2005). If there are too few, broaden your search by using fewer or different keywords.

6. *When you think you are done, start over.* Choose another search engine or directory and perform your search again. Why? Because different systems access different sites and sources.

## Use Analytical Thinking to Evaluate Every Source

It is up to you to evaluate the truth and usefulness of Internet information. Because the Internet is largely uncensored and unmonitored—a kind of "information free-for-all"—you must decide which sources to value and which to ignore. Use the following strategies to analyze the validity and usefulness of each source.[7]

- **Ask questions about the source.** Is the author a recognized expert? Does he or she write from a particular perspective that may bias the presentation? Is the source recent enough for your purposes? Where did the author get the information?

    Note also the website's name and the organization that creates and maintains the site. Is the organization reputable? Is it known as an authority on the topic you are researching? If you are not sure of the source, the URL may give you a clue. For example, URLs ending in .edu originate at an educational institution, and .gov sites originate at government agencies.

- **Evaluate the material.** Evaluate Internet sources the way you would other material. Is the source a published document (newspaper article, professional journal article, etc.), or is it simply one person's views? Can you verify the data by comparing it to other material? Pay attention, also, to writing quality. Texts with grammatical and spelling errors, poor organization, or factual errors are likely to be unreliable.

Take advantage of the wealth of material the Internet offers—but be picky. Always remember that your research will only be as strong as your thinking. If you work hard to ensure that your research is solid and comprehensive, the product of your efforts will speak for itself.

Library and Internet research is often done as a step in writing a research paper. The success of your paper depends on the quality of your research and on your ability to write.

# What Is the *Writing Process?*

Knowing how to write well is so important for success—academic and otherwise—that most schools require students to pass a semester- or yearlong writing course. Many schools also have self-directed writing labs where students can practice and hone specific skills. This overview is intended to reinforce some of the basics you will learn in these settings.

The writing process for research papers and essays allows you to get your thoughts down on paper and rework them until you express yourself clearly. The four main parts of the process are planning, drafting, revising, and editing. Analytical, creative, and practical thinking play important roles throughout.

## Planning

PREWRITING
STRATEGIES
Techniques for generating ideas about a topic and finding out how much you already know before you start your research and writing.

Planning gives you a chance to think about what to write and how to write it. Planning involves brainstorming for topic ideas, using **prewriting strategies** to define and narrow your topic, conducting research, writing a thesis statement, and writing a working outline. Although these steps are listed in sequence, in real life they overlap one another as you plan your document.

FIGURE 9.3

## Brainstorm your topic and organize ideas in an outline

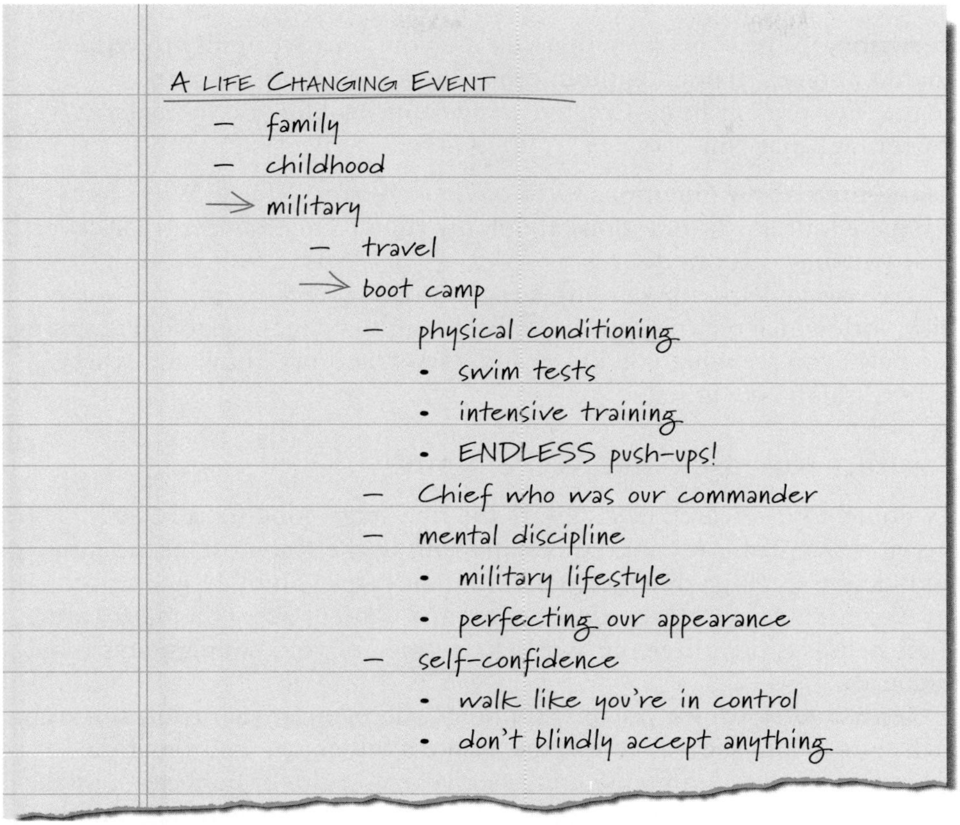

```
A LIFE CHANGING EVENT
     — family
     — childhood
  ⟶ military
         — travel
         ⟶ boot camp
              — physical conditioning
                   • swim tests
                   • intensive training
                   • ENDLESS push-ups!
              — Chief who was our commander
              — mental discipline
                   • military lifestyle
                   • perfecting our appearance
              — self-confidence
                   • walk like you're in control
                   • don't blindly accept anything
```

## Open Your Mind Through Brainstorming

Brainstorming is a creative technique that involves generating ideas about a subject without making judgments (see Chapter 4). To begin brainstorming, write down anything on the assigned subject that comes to mind, in no particular order. Then, organize that list into an outline or think link that helps you see the possibilities more clearly. To make the outline or think link, separate the items you've listed into general ideas or categories and subideas or examples. Then, associate the subideas or examples with the ideas they support or fit.

Figure 9.3 shows a portion of an outline that student Michael B. Jackson constructed from a brainstorming list. The assignment is a five-paragraph essay on a life-changing event. Here Michael brainstorms the topic of "boot camp"; then he organizes his ideas into categories.

## Narrow Your Topic Through Prewriting Strategies

Next, use one or more of the following prewriting strategies to narrow your topic, focusing on the specific subideas and examples from your brainstorming session.[8] As you prewrite, keep paper length, due date, and other requirements (such as topic area or purpose) in mind. These requirements influence your choice of a final topic.

**Brainstorming.** The same process you used to generate ideas also helps you narrow your topic. Write down your thoughts about the possibility you have chosen, and then organize them into categories. See if any of the subideas or examples might make good topics.

**Freewriting.** When you freewrite, you use your creative ability to write whatever comes to mind without censoring ideas or worrying about language or organization. Creative freewriting enables you to begin integrating what you know.

**Asking Journalists' Questions.** Who? What? Where? When? Why? How? Ask these journalists' questions about any subidea or example to discover what you may want to discuss.

Prewriting helps you develop a topic broad enough to give you something with which to work but narrow enough to be manageable. Prewriting also helps you see what you know and what you don't know and where more research is required.

## Conduct Research and Make Notes

Try doing your research in stages. In the first stage, look for a basic overview that can lead to a thesis statement. In the second stage, go into more depth, tracking down information that helps you fill in gaps.

As you research, create source notes and content notes on index cards. These help you organize your work, keep track of your sources, and avoid plagiarism.

*Source notes* are the preliminary notes you take as you review research. Each source note should include the author's full name; the title of the work; the edition (if any); the publisher, year, and city of publication; issue and/or volume number when applicable (such as for a magazine); and the page numbers you consulted. After this bibliographic information, write a short summary and a critical evaluation of the work. Figure 9.4 shows an example of how you can write source notes on index cards.

*Content notes*, written on large index cards, in a notebook, or on your computer, are taken during a thorough reading and provide an in-depth look at sources. Use them to record the information you need to write your draft. To supplement your content notes, make notations— marginal notes, highlighting, and underlining—directly on photocopies of sources.

When research-based writing projects involve teamwork, you may need to adjust to the differences in how team members work. If you are collaborating with a student from a high-context culture such as Indonesia or the Philippines, for example, the student may hesitate to express an opinion in writing that differs from the instructor's. Because these cultures value respect to people in authority, disagreeing with the instructor is often considered rude. (For more on high- and low-context cultures, see Chapter 2.)

**WRITING PURPOSE**
The point of a paper, which is usually to inform or persuade readers.

**AUDIENCE**
The readers of your work for whom your purpose and content must be clear.

## Write a Thesis Statement

Your work has prepared you to write a *thesis statement*, the central message you want to communicate. The thesis statement states your subject and point of view, reflects your **writing purpose** and **audience**, and acts as the organizing principle of your paper.

| FIGURE 9.4 | Create source note cards as you review research |
| --- | --- |

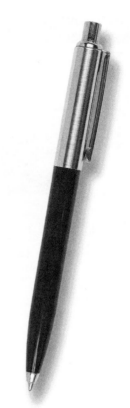

> LORENZ, KONRAD. *King Solomon's Ring*, New York: Crowell, 1952, pp. 102–122.
>
> Summary: Descriptions of the fascinating habits of various animals and birds.
>
> Evaluation: Although this book is old., it's a classic! Added pluses: the author can be funny and provocative.

## Write a Working Outline

The final step in the preparation process is writing a working outline or think link. Use this outline as a loose guide instead of a final structure. Only by allowing changes to occur do you get closer to what you really want to say.

## Create a Checklist

Use the checklist in Figure 9.5 to make sure your preparation is complete. Under Date Due, create your own writing schedule, giving each task an intended completion date. Work backward from the date the assignment is due and estimate how long it will take to complete each step. Keep in mind that you'll probably move back and forth among the tasks on the schedule.

| FIGURE 9.5 | Use a preparation checklist to complete tasks and stay on schedule |
| --- | --- |

| DATE DUE | TASK | IS IT COMPLETE? |
| --- | --- | --- |
| | Brainstorm | |
| | Define and narrow | |
| | Use prewriting strategies | |
| | Conduct research if necessary | |
| | Write thesis statement | |
| | Write working outline | |
| | Complete research | |

**FIGURE 9.6**   Think of the parts of your draft as a "writing sandwich"

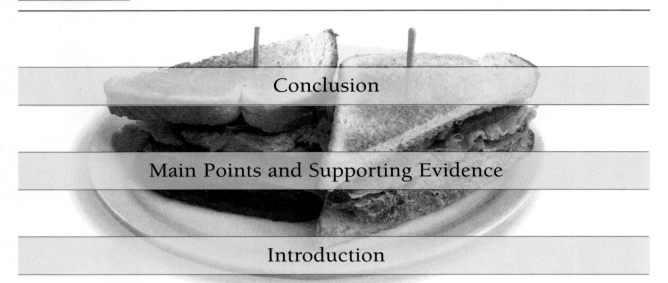

## Drafting

A first draft involves putting ideas down on paper for the first time—but not the last. You may write many versions of the assignment until you are satisfied. Each version moves you closer to saying exactly what you want in the way you want to say it.

When you think of drafting, it might help to imagine that you are creating a kind of "writing sandwich." The bottom slice of bread is the introduction, the top slice is the conclusion, and the sandwich stuffing is made of central ideas and supporting evidence (see Figure 9.6).

### Freewriting Your Rough Draft

Take everything that you have developed in the planning stages and freewrite a rough draft. For now, don't consciously think about your introduction, conclusion, or the structure within the paper's body. Simply focus on getting your ideas out onto paper. When you have something written, you can start to give it a more definite form. First, work on how you want to begin.

### Writing an Introduction

The introduction tells readers what the rest of the paper contains and includes a thesis statement. Take a look at this draft of an introduction for Michael's paper about the Coast Guard. The thesis statement is underlined at the end of the paragraph.

### Creating the Body of a Paper

The body of the paper contains your central ideas and supporting evidence. *Evidence* consists of facts, statistics, examples, and expert opinions. Think about how you might group the evidence with the particular ideas it supports.

## FIGURE 9.7 — Find the best way to organize the body of the paper

| ORGANIZATIONAL STRUCTURE | WHAT TO DO |
| --- | --- |
| Arrange ideas by time | Describe events in order or in reverse order. |
| Arrange ideas according to importance | Start with the idea that carries the most weight and move to less important ideas. Or move from the least to the most important ideas. |
| Arrange ideas by problem and solution | Start with a problem and then discuss solutions. |
| Arrange ideas to present an argument | Present one or both sides of an issue. |
| Arrange ideas in list form | Group a series of items. |
| Arrange ideas according to cause and effect | Show how events, situations, or ideas cause subsequent events, situations, or ideas. |
| Arrange ideas through the use of comparisons | Compare and contrast the characteristics of events, people, situations, ideas. |

Then, try to find a structure that helps you organize your ideas and evidence into a clear pattern. Figure 9.7 presents several organizational options.

## Writing the Conclusion

A conclusion summarizes the information that is in the body of your paper and critically evaluates what is important about it. Think about using one of the following strategies to conclude a paper:

- Summarize main points (if material is longer than three pages).
- Relate a provocative story, statistic, quote, or question.
- Call the reader to action.
- Look to the future.

Avoid introducing new facts or restating what you've already proved. Let your ideas in the body of the paper speak for themselves. Readers should feel that they have reached a natural point of completion.

## Avoiding Plagiarism: Crediting Authors and Sources

When you incorporate ideas from other sources into your work, you are using other writers' *intellectual property*. Using another writer's words, content, unique approach, or illustrations without crediting the author is called **plagiarism** and is illegal and unethical. The following techniques will help you properly credit sources and avoid plagiarism:

PLAGIARISM
The act of using someone else's exact words, figures, unique approach, or specific reasoning without giving appropriate credit.

- **Make source notes as you go.** Plagiarism often begins accidentally during research. You may forget to include quotation marks around a quotation, or you may intend to cite or paraphrase a source but never do. To avoid forgetting, write detailed source and content notes as you research. Try writing something like "Quotation from original; rewrite later" next to quoted material you copy into notes, and add bibliographic information (title, author, source, page number, etc.) so you don't spend hours trying to locate it later.

- **Learn the difference between a quotation and a paraphrase.** A *quotation* repeats a source's exact words, which are set off from the rest of the text by quotation marks. A *paraphrase* is a restatement of the quotation in your own words. A restatement requires that you completely rewrite the idea, not just remove or replace a few words. As Figure 9.8 illustrates, a paraphrase may not be acceptable if it is too close to the original.

- **Use a citation even for an acceptable paraphrase.** Take care to credit any source that you quote, paraphrase, or use as evidence. To credit a source, write a footnote or endnote that describes it, using the format preferred by your instructor. Writing handbooks explain the two standard documentation styles from the American Psychological Association (APA) and the Modern Language Association (MLA).

- **Understand that lifting material off the Internet is plagiarism.** Words in electronic form belong to the writer just as words in print form do. If you cut and paste sections from a source document onto your draft, you are committing plagiarism.

**FIGURE 9.8** Avoid plagiarism by learning how to paraphrase

---

**QUOTATION**

"The most common assumption that is made by persons who are communicating with one another is . . . that the other perceives, judges, thinks, and reasons the way he does. Identical twins communicate with ease. Persons from the same culture but with a different education, age, background, and experience often find communication difficult. American managers communicating with managers from other cultures experience greater difficulties in communication than with managers from their own culture."*

**UNACCEPTABLE PARAPHRASE** (THE UNDERLINED WORDS ARE TAKEN DIRECTLY FROM THE QUOTED SOURCE.)

When we communicate, we assume that the person to whom we are speaking perceives, judges, thinks, and reasons the way we do. This is not always the case. Although identical twins communicate with ease, persons from the same culture but with a different education, age, background, and experience often encounter communication problems. Communication problems are common among American managers as they attempt to communicate with managers from other cultures. They experience greater communication problems than when they communicate with managers from their own culture.

**ACCEPTABLE PARAPHRASE**

Many people fall into the trap of believing that everyone sees the world exactly as they do and that all people communicate according to the same assumptions. This belief is difficult to support even within our own culture as African-Americans, Hispanic-Americans, Asian-Americans, and others often attempt unsuccessfully to find common ground. When intercultural differences are thrown into the mix, such as when American managers working abroad attempt to communicate with managers from other cultures, clear communication becomes even harder.

---

*Source of quotation: Lynn Quitman Troyka, *Simon & Schuster Handbook for Writers* (Upper Saddle River, NJ: Prentice Hall, 1996).

Instructors consider work to be plagiarized when a student

- Submits a paper from a website that sells or gives away research papers.
- Buys a paper from a non-Internet service.
- Hands in a paper written by a fellow student or a family member.
- Copies material in a paper directly from a source without proper quotation marks or source citation.
- Paraphrases material in a paper from a source without proper source citation.

Students who plagiarize place their academic careers at risk, in part because the cheating is easy to discover. Increasingly, instructors are using anti-plagiarism software to investigate whether strings of words in student papers match those in a database.

Make a commitment to hand in your own work and to uphold the highest standards of academic integrity. The potential consequences of cheating are not worth the risk.

### Continue your Checklist

Create a checklist for your first draft (see Figure 9.9). The elements of a first draft do not have to be written in order. In fact, many writers prefer to write the introduction after the body of the paper, so the introduction reflects the paper's content and tone. Whatever order you choose, make sure your schedule gives you enough time for revisions.

## Revising

When you revise, you critically evaluate the word choice, paragraph structure, and style of your first draft. Be thorough as you add, delete, replace, and

**FIGURE 9.9**    Update your checklist for the first draft

| DATE DUE | TASK | IS IT COMPLETE? |
|---|---|---|
| | Freewrite a draft | |
| | Plan and write the introduction | |
| | Organize the body of the paper | |
| | Include research evidence in the body | |
| | Plan and write the conclusion | |
| | Check for plagiarism and rewrite passages to avoid it | |
| | Credit your sources | |
| | Solicit feedback | |

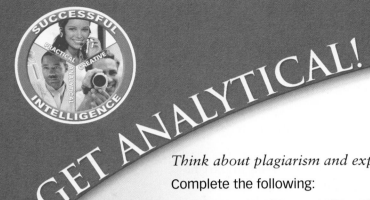

# Avoid Plagiarism

*Think about plagiarism and explore your views on this growing problem.*

Complete the following:

- Why is plagiarism considered an offense that involves both stealing and lying? Describe how you look at it.

- Citing sources indicates that you respect the ideas of others. List two additional ways that accurate source citation strengthens your writing and makes you a better student.

  1.

  2.

- What specific penalties for plagiarism are described in your college handbook? Explain whether you feel that these penalties are reasonable or excessive and whether they will keep students from plagiarizing.

- Many experts believe that researching on the Internet is behind many acts of plagiarism. Do you agree? Why or why not?

reorganize words, sentences, and paragraphs. If your instructor evaluates an early draft of your paper, incorporate his or her ideas into the final product. If you disagree with a point, schedule a conference to talk it over.

Some classes include a peer review process in which students critique each other's work. Many schools also have tutors in writing or learning centers who can act as peer readers of a draft. Figure 9.10 shows a paragraph from Michael's first draft, with revision comments added.

During the revision process, you assess what you have done and revisit any part of your work that is off the mark. The best time to critically evaluate your writing is after you let it sit for a while, says Dr. Mel Levine, author of *The Myth of Laziness*. "The writing experience needs time to incubate. It is preferable to check something several days later or the night after it came to be. With time, it is much easier to evaluate your own work, to detect and correct its flaws with some objectivity, and to deftly surmount the impasses that felt insurmountable while you were immersed in the act of writing."[9]

## Using Analytical Abilities as You Revise

Engage your analytical thinking to evaluate the content and form of your paper. Ask yourself these questions as you revise:

- Does the paper fulfill the requirements of the assignment?
- Will my audience understand my thesis and how I've supported it?
- Does the introduction prepare the reader and capture attention?

**FIGURE 9.10**   Sample first draft with revision comments

Of the changes that ~~happened to us,~~ [military recruits undergo,] the physical transformation is the ~~biggest.~~ [most evident] ~~When~~ [Too much] ~~we arrived at the training facility, it was January, cold and cloudy. At the time,~~ [Maybe— upon my January arrival at the training facility,] I was a

little thin, but I had been working out and thought that I could physically do anything.

Oh boy, was I wrong! The Chief said to us right away: "Get down, maggots!" [his trademark phrase] Upon this

command, we [were] all to drop to the ground and do [endless] military-style push-ups. Water survival

tactics were also part of the training ~~that we had to complete.~~ [unnecessary] Occasionally, my dreams of

home were interrupted at 3 a.m. when we had a surprise aquatic test. Although we ~~didn't~~ [resented]

~~feel too happy about~~ this sub-human treatment at the time, we learned to appreciate how [mention how chief was involved]

the conditioning was turning our bodies into fine-tuned machines. [say more about this (swimming in uniform incident?)]

- Is the body of the paper organized effectively?
- Is each idea fully developed, explained, and supported by examples?
- Are my ideas connected to one another through logical transitions?
- Do I have a clear, concise, simple writing style?
- Does the conclusion provide a natural ending to the paper?

## Evaluating Paragraph Structure

Make sure that each paragraph has a *topic sentence* that states the paragraph's main idea (a topic sentence does for a paragraph what a thesis statement does for an entire paper). The remainder of the paragraph should support the idea with evidence. Most topic sentences are at the beginning of the paragraph, although sometimes topic sentences appear elsewhere.

In addition, examine how paragraphs flow into one another by evaluating transitions—the words, phrases, or sentences that connect ideas.

## Checking for Clarity and Conciseness

Rewrite wordy phrases in a more straightforward, conversational way. For example, write "if" instead of "in the event that," and "now" instead of "at this point in time."

# Editing

*Editing* involves correcting technical mistakes in spelling, grammar, and punctuation, as well as checking for consistency in such elements as abbreviations and capitalization. Editing comes last, after you are satisfied with your ideas, organization, and writing style. If you use a computer, start with the grammar check and spell check to find mistakes, realizing that you still need to check your work manually. Although a spell checker won't pick up the mistake in the sentence, "They are not hear on Tuesdays," someone who is reading for sense will.

Peer editing can sharpen your writing. Kristina Torres, a senior at Susquehanna University in Selinsgrove, Pennsylvania, is convinced that her relationship with Adam Cole helped make her a better writer. A senior, she has worked with Adam for more than three years to fine-tune her work. In one case, Adam helped Kristina cut a 40-page paper in half. "It's hard to do that on your own," she said, "because you get really attached to a line or a section. You need to have someone who can help you step back and take another look at it."[10]

*Proofreading* is the last editing stage and happens once your paper reaches its final form. Proofreading means reading every word and sentence for accuracy. Look for technical mistakes, run-on sentences, and sentence fragments. Look for incorrect word usage and unclear references.

## A Final Checklist

You are now ready to complete your revising and editing checklist. All the tasks listed in Figure 9.11 should be complete before you submit your paper. Figure 9.12 shows the final version of Michael's paper.

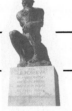

Writing is rewriting.

ERNEST HEMINGWAY

**FIGURE 9.11** Use a revising and editing checklist to finalize your paper

| DATE DUE | TASK | IS IT COMPLETE? |
|---|---|---|
| | Check the body of the paper for clear thinking and adequate support of ideas | |
| | Finalize introduction and conclusion | |
| | Check word spelling, usage, and grammar | |
| | Check paragraph structure | |
| | Make sure language is familiar and concise | |
| | Check punctuation and capitalization | |
| | Check transitions | |
| | Eliminate sexist language | |
| | Get feedback from peers and/or instructor | |

**FIGURE 9.12** Sample final version of paper incorporates all changes

Michael B. Jackson                                                                                                    March 19, 2006

## BOYS TO MEN

His stature was one of confidence, often misinterpreted by others as cockiness. His small frame was lean and agile, yet stiff and upright, as though every move were a calculated formula. For the longest eight weeks of my life, he was my father, my instructor, my leader, and my worst enemy. His name is Chief Marzloff, and he had the task of shaping the lives and careers of the youngest, newest members of the U.S. Coast Guard. As our Basic Training Company Commander, he took his job very seriously and demanded that we do the same. Within a limited time span, he conditioned our bodies, developed our self-confidence, and instilled within us a strong mental discipline.

Of the changes that recruits in military basic training undergo, the physical transformation is the most immediately evident. On my January arrival at the training facility, I was a little thin, but I had been working out and thought that I could physically do anything. Oh boy, was I wrong! The Chief wasted no time in introducing me to one of his trademark phrases: "Get down, maggots!" Upon this command, we were all to drop to the ground and produce endless counts of military-style push-ups. Later, we found out that exercise prepared us for hitting the deck in the event of enemy fire. Water survival tactics were also part of the training. Occasionally, my dreams of home were interrupted at about 3 A.M. when our company was selected for a surprise aquatic test. I recall one such test that required us to swim laps around the perimeter of a pool while in full uniform. I felt like a salmon swimming upstream, fueled only by natural instinct. Although we resented this subhuman treatment at the time, we learned to appreciate how the strict guidance of the Chief was turning our bodies into fine-tuned machines.

Beyond physical ability, Chief Marzloff also played an integral role in the development of our self-confidence. He would often declare in his raspy voice, "Look me in the eyes when you speak to me! Show me that you believe what you're saying!" He taught us that anything less was an expression of disrespect. Furthermore, he appeared to attack a personal habit of my own. It seemed that whenever he would speak to me individually, I would nervously nod my head in response. I was trying to demonstrate that I understood, but to him, I was blindly accepting anything that he said. He would roar, "That is a sign of weakness!" Needless to say, I am now conscious of all bodily motions when communicating with others. The Chief also reinforced self-confidence through his own example. He walked with his square chin up and chest out, like the proud parent of a newborn baby. He always gave the appearance that he had something to do, and that he was in complete control. Collectively, the methods that the Chief used were all successful in developing our self-confidence.

Perhaps the Chief's greatest contribution was the mental discipline that he instilled in his recruits. He taught us that physical ability and self-confidence were nothing without the mental discipline required to obtain any worthwhile goal. For us, this discipline began with adapting to the military lifestyle. Our day began promptly at 0500 hours, early enough to awaken the oversleeping roosters. By 0515 hours, we had to have showered, shaved, and perfectly donned our uniforms. At that point, we were marched to the galley for chow, where we learned to take only what is necessary, rather than indulging. Before each meal, the Chief would warn, "Get what you want, but you will eat all that you get!" After he made good on his threat a few times, we all got the point. Throughout our stay, the Chief repeatedly stressed the significance of self-discipline. He would calmly utter, "Give a little now, get a lot later." I guess that meant different things to all of us. For me, it was a simple phrase that would later become my personal philosophy on life. The Chief went to great lengths to ensure that everyone under his direction possessed the mental discipline required to be successful in boot camp or in any of life's challenges.

Chief Marzloff was a remarkable role model and a positive influence on many lives. I never saw him smile, but it was evident that he genuinely cared a great deal about his job and all the lives that he touched. This man single-handedly conditioned our bodies, developed our self-confidence, and instilled a strong mental discipline that remains in me to this day. I have not seen the Chief since March 28, 1995, graduation day. Over the years, however, I have incorporated many of his ideals into my life. Above all, he taught us the true meaning of the U.S. Coast Guard slogan, "Semper Paratus" (Always Ready).

Your final paper reflects your efforts. Ideally, you have a piece of work that shows how you used your analytical, creative, and practical thinking to communicate ideas.

# How Can You Do an *Effective* Presentation?

One key way to communicate with others is through an effective presentation. In school, you may be asked to deliver a speech, take an oral exam, or present a team project. When you ask a question or make a comment in class, you are using public-speaking skills. On the job, you will need to deliver presentations to colleagues, run meetings, and provide information to patients.

The public-speaking skills that you learn for presentations will help you make a favorable impression in *any* setting such as when you meet with an instructor, summarize a reading for your study group, or have a planning session at work. When you are articulate, others take notice. You do not have to speak perfect English, just be prepared.

## Prepare

Speaking in front of others involves preparation, strategy, and confidence. Planning a speech is similar to planning a piece of writing; you must know your topic and audience and think about presentation strategy, organization, and word choice. Specifically, you should do the following:

- **Think through what you wish to say and why.** What is your purpose—to make or refute an argument, present information, entertain? Have a goal for your speech.
- **Plan.** Take time to think about who your listeners are and how they are likely to respond. Then, get organized. Brainstorm your topic—narrow it with prewriting strategies, determine your thesis, write an outline, and do research.
- **Draft your thoughts.** Draft your speech. Illustrate ideas with examples, and show how examples lead to ideas. As in writing, have a clear beginning and an end. Start with an attention getter and conclude with a wrap-up that summarizes your thoughts and leaves your audience with something to remember.
- **Integrate visual aids.** Think about building your speech around visual aids including charts, maps, slides and photographs, and props. Learn software programs to create presentation graphics.

## Practice Your Performance

The element of performance distinguishes speaking from writing. Here are tips to keep in mind:

- **Know the parameters.** How long do you have? Where are you speaking? Be aware of the setting—where your audience will be and available props (e.g., a podium, a table, a blackboard).

- **Pay attention to the physical.** Your body position, voice, and clothing contribute to the impression you make. Your goal is to look and sound good and to appear relaxed. Try to make eye contact with your audience, and walk around if you are comfortable presenting in that way.

- **Practice ahead of time.** Do a test run with friends or alone. If possible, practice in the room where you will speak. Audiotape or videotape your practice sessions and evaluate your performance.

- **Be yourself.** When you speak, you express your personality through your words and presence. Don't be afraid to add your own style to the presentation. Take deep breaths. Smile. Know that you can speak well and that your audience wants to see you succeed. Finally, envision your own success.

---

## *The Best All-Purpose Presentation Format You Will Ever Find*

The presentation has three parts:

1. The introduction
2. The discussion (content or information you wish to convey)
3. The conclusion

Each of these parts can be broken down:

I. Introduction
   a. Attention-getting opener (question, statistics)
   b. Agenda, or preview, of what you will cover

II. Discussion
   a. Main points
   b. Logical order (chronological, problem to solution)
   c. Data to support the points (use research to support your points)

III. Conclusion
   a. Summary, or review, of your presentation (don't add anything new here!)
   b. Memorable ending (quote, point of emphasis, the one thing you absolutely want your audience to take away)

The timing of each section is easy too.

   15% on the introduction
   75% on the discussion
   10% on the conclusion

Timing may vary depending on the audience. If you are talking to a group of teenagers or children you may spend 75% on the attention getter and 15% or less on the discussion—making just one point. That one point might be don't smoke or don't take drugs.

Use this format for any presentation. You can add PowerPoint slides, overheads, flip charts, or other visual aids during the presentation to add emphasis and interest. You may also add music if that fits the situation.

### Stage Fright

Preparing and practicing are the best ways to counter stage fright. Remember that the more often you make yourself talk in front of other people the faster you will get over fear of public speaking. It can be done. One of this book's authors, Janet Katz, was so afraid of public speaking that she only took science classes in college to avoid speeches. Later, she found out she loved science and that led to nursing. But she found out in nursing school and as a nurse that speaking was unavoidable. Nurses do lots of patient and family teaching, and they teach their colleagues as well. Janet started with short, easy presentations and worked her way up. She says, "Look upon giving a presentation as a performance and most of all have fun—do it for yourself. If I could get over my fear, you can too—I was terrified; now I love it. I still get nervous but know that nervousness is just a part of the presentation."

Here are a few tips:

- Almost everyone has a fear of public speaking—you are not alone.
- Take focus off yourself by focusing on the audience and/or focusing on the message you wish to get across.
- Use your slides or other visual aids to take the audience's attention off you.
- Remember that the audience wants you to succeed, not to fail.
- Experience over time will reduce stage fright.
- Even the most successful public figures get stage fright.

Adapted from Leon Fletcher, *How to Speak Like a Pro* (New York: Ballantine Books, 1983).

# *Sùa*

*Sùa* is a Shoshone Indian word, derived from the Uto-Aztecna language, that means "to think." Use your thinking skills to evaluate research sources as the basis for your positions and communicate your conclusions effectively through writing and speaking. Through the power of thought, you will choose sources that support your thesis and express your insights.

# Building World-Class Skills

## for College, Career, and Life Success

## Create Your Future

## DEVELOPING SUCCESSFUL INTELLIGENCE

### *Putting It All Together*

**Be a Planner.** Engage analytical, creative, and practical skills as you work through the planning stage of writing.

**Step 1. Think it through:** *Analyze your writing goal.* Imagine that you have been asked to write an essay on a time when you turned a difficulty into an opportunity. First, write a brief description of your topic:

Next, think about your purpose and audience. How might you frame your purpose if you were writing to a person who is going through a tough time and needs inspiration? How would your purpose change if you were writing to an instructor who wanted to know what you learned from a difficult experience? Write your purpose and intended audience here.

**Step 2. Think out of the box:** *Prewrite to create ideas.* On a separate sheet of paper, use prewriting strategies to start the flow of ideas.

- Brainstorm your ideas.
- Freewrite.
- Ask journalists' questions.

**Step 3. Make it happen:** *Write a thesis statement.* With the thesis statement, you make your topic as specific as possible and you clearly define your purpose. Write your thesis statement here:

## TEAM BUILDING

### *Collaborative Solutions*

**Team Research.** Join with three other classmates and decide on two relatively narrow research topics that interest all of you and that you can investigate by

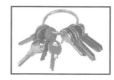

spending no more than an hour in the library. The first topic should be current and in the news—for example, safety problems in sport utility vehicles (SUVs), body piercing, or the changing U.S. family. The second topic should be more academic and historical—for example, the polio epidemic in the 1950s, the Irish potato famine, or South African apartheid.

Working alone, team members will use the college library and the Internet to research both topics. Set a research time limit of no more than one hour per topic. The goal should be to collect a list of sources for later investigation. When everyone is through, the group should come together to discuss the research process. Ask each other questions such as:

- How did you attack and organize your research for each topic?
- What research tools did you use to investigate each topic?
- How did your research differ from topic to topic? Why do you think this was the case?
- How did your use of library and Internet resources differ from topic to topic?
- Which research techniques yielded the best results? Which techniques led to dead ends?

Next, compare the specific results of everyone's research. Analyze each source for what it is likely to yield in the form of useful information. Finally, come together as a group and discuss what you learned that might improve your approach to library and Internet research.

## WRITING
### *Discovery Through Journaling*

*Record your thoughts on a separate piece of paper or in a journal.*

**Learning from Other Writers.** Identify a piece of powerful writing that you have recently read. (It could be a work of literature, a biography, a magazine or newspaper article, or even a section from one of your college texts.) Describe, in detail, why it was powerful. Did it make you feel something, think something, or take action? Why? What can you learn about writing from this piece that you can apply to your own writing?

## CAREER PORTFOLIO
### *Plan for Success*

**Writing Sample: A Job Interview Cover Letter.** To secure a job interview, you will, at some point, have to write a letter describing your background and explaining your value to the company. For your portfolio, write a one-page, three-paragraph cover letter to a prospective employer. (The letter will accompany your résumé.) Be creative—you may use fictitious names, but select a career and industry that interest you. Use the format shown in the sample letter in Figure 9.13.

First name Last name
1234 Your Street
City, ST 12345

November 1, 2005

Ms. Prospective Employer
Prospective Company
5432 Their Street
City, ST 54321

Dear Ms. Employer:

On the advice of Mr. X, career center adviser at Y College, I am writing to inquire about the position of production assistant at XYZ Radio. I read the description of the job and your company on the career center's employment-opportunity bulletin board, and I would like to apply for the position.

I am a senior at Y College and will graduate this spring with a degree in communications. Since my junior year when I declared my major, I have wanted to pursue a career in radio. For the last year I have worked as a production intern at WCOL Radio, the college's station, and have occasionally filled in as a disc jockey on the evening news show. I enjoy being on the air, but my primary interest is production and programming. My enclosed résumé will tell you more about my background and experience.

I would be pleased to talk with you in person about the position. You can reach me anytime at 555/555-5555 or by e-mail at xxxx@example.com. Thank you for your consideration, and I look forward to meeting you.

Sincerely,

*Sign Your Name Here*

First name Last name

Enclosure(s) *(use this notation if you have included a résumé or other item with your letter)*

- **Introductory paragraph.** Start with an attention getter, a statement that convinces the employer to read on. For example, name a person the employer knows who told you to write, or refer to something positive about the company that you read in the paper. Identify the position for which you are applying, and tell the employer that you are interested in working for the company.

- **Middle paragraph.** Sell your value. Try to convince the employer that hiring you will help the company in some way. Center your sales effort on your experience in school and the workplace. If possible, tie your qualifications to the needs of the company. Refer indirectly to your enclosed résumé.

- **Final paragraph.** Close with a call to action. Ask the employer to call you, or tell the employer to expect your call to arrange an interview.

Exchange your first draft with a classmate. Read each other's letter and make notes in the margins that try to improve the letter's impact and persuasiveness, as well as its writing style, grammar, punctuation, and spelling. Discuss each letter and make whatever corrections are necessary to produce a well-written, persuasive letter. Create a final draft for your portfolio.

# JOIN A NURSING HONOR SOCIETY

An international student honor society based on scholarship and research is Sigma Theta Tau. When you become a successful nursing student you can ask a faculty member to nominate you. Following is an overview from its website, www.nursingsociety.org:

- Sigma Theta Tau International is dedicated to improving the health of people worldwide by increasing the scientific base of nursing practice.

- Members are nursing scholars committed to the pursuit of excellence in clinical practice, education, research and leadership.

- We believe that broadening the base of nursing knowledge through knowledge development, dissemination and use offers great promise for promoting a healthier populace.

- We are committed to furthering nursing research in health care delivery and public policy.

- We sustain and support nursing's development and provide vision for the future of nursing and health care through our network of worldwide community of nurse scholars.

- We make available our diverse resources to all people and institutions interested in the scientific knowledge base of the nursing profession.

## Suggested Readings

Becker, Howard S. *Tricks of the Trade: How to Think About Your Research While You're Doing It*. Chicago: University of Chicago Press, 1998.

Booth, Wayne C., Gregory G. Columb, and Joseph M. Williams. *The Craft of Research*, 2nd ed. Chicago: University of Chicago Press, 2003.

Cameron, Julia. *The Right to Write: An Invitation into the Writing Life*. New York: Putnam, 2000.

Gibaldi, Joseph, and Phyllis Franklin. *MLA Handbook for Writers of Research Papers*, 6th ed. New York: Modern Language Association of America, 2003.

LaRocque, Paula. *Championship Writing: 50 Ways to Improve Your Writing*. Oak Park, IL: Marion Street Press, 2000.

Markman, Peter T., and Roberta H. Markman. *10 Steps in Writing the Research Paper*, 6th ed. New York: Barron's Educational Series, 2001.

Strunk, William, Jr., and E. B. White. *The Elements of Style*, 4th ed. New York: Allyn & Bacon, 2000.

Troyka, Lynn Quitman. *Simon & Schuster Handbook for Writers*, 7th ed. Upper Saddle River, NJ: Prentice Hall, 2004.

Walsch, Bill. *Lapsing into a Comma: A Curmudgeon's Guide to the Many Things That Can Go Wrong in Print—and How to Avoid Them*. New York: Contemporary Books, 2000.

Williams, Joseph M. *Style: Ten Lessons in Clarity and Grace*. Chicago: University of Chicago Press, 2003.

## Internet Resources

Prentice Hall Student Success SuperSite—study skills section (valuable information on writing and research): **www.prenhall.com/success**

National Writing Centers Association (a collection of writing labs and writing centers on the Web): **http://iwca.syr.edu**

Online Writing Lab—Purdue University: **http://owl.english.purdue.edu**

How to Organize a Research Paper and Document It with MLA Citations (specific citation rules from the Modern Language Association): **www.geocities.com/Athens/Oracle/4184**

A Student's Guide to WWW Research: Web Searching, Web Page Evaluation, and Research Strategies (a comprehensive site developed at St. Louis University): **www.slu.edu/departments/english/research**

## Endnotes

[1] Scott Carlson, "The Deserted Library: As Students Work Online, Reading Rooms Empty Out—Leading Some Campuses to Add Starbucks," *The Chronicle of Higher Education* (November 16, 2001). Retrieved March 2004, from: http://chronicle.com/weekly/v48/i12/12a03501.htm.

[2] Indiana University website, "Amazing Student, Chad Clunie: On a Knowledge Quest." Available: http://excellence.indiana.edu/clunie/.

[3] Joyce Kasman Valenza, "Skills That College Freshmen Need," *Philadelphia Inquirer*, April 26, 2001, p. NA.

[4] Jeffrey R. Young, "Libraries Try to Widen Google's Eyes," *The Chronicle of Higher Education*, May 21, 2004, p. A1.

[5] Lori Leibovich, "Choosing Quick Hits Over the Card Catalog," *New York Times*, August 10, 2000, p. 1.

[6] David Hochman, "In Searching We Trust," *New York Times*, March 14, 2004, Section 9, p. 1.

[7] Floyd H. Johnson, "The Internet and Research: Proceed with Caution" (May 1996). Retrieved August 2000, from: www.lanl.gov/SFC/96/posters.html#johnson.

[8] Analysis based on Lynn Quitman Troyka, *Simon & Schuster Handbook for Writers* (Upper Saddle River, NJ: Prentice Hall, 1996), pp. 22–23.

[9] Mel Levine, *The Myth of Laziness* (New York: Simon & Schuster, 2003, p. 183).

[10] Thomas Bartlett, "Undergraduates Heed the Writer's Muse: English Departments Add Programs as More Students Push to Write Fiction and Poetry," *The Chronicle of Higher Education* (March 15, 2002). Retrieved March 2004, from: http://chronicle.com/weekly/v48/i27/2703901.htm.

# Slay the Math Anxiety Dragon

A special form of test anxiety, math anxiety is based on common misconceptions about math, such as the notion that people are born with or without an ability to think quantitatively or that men are better at math than women. Students who feel they can't do math may give up without asking for help. On exams, these students may experience a range of physical symptoms—including sweating, nausea, dizziness, headaches, and fatigue—that reduce their ability to concentrate and leave them feeling defeated.

The material in this Study Break is designed to help you deal with the kind of math-related anxiety that affects your grades on exams. As you learn concrete ways to calm your nerves and discover special techniques for math tests, you will feel more confident in your ability to succeed.

These test-taking tips supplement what you learned in Chapter 7, "Test Taking: Showing What You Know," in which you studied test taking in depth and generalized test anxiety. Chapter 7 also includes valuable information on test preparation, general test-taking strategies, strategies for handling different types of test questions, and learning from test mistakes.

## Use Special Techniques for Math Tests

Use the general test-taking strategies presented in Chapter 7 as well as the techniques here to achieve better results on math exams.

- **Read through the exam first.** When you first get an exam, read through every problem quickly and make notes on how you might attempt to solve the problems.

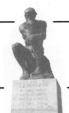

Do not worry about your difficulties in mathematics; I assure you that mine are greater.

ALBERT EINSTEIN

- **Analyze Problems Carefully.** Categorize problems according to type. Take the "givens" into account, and write down any formulas, theorems, or definitions that apply before you begin. Focus on what you want to find or prove.

- **Estimate Before You Begin to Come Up With a Ballpark Solution.** Work the problem and check the solution against your estimate. The two answers should be close. If they're not, recheck your calculations. You may have made a calculation error.

## Gauge Your Level of Math Anxiety

Use the questionnaire on the next page to get an idea of your math anxiety level.

- **Break the Calculation into the Smallest Possible Pieces.** Go step by step, and don't move on to the next step until you are clear about what you've done so far.
- **Recall How You Solved Similar Problems.** Past experience can provide valuable clues.
- **Draw a Picture to Help You See the Problem.** Visual images such as a diagram, chart, probability tree, or geometric figure may help clarify your thinking.
- **Be Neat.** Sloppy numbers can mean the difference between a right and a wrong answer. A 4 that looks like a 9 will be marked wrong.
- **Use the Opposite Operation to Check Your Work.** Work backward from your answer to see if you are right.
- **Look Back at the Question to Be Sure You Did Everything.** Did you answer every part of the question? Did you show all required work?

## Decide How Well These Techniques Work for You

Use what you just learned about yourself and math to answer the following questions:

- What did you learn from the math anxiety questionnaire? Describe your current level of math anxiety.
- What effect do you think your attitude toward math will have on your future?
- Which suggestions for reducing math anxiety are you likely to use? How do you think they will help you feel more comfortable with math?
- Which suggestions for improving your performance on math tests are you likely to use?
- What other ways can you think of to improve your math performance?

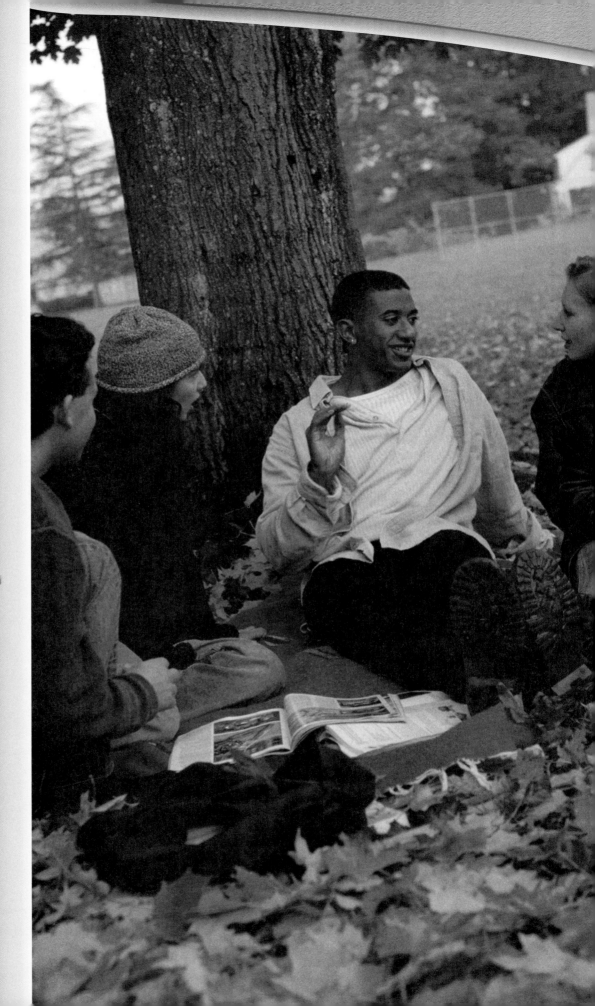

# CONNECT: RELATING TO OTHERS

*COMMUNICATING IN A DIVERSE WORLD*

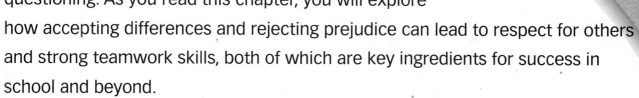

A mong your most meaningful, life-changing experiences at college will be those that take you out of your comfort zone and force you to question your thinking and even your basic beliefs. Encountering the diversity of the people around you can inspire this kind of questioning. As you read this chapter, you will explore how accepting differences and rejecting prejudice can lead to respect for others and strong teamwork skills, both of which are key ingredients for success in school and beyond.

In this chapter, you will investigate how analytical, creative, and practical abilities can help you build the cultural competence that will allow you to relate successfully to others. You will explore how to communicate effectively, investigating different communication styles and methods for handling conflict. Finally, you will look at how your personal relationships can inspire you and enhance your college and life experience.

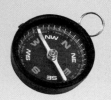

# Q & A BLUE SKY QUESTIONS DOWN-TO-EARTH ANSWERS

### *How can being bilingual help me as a nurse? How can I adjust to a new society and connect to my college fellows and people of my community?*

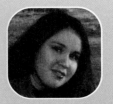

Liduvina Perez
Senior, Arizona State
University, Tempe, Arizona

I've been a translator for as long as I can remember. My mother suffered from heart disease, and she didn't speak English. Because I knew both English and Spanish, I served as the interpreter for my mother and explained what the doctors and nurses said. Every other Tuesday I would have to miss school so that I could go with my mother to the clinic and translate for her. It became routine for me to fall behind in school, but I worked hard to stay caught up.

When you're only 6 years old, it's difficult to translate medical terms and procedures correctly, so I'm sure I made mistakes at times. This role put me under a lot of pressure, but I also felt good about helping my mom. Not long after she had a pacemaker put in, my mother died of a heart attack. I was 12 years old. After that I went to live with my godparents, and they encouraged me to pursue an education. Taking care of my mother is the main reason I decided to train for a career in nursing.

Now that I'm in clinicals, I see many non-English-speaking patients struggle, as my mother did, to grasp what is happening to them. For instance, during my medical-surgical rotation, I had a Mexican patient with tuberculosis. He didn't understand his disease or how to help himself recover. There are many patients like him, and I see fear and confusion on their faces, too. We have a large Hispanic population in Arizona, and I can tell it really helps when I step in and explain things to them in their language.

During my community health rotation I saw a little Asian girl begin her eye-screening test with a school nurse, but the child didn't know English. Then the nurse did something that I thought was very smart and sensitive. She pulled out picture cards that showed children doing different things related to an eye exam. The nurse pointed to the cards to demonstrate what she wanted the little girl to do. The child did it, and the eye exam was successfully completed. I found that very inspiring.

I will be the first person in my family to graduate from college. I'm also considering graduate school to become a nurse practitioner. As I prepare to enter the diverse world of nursing, what can I do to fulfill my role as a bilingual professional?

## PRACTICAL ANSWERS

### *People will trust you and may receive better care.*

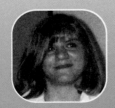

Elda G. Ramirez
Assistant Professor of
Clinical Nursing, University
of Texas Health Science
Center, Houston, Texas

I can certainly appreciate your question because I grew up in a barrio near the border of Mexico. Some of us spoke better English than others, but there was a barrier even more profound than language: the barrier of social class. When I revisit my old neighborhood, I see barefoot kids play outside even on cold days, and they live in houses that are not up to building code. Yet these same children have the latest toys and their parents drive new cars. The dichotomy is almost unbelievable as I watch these families struggle to fit into the American way of life.

When I was 13 I volunteered in emergency care at the local hospital, so I've had the desire to be a nurse for a long time. I didn't grow up experiencing prejudice because I was only around my own people, and I never thought much about ethnicity. But when I arrived in Houston to attend college, all of a sudden I was referred to as "this Mexican girl." When people met me, my being Hispanic seemed to be at the forefront of their mind.

When I started seeing Hispanic patients during my clinical rotations, I was angry because they weren't taking care of themselves. They came in with conditions that should have been taken care of a long time ago. Many of these patients had put off their health care needs to avoid interacting with people who don't speak their language. I criticized and even yelled at them for eating *menudo* and corn tortillas. At this point I began to face an identity crisis. I realized I had been educated by a Westernized force of knowledge that didn't fit my people.

A personal breakthrough occurred when I met Dr. Dalhia Rojas, and she became my mentor. She asked me two questions: "What are you doing for your people, and do you like who you are becoming?" She also asked me if I was condescending to the very people I was trying to help. Thinking through these questions prompted me to choose a direction for my career. For my undergraduate community experience project, I decided to work at an impoverished apartment complex where several Hispanic families lived. When I walked into that community I found myself. Today I feel privileged to be highly educated, and I also feel privileged to be Hispanic. I am them and they are me.

My suggestion to you is to find out what you love and what you believe in. Also, I think it's important to understand that when you change one person you really do change the world. With my patients and my students I try to break the stereotypical visions they have of other cultures. If you attack the patient's inner self, they become defensive. But when you identify with them, perhaps by saying, "I like that food too, but I've tried this as an alternative," you become the strongest tool to better that society. Being a bilingual professional is about embracing the culture and incorporating health care knowledge into that tradition.

One final piece of advice. As a nursing professional, it's easy to become overwhelmed. When I find myself getting off balance I go back to my roots by refocusing on the three things that matter most to me: Family, God, and self. You need to take care of yourself, too. You can't give something away that you don't have. Providing health care isn't only about healing the physical. True healing is what you give of yourself to your patients: a smile, reassuring words, a hug when they leave. My patients often bless me by expressing their thanks or by saying, "God bless you for what you've done for me." We touch people when we keep the whole person in mind.

# How Do You Experience *Diversity?*

A century ago it was possible to live an entire lifetime knowing no one from a culture different from your own. Not so today. With waves of new immigrants continually arriving, just as they have done throughout U.S. history, American society consists of people from a multitude of countries and cultural backgrounds.

The speed of cultural change is dramatic: In the 2000 census, American citizens described themselves in terms of 63 different racial categories, compared with only 5 in 1990.[1] Technology and economic interdependence add to our growing cultural awareness. Cable television, the Internet, and the global marketplace link people from all over the world in ways that were unimaginable less than a decade ago. You have unprecedented access to information about what people do and how they live in nearly every corner of the globe.

## Diversity Affects Everyone

As you read in Chapter 1, diversity exists both within each person and among all people:

- **The diversity within each person.** Your physical being, personality, learning style, talents and skills, and analytical, creative, and practical abilities set you apart from everyone else. *No one else has been or will ever be exactly like you.*

- **The diversity among people.** Differences in skin color, gender, ethnicity and national origin, age, physical characteristics and abilities, and sexual orientation are among the major differences that exist among people. Differences in cultural and religious beliefs and practices, education and socioeconomic status, family background, and marital and parental status add to our country's cultural mosaic.

You may work with people from different backgrounds. You may encounter all kinds of people as you attend religious services, buy groceries and stamps, swim at a pool, or socialize. You may experience diversity within your family—often the kind of diversity that is not visible. Even if friends or family members have the same racial and ethnic background as you do, they might be completely different in how they learn, the way they communicate, what they value, and what they do well.

## Diversity on Campus

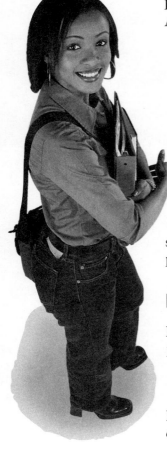

In college you are likely to meet classmates or instructors who reflect America's growing diversity, including

- Bi- or multiracial individuals or those who come from families with more than one religious tradition.

- English-learning speakers who may have immigrated from countries outside the United States.

- People older than "traditional" 18- to 22-year-old students.

- Persons living with various kinds of disabilities.

- Persons practicing different lifestyles—often expressed in the way they dress, their interests, their sexual orientation, and their leisure activities.

Being able to appreciate and adjust to differences among people is crucial to your success at school, at work, and in your personal relationships. You can accomplish this goal by using your analytical, creative, and practical abilities to develop cultural competence.

## Diversity in Nursing

For you as a nursing student, diversity in nursing means that you will be a part of a global structure. As a nurse of any kind, you will not be working in a vacuum; you will have contact with a variety of people, even if you work in a small clinic miles from anyone or anything. You will still need to write grants, present your findings, and communicate to get supplies. Furthermore, the people you contact will not always be from the same culture as you. This is not a choice anymore, but a reality. Part of your education is learning about diversity and, more important, participating in it. You can accomplish this by

- Meeting and working with other students in your classes who are from ethnic or cultural backgrounds different from yours.
- Taking courses on multiculturalism.
- Traveling to other countries to study or to visit.
- Reading books, fiction and nonfiction, that describe the perspectives of people who have grown up in different circumstances from yours.
- Watching foreign movies or those made by minority groups (e.g., *Smoke Signals*, 1998, an award-winning movie produced, directed, written, and acted by American Indians; and *Rabbit Proof Fence*, 2003, about indigenous people in Australia).
- Keeping up with international news.
- Learning a foreign language.

# What Is *Cultural* Competence in Nursing?

As you learned in Chapter 2, *cultural competence* refers to the ability to understand and appreciate differences among people and change your behavior in a way that enhances, rather than detracts from, relationships and communication. First, cultural competence means understanding your own culture including how you view the world, your values, and your traditions. Second, it means understanding others' cultures and using this understanding to provide patient care that is meaningful and appropriate. To do this you must not only have information about other cultures, but you must also learn to respect other viewpoints. You must also be flexible so you can adapt to change.

T. Cross and colleagues list five factors that contribute to cultural competence, and although this is an older reference, it is still frequently used in current readings about cultural competence:[2]

1. Valuing diversity;
2. Having the capacity for cultural self-assessment (knowing what your culture is);
3. Being conscious of the dynamics inherent when cultures interact;
4. Having institutionalized cultural knowledge; and
5. Having developed adaptations of service delivery reflecting an understanding of cultural diversity.

Cultural competence is growing in importance in all of the health sciences. As a nurse, as noted in this chapter, you will be working with many different people. Although international travel is one good way to gain cultural competence, it is possible to gain these experiences in the United States. There are many different cultures right here. You can learn from meeting people, reading books, watching movies, and going to different places to eat. One book you might like to read is *The Spirit Catches You and You Fall Down* by Anne Fadiman. This book will open your eyes to how someone of another culture does not receive the care needed because of misunderstandings within the American health care system. How someone views illness, its causes, and its treatments is affected by the person's culture. Cultural competence is the ability to take your knowledge and apply it such that your practice and the policies of your workplace are not creating barriers to quality health care for all.

Because the perception of illness and disease and their causes varies by culture, health care may be affected. Culture influences how people seek health care and how they behave toward health care providers. How we care for patients and how patients respond to this care are greatly influenced by culture. Health care providers must have the ability and knowledge to communicate and understand culturally influenced health behaviors. Having this ability and knowledge can eliminate barriers to health care. Nurses and health care organizations need to develop policies, practices, and procedures to deliver culturally competent care.

As a resource for working with patients and their families from other countries, you may want to check out the Nursing Students Without Borders website: www.nswb.org.

The Transcultural Nursing Association says this about cultural competence on its website (www.culturediversity.org):

> As individuals, nurses and health care providers, we need to learn to ask questions sensitively and to show respect for different cultural beliefs. Most important, we must listen to our patients carefully. The main source of problems in caring for patients from diverse cultural backgrounds is the lack of understanding and tolerance. Very often, neither the nurse nor the patient understands the other's perspective.

You might also go to the Office on Minority Health (www.omh.gov) for cultural competency standards and information on health disparities.

## Communicating Respect to Patients: The Top-10 Questions

The most common advice given by health care providers who are successfully providing culturally competent care is to show respect. One way is to ask patients for their opinions. These 10 questions can improve and convey respect in patient encounters. (Department of Health and Human Services, 2003):[3]

1. What do you think caused your problem?
2. Why do you think it started when it did?
3. What do you think your sickness does to your body? How does it work?
4. How severe is your sickness? How long do you think it will last?
5. What are the main problems your sickness has caused you?
6. Do others you know have this problem? What did they do to treat it?
7. Did you discuss the problem with any relatives or friends? What did they say?
8. What kinds of medicines, home remedies, or treatments have you tried? Did they help?

9. What type of treatment do you think you should receive? What are the most important results you hope to receive from this treatment?

10. Do you think there is anyway to prevent this problem in the future? How?

Visit the U.S. Department of Health and Human Services Office of Minority Health website. There you will find the National Standards on Culturally and Linguistically Appropriate Services (CLAS). The CLAS standards demonstrate the legal obligations organizations may have in regard to being culturally competent. (http://www.omhrc.gov/templates/browse.aspx?lvl=1&lvlID=3).

# How Can You Develop *Cultural Competence?*

As you develop cultural competence, you heighten your ability to analyze how people relate to one another. Most important, you develop practical skills that enable you to connect to others by bridging the gap between who you are and who they are.[4]

Following are specific strategies for developing your cultural competence.

## Value Diversity

Valuing diversity means having a basic respect for, and acceptance of, the differences among people. Every time you meet someone new, you have a choice about how to relate. If you value diversity, you will choose to treat people with tolerance and respect, granting them the right to think, feel, and believe without being judged.

Being open-minded in this way will help your relationships thrive, as shown in Figure 10.1. Even though you won't like every person you meet, you can make an effort to show respect while focusing on the person as an individual.

## Identify and Evaluate Personal Perceptions and Attitudes

Whereas people may value the *concept* of diversity, attitudes and emotional responses may influence how they act when they confront the *reality* of diversity in their own lives. As a result, many people have prejudices that lead to damaging stereotypes.

### Prejudice

Almost everyone has some level of **prejudice**, meaning that they prejudge others, usually on the basis of characteristics such as gender, race, sexual orientation, and religion. People judge others without knowing anything about them because of

PREJUDICE
A preconceived judgment or opinion, formed without just grounds or sufficient knowledge.

- **Influence of family and culture.** Children learn attitudes, including intolerance, superiority, and hate, from their parents, peers, and community.

FIGURE 10.1 Approaching diversity with an open mind builds relationships

| YOUR ROLE | SITUATION | CLOSED-MINDED ACTIONS | OPEN-MINDED ACTIONS |
|---|---|---|---|
| Fellow student | For an assignment, you are paired with a student old enough to be your mother. | You assume the student will be clueless about the modern world. You think she might preach to you about how to do the assignment. | You get to know the student as an individual. You stay open to what you can learn from her experiences and knowledge. |
| Friend | You are invited to dinner at a friend's house. When he introduces you to his partner, you realize that he is gay. | You are turned off by the idea of two men in a relationship. You make an excuse to leave early. You avoid your friend after that. | You have dinner with the two men and make an effort to get to know more about them, individually and as a couple. |
| Employee | Your new boss is of a different racial and cultural background than yours. | You assume that you and your new boss don't have much in common. You think he will be distant and uninterested in you. | You rein in your stereotypes. You pay close attention to how your new boss communicates and leads. You adapt to his style and make an effort to get to know him better. |

- **Fear of differences.** It is human to fear, and to make assumptions about, the unfamiliar.
- **Experience.** One bad experience with a person of a particular race or religion may lead someone to condemn all people with the same background.

## Stereotypes

STEREOTYPE
A standardized mental picture that represents an oversimplified opinion or uncritical judgment.

Prejudice is usually based on **stereotypes**—assumptions made, without proof or critical thinking, about the characteristics of a person or group of people. Stereotyping emerges from

- **A desire for patterns and logic.** People often try to make sense of the world by using the labels, categories, and generalizations that stereotypes provide.
- **Media influences.** The more people see stereotypical images—the airhead beautiful blonde, the jolly fat man—the easier it is to believe that stereotypes are universal.
- **Laziness.** Labeling group members according to a characteristic they seem to have in common takes less energy than exploring the qualities of individuals.

Stereotypes stall the growth of relationships because pasting a label on a person makes it hard for you to see the real person underneath. Even stereotypes that seem positive may not be true and may get in the way of perceiving people as individuals. Figure 10.2 shows some so-called "positive" and negative stereotypes.

Use your analytical abilities to question your own ideas and beliefs and to weed out the narrowing influence of prejudice and stereotyping. Giving

## FIGURE 10.2 Stereotypes involve generalizations that may not be accurate

| POSITIVE STEREOTYPE | NEGATIVE STEREOTYPE |
| --- | --- |
| Women are nurturing. | Women are too emotional for business. |
| African Americans are great athletes. | African Americans struggle in school. |
| Hispanic Americans are family oriented. | Hispanic Americans have too many kids. |
| White people are successful in business. | White people are cold and power hungry. |
| Gay men have a great sense of style. | Gay men are sissies. |
| People with disabilities have strength of will. | People with disabilities are bitter. |
| Older people are wise. | Older people are set in their ways. |
| Asian Americans are good at math and science. | Asian Americans are poor leaders. |

honest answers to questions like the following is an essential step in the development of cultural competence:

- How do I react to differences?
- What prejudices or stereotypes come to mind when I see people, in real life or the media, who are a different color than I am? From a different culture? Making different choices?
- Where did my prejudices and stereotypes come from?
- Are these prejudices fair? Are these stereotypes accurate?
- What harm can having these prejudices and believing these stereotypes cause?

With the knowledge you build as you answer these questions, move on to the next stage: looking carefully at what happens when people from different cultures interact.

## Be Aware of What Happens When Cultures Interact

As history has shown, when people from different cultures interact, they often experience problems caused by lack of understanding, prejudice, and stereotypic thinking. At their mildest, these problems create roadblocks that obstruct relationships and communication. At their worst, they set the stage for acts of discrimination and hate crimes.

### Discrimination

Discrimination refers to actions that deny people equal employment, educational, and housing opportunities, or treat people as second-class citizens. Federal law says that you cannot be denied basic opportunities and

# Expand Your Perception of Diversity

*get creative!*

*Heighten your awareness of diversity by examining your own uniqueness.*

Being able to respond to people as individuals requires that you become more aware of the diversity that is not always on the surface. Brainstorm 10 words or phrases that describe you. The challenge: Keep references to your ethnicity or appearance (brunette, Cuban American, wheelchair dependent, and so on) to a minimum, and fill the rest of the list with characteristics others can't see at a glance (laid-back, only child, 24 years old, drummer, marathoner, interpersonal learner, and so on).

1.                                     6.

2.                                     7.

3.                                     8.

4.                                     9.

5.                                     10.

Use a separate piece of paper to make a similar list for someone you know well—a friend or family member. Again, stay away from the most obvious visible characteristics. See if anything surprises you about the different image you create of this familiar person.

rights because of your race, creed, color, age, gender, national or ethnic origin, religion, marital status, potential or actual pregnancy, or potential or actual illness or disability (unless the illness or disability prevents you from performing required tasks and unless accommodations are not possible).

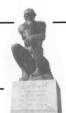

Minds are like parachutes. They only function when they are open.

SIR JAMES DEWAR

Despite these legal protections, discrimination is common and often appears on college campuses. Students may not want to work with students of other races. Members of campus clubs may reject prospective members because of religious differences. Outsiders may harass students attending gay and lesbian alliance meetings. Instructors may judge students according to their weight, accent, or body piercings.

## Hate Crimes

When prejudice turns violent, it often manifests itself in **hate crimes** directed at racial, ethnic, and religious minorities and homosexuals:

**HATE CRIME**
A crime motivated by a hatred of a specific characteristic thought to be possessed by the victim.

- In Wyoming in 1998, Matthew Shepard, a gay college student, was kidnapped and tied to a fence where his captors beat and abandoned him. He died of his injuries.
- In California in 1999, Buford O. Furrow Jr. entered a community center and shot five people because they were Jewish. He then shot and killed a Filipino-American letter carrier.

The increase in hate crimes in recent years is alarming. According to FBI statistics, reported hate crimes more than doubled from 1991 to 2001.[5] Incidents categorized as hate crimes include simple assault (the most common hate crime), aggravated assault, forcible sex offenses, arson, manslaughter, and murder. Because the statistics include only reported incidents, they tell only a part of the story. Many more crimes likely go unreported by victims fearful of what might happen if they contact authorities.

## Build Cultural Knowledge

The successfully intelligent response to discrimination and hate, and the next step in your path toward cultural competence, is to gather knowledge. You have a personal responsibility to learn about people who are different from you, including those you are likely to meet on campus.

What are some practical ways to begin?

- *Read* newspapers, books, magazines, and websites.
- *Ask questions* of all kinds of people, about themselves and their traditions.
- *Observe* how people behave, what they eat and wear, how they interact with others.
- *Travel internationally* to unfamiliar places where you can experience different ways of living firsthand.
- *Travel locally* to equally unfamiliar, but close-by, places where you will encounter a variety of people.
- *Build friendships* with fellow students or coworkers you would not ordinarily approach.

Some colleges have international exchange students who can help you appreciate the world's cultural diversity. When Yiting Liu left China to study mathematics and economics at a U.S. college, she knew little about the United States. Dorothy Smith, her African American roommate, helped her adjust. "Yiting didn't know much about race relations when she first got to America," explained Dorothy, "but from hanging around us, she's been able to get an interpretive experience." Also, said Dorothy, when Yiting "first came here, she was an outsider. She didn't know what the taboos were. Now she's able to cross into different groups."[6]

Building knowledge also means exploring yourself. Talk with family, read, seek experiences that educate you about your own cultural heritage. Then share what you know with others.

## Adapt to Diverse Cultures

Here's where you take everything you have gathered—your value of diversity, your self-knowledge, your understanding of how cultures interact, your information about different cultures—and put it to work with practical actions. With these actions you can improve how you relate to others, and perhaps even change how people relate to one another on a larger scale. Think carefully, and creatively, about what kinds of actions feel right to you. Make choices that you feel comfortable with, that cause no harm, and that may make a difference, however small.

Martin Luther King Jr. believed that careful thinking could change attitudes. He said,

> The tough-minded person always examines the facts before he reaches conclusions: in short, he postjudges. The tender-minded person reaches conclusions before he has examined the first fact; in short, he prejudges and is prejudiced. . . . There is little hope for us until we become tough minded enough to break loose from the shackles of prejudice, half-truths, and down-right ignorance.[7]

Try the following suggestions. In addition, let them inspire your own creative ideas about what else you can do in your daily life to improve how you relate to others.

### Look Past External Characteristics

If you meet a woman with a disability, get to know her. She may be an accounting major, a daughter, and a mother. She may love baseball, politics, and science fiction novels. These characteristics—not just her physical person—describe who she is.

### Put Yourself in Other People's Shoes

Shift your perspective and try to understand what other people feel, especially if there's a conflict. If you make a comment that someone interprets as offensive, for example, think about why what you said was hurtful. If you can talk about it with the person, you may learn even more about how he or she heard what you said and why.

### Adjust to Cultural Differences

When you understand someone's way of being and put it into practice, you show respect and encourage communication. If a friend's family is formal at home, dress appropriately and behave formally when you visit. If an instructor maintains a lot of personal space, keep a respectful distance when you visit during office hours. If a study group member takes offense at a particular kind of language, avoid it when you meet.

### Help Others in Need

Newspaper columnist Sheryl McCarthy wrote about an African American who, in the midst of the 1992 Los Angeles riots, saw an Asian American man being beaten and helped him to safety: "When asked why he risked grievous harm to save an Asian man he didn't even know, the African American man said, 'Because if I'm not there to help someone else, when the mob comes for me, will there be someone there to save me?'"[8]

## Stand up Against Prejudice, Discrimination, and Hate

When you hear a prejudiced remark or notice discrimination taking place, think about what you can do to encourage a move in the right direction. You may choose to make a comment, or to get help by approaching an authority such as an instructor or dean. Sound the alarm on hate crimes: Let authorities know if you suspect that a crime is about to occur, join campus protests, support organizations that encourage tolerance.

## Recognize That People Everywhere Have the Same Basic Needs

Everyone loves, thinks, hurts, hopes, fears, and plans. When you are trying to find common ground with diverse people, remember that you are united first through your essential humanity.

When people use successful intelligence to work through problems, changes can happen. After a gay tutor left a job at a university rather than face harassment, his friends organized an intercollegiate meeting on intolerance. Chandra J. Johnson, assistant to the president at the University of Notre Dame, asked participants to start by examining themselves: "This is an opportunity to see how our own biases have been formed," she said. "We are not born with notions of racism. These kinds of social ills have been projected onto us. . . . These things are very, very real and people's spirits are destroyed every day as a result of a bias or a misconception."

Ada Maxwell, a student attendee, believes that talking about intolerance is the key to eliminating it. "It doesn't have to be taboo," she said. "Half of the education . . . is the classes and the professors, but the other half—and it's a really important half—is what you can learn from other people. Your thinking can change and other people's thinking can change."[9]

Many minority students experience a dimension to college life unknown to majority students. Examining their experiences and choices will help *all* students understand the complexity of what it means to be a minority in America.

# How Can *Minority Students* Make the Most of College?

Who fits into the category of "minority student" at your school? The term *minority* includes students of color; students who are not part of the majority Christian sects; and gay, lesbian, and bisexual students. However, even for members of these groups, there is no universal minority experience. Each person's experiences are unique.

If you are a minority student, two actions will help you make the most of college: defining your perspective and defining your experience.

## Define Your Perspective

You have a choice about what perspective to bring to your new relationships. Do you expect others to stereotype you right away, or do you expect that they will be open to getting to know you as an individual?

What might be the consequences of each perspective? For your part, do you plan to try to approach each person as an individual rather than to type them according to their ethnic or cultural status, age or gender, values or choices?

Part of getting off to a positive and productive start at college means being open-minded and avoiding assumptions as you get to know people. Yes, everyone will have their own ideas, values, and ways of living. It is possible, however—as well as productive—to get to know these ideas and values in the people you encounter without immediately making assumptions or placing judgments. Working toward understanding is the key. As Paul Barrett Jr., political science major at Earlham College, says,

> As a black male, I am faced with situations very different from that of a white male, a white female, a black female, an Asian-American male, and so on. We must have the ability to approach situations with a panoramic perspective rather than the narrow scope of our own worlds. Is that not the very essence of diversity? Is it not the ability to at least try to understand differences in culture and understand what makes a person act or think the way that he or she does?[10]

University of Michigan student Fiona Rose describes the benefits of a positive approach to diversity this way:

> My years at U-M have been enhanced by relationships with men and women from all cultures, classes, races, and ethnicities. Such interactions are essential to an education. While courses teach us the history and academic value of diversity, friendships prepare us to survive and thrive in our global community. Good institutions consider not only what a potential student will gain from classes and course work, but what he or she will bring to the campus community.[11]

Consider the mind-set you want to take as you begin college. Adopt the perspective that will open you to new friendships and horizon-broadening experiences.

## Define Your Experience

When you start school, it's natural to want to live with, sit next to, or socialize with people similar to you. However, if you define your entire college experience by these ties, you may limit your understanding of others and your opportunities for growth.

Along with activities that appeal to the general student population, most colleges have organizations and services that support minority groups. Among these are specialized student associations, cultural centers, arts groups with a minority focus, minority fraternities and sororities, and political-action groups. Many minority students look for a balance, involving themselves in activities with members of their group as well as with the college mainstream. For example, a student may join the African American Students Association as well as clubs for all students such as the campus newspaper or an athletic team.

# Make a Difference

*Find personal ways to connect with other cultures.*

Rewrite three strategies in the "Adapt to Diverse Cultures" section on pages 312–313 as specific actions to which you commit. For example, "Help others in need" might become "Sign up to tutor in the Writing Center." Circle or check the number when you have completed each task or, if it is ongoing, when you have begun the change.

1.

2.

3.

To make choices as a minority student on campus, ask yourself these questions:

- How much time do I want to spend pursuing minority-related activities? Do I want to focus my studies on a minority-related field, such as African American studies?

- Do I want to minimize my ties with my minority group? Will I care if other minority students criticize my choices?

- Do I want to spend part of my time among people who share my background and part with students from other groups?

The attitudes and habits you develop now may have implications for the rest of your life—in your choice of friends, where you decide to live, your work, and even your family. Think carefully about the path you take, and follow your head and heart.

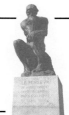

I have a dream that one day on the red hills of Georgia the sons of former slaves and the sons of former slave owners will be able to sit down together at the table of brotherhood.

MARTIN LUTHER KING, JR.

So far, the chapter has focused on the need to accept and adapt to diversity in its many forms. Just as there is diversity in skin color and ethnicity, there is also diversity in the way people communicate. Effective communication helps people of all cultures understand one another and make connections.

# How Can You *Communicate Effectively?*

Clear-spoken communication promotes success at school, at work, and in personal relationships. Successfully intelligent communicators analyze and adjust to communication styles, learn to give and receive criticism, analyze and make practical use of body language, and work through communication problems.

## Adjust to Communication Styles

When you speak, your goal is for listeners to receive the message as you intended. Problems arise when one person has trouble translating a message coming from someone using a different communication style. Your knowledge of the Personality Spectrum (see Chapter 3) will help you understand and analyze the ways diverse people communicate.

### Identifying Your Styles

Following are some communication styles that tend to be associated with the four dimensions in the Personality Spectrum. No one style is better than another. Successful communication depends on understanding your personal style and becoming attuned to the styles of others.

**Thinker-Dominant Communicators Focus on Facts and Logic.** As speakers, they tend to rely on logical analysis to communicate ideas and prefer quantitative concepts to those that are conceptual or emotional. As listeners, they often do best with logical messages. Thinkers may also need time to process what they have heard before responding. Written messages—on paper or via e-mail—are often useful for these individuals because writing can allow for time to put ideas together logically.

**Organizer-Dominant Communicators Focus on Structure and Completeness.** As speakers, they tend to deliver well-thought-out, structured messages that fit into an organized plan. As listeners, they often appreciate a well-organized message that defines practical tasks in concrete terms. As with Thinkers, a written format is often an effective form of communication to or from an Organizer.

**Giver-Dominant Communicators Focus on Concern for Others.** As speakers, they tend to cultivate harmony, analyzing what will promote closeness in relationships. As listeners, they often appreciate messages that emphasize personal connection and address the emotional side of an issue. Whether speaking or listening, Givers often favor in-person talks over written messages.

**Adventurer-Dominant Communicators Focus on the Present.** As speakers, they focus on creative ideas, tending to convey a message as soon as the idea arises and move on to the next activity. As listeners, they appreciate up-front, short, direct messages that don't get sidetracked. Like Givers, Adventurers tend to communicate and listen more effectively in person.

Use this information as a jumping-off point for your self-exploration. Just as people tend to demonstrate characteristics from more than one Personality Spectrum dimension, communicators may demonstrate different styles. Analyze your style by thinking about the communication styles associated with your dominant Personality Spectrum dimensions. Compare them to how you tend to communicate and how others seem to respond to you. Then, use creative and practical thinking skills to decide what works best for you as a communicator.

## Speakers Adjust to Listeners

Listeners may interpret messages in ways you never intended. Think about practical solutions to this kind of problem as you read the following example involving a Giver-dominant instructor and a Thinker-dominant student (the listener):

*Instructor:* "Your essay didn't communicate any sense of your personal voice."

*Student:* "What do you mean? I spent hours writing it. I thought it was on the mark."

- **Without adjustment:** The instructor ignores the student's need for detail and continues to generalize. Comments like, "You need to elaborate. Try writing from the heart. You're not considering your audience" might confuse or discourage the student.

- **With adjustment:** Greater logic and detail will help. For example, the instructor might say, "You've supported your central idea clearly, but you didn't move beyond the facts into your interpretation of what they mean. Your essay reads like a research paper. The language doesn't sound like it is coming directly from you."

## Listeners Adjust to Speakers

As a listener, improve understanding by being aware of stylistic differences and translating the message into one that makes sense to you. The following example of an Adventurer-dominant employee speaking to an Organizer-dominant supervisor shows how adjusting can pay off.

*Employee:* "I'm upset about the e-mail you sent me. You never talked to me directly and you let the problem build into a crisis. I haven't had a chance to defend myself."

- **Without Adjustment:** If the supervisor is annoyed by the employee's insistence on direct personal contact, he or she may become defensive: "I told you clearly what needs to be done. I don't know what else there is to discuss."

- **With Adjustment:** In an effort to improve communication, the supervisor responds by encouraging the in-person exchange that is best for the employee. "Let's meet after lunch so you can explain to me how you believe we can improve the situation."

Although adjusting to communication styles helps you speak and listen more effectively, you also need to understand, and learn how to effectively give and receive, criticism.

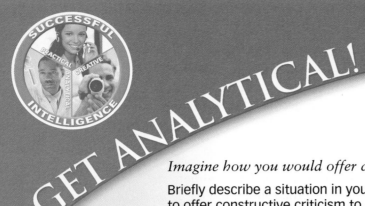

# GET ANALYTICAL!

# Give Constructive Criticism

*Imagine how you would offer constructive criticism.*

Briefly describe a situation in your life that could be improved if you were able to offer constructive criticism to a friend or family member. Describe the improvement you want:

Imagine that you have a chance to speak to this person. First describe the setting—time, place, atmosphere—where you think you would be most successful:

Now develop your "script." Keeping in mind what you know about constructive criticism, analyze the situation and decide on what you think would be the best approach. Freewrite what you would say. Keep in mind the goal you want your communication to achieve.

Finally, if you can, make your plan a reality. Will you do it?　　Yes　　No

If you do have the conversation, note here: Was it worth it?　　Yes　　No

## Know How to Give and Receive Criticism

CONSTRUCTIVE
*Promoting improvement or development.*

Criticism can be either **constructive** or nonconstructive. Constructive criticism is a practical problem-solving strategy, involving goodwill suggestions for improving a situation. In contrast, nonconstructive criticism focuses on what went wrong, doesn't offer alternatives or help that might help solve the problem, and is often delivered negatively, creating bad feelings.

When offered constructively and carefully, criticism can help bring about important changes. Consider a case in which someone has continually been late to study group sessions. The group leader can comment in one of two ways. Which comment would encourage you to change your behavior?

- **Constructive.** The group leader talks privately with the student: "I've noticed that you've been late a lot. We count on you because our success depends on what each of us contributes. Is there a problem that is keeping you from being on time? Can we help?"

- **Nonconstructive.** The leader watches the student arrive late and says, in front of everyone, "If you can't start getting here on time, there's really no point in your coming."

While at school, your instructors will criticize your class work, papers, and exams. On the job, criticism may come from supervisors, coworkers, or customers. No matter the source, constructive comments can help you grow as a person. Be open to what you hear, and always remember that most people want to help you succeed.

## Offering Constructive Criticism

When offering constructive criticism, use the following strategies to be effective:

- **Criticize the behavior rather than the person.** Avoid personal attacks. "You've been late to five group meetings" is much preferable to "You're lazy."

- **Define the problematic behavior specifically.** Try to focus on the facts, substantiating with specific examples and minimizing emotions. Avoid additional complaints: People can hear criticisms better if they are discussed one at a time.

- **Suggest new approaches and offer help.** Talk about practical ways of handling the situation. Work with the person to develop creative options. Help the person feel supported.

- **Use a positive approach and hopeful language.** Express the conviction that changes will occur and that the person can turn the situation around.

## Receiving Criticism

When you find yourself on criticism's receiving end, use the following techniques:

- **Analyze the comments.** Listen carefully; then evaluate what you heard. What does it mean? What is the intent? Try to let nonconstructive comments go without responding.

- **Request suggestions on how to change your behavior.** Ask, "How would you like me to handle this in the future?"

- **Summarize the criticism and your response to it.** Make sure everyone understands the situation.

- **Use a specific strategy.** Use problem-solving skills to analyze the problem, brainstorm ways to change, choose a strategy, and take practical action to make it happen.

Criticism, as well as other thoughts and feelings, may be communicated nonverbally. You will become a more effective communicator if you understand body language.

# Understand Body Language

Body language has an extraordinary capacity to express people's real feelings through gestures, eye movements, facial expressions, body positioning and posture, touching behaviors, vocal tone, and use of personal space. Why is it important to know how to analyze body language?

## Nonverbal Cues Shade Meaning

What you say can mean different things depending on body positioning or vocal tone. The statement "That's a great idea" sounds positive. However, said while sitting with your arms and legs crossed and looking away, it may communicate that you dislike the idea. Said sarcastically, the tone may reveal that you consider the idea a joke.

### Culture Influences How Body Language Is Interpreted

For example, in the United States, looking away from someone may be a sign of anger or distress; in Japan, the same behavior is usually a sign of respect.

### Nonverbal Communication Strongly Influences First Impressions

First impressions emerge from a combination of verbal and nonverbal cues. Nonverbal elements, including tone of voice, posture, eye contact, and speed and style of movement, usually come across first and strongest.

Although reading body language is not an exact science, the following practical strategies will help you use it to improve communication.

- **Pay attention to what is said through nonverbal cues.** Focus on your tone, your body position, whether your cues reinforce or contradict your words. Then do the same for those with whom you are speaking. Look for the level of meaning in the physical.

- **Note cultural differences.** Cultural factors influence how an individual interprets nonverbal cues. In cross-cultural conversation, discover what seems appropriate by paying attention to what the other person does on a consistent basis, and by noting how others react to what you do.

- **Adjust body language to the person or situation.** What body language might you use when making a presentation in class? Meeting with your adviser? Confronting an angry coworker? Think through how to use your physicality to communicate successfully.

## Communicate Across Cultures

As you meet people from other countries and try to form relationships with them, you may encounter communication issues that are linked to cultural differences.[12] As you recall from Chapter 2, these problems often stem from the different communication styles that are found in high-context and low-context cultures.

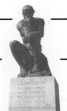

You cannot shake hands with a clenched fist.

INDIRA GANDHI

In the United States and other low-context cultures, communication is linked primarily to words and to the explicit messages sent through these words. In contrast, in high-context cultures, such as those in the Middle and Far East, words are often considered less important than such factors as context, situation, time, formality, personal relationships, and nonverbal behavior.

Figure 10.3 will help you see how 12 world cultures fit on the continuum of high- to low-context communication styles. Figure 10.4 summarizes some major communication differences you should be aware of when talk-

## FIGURE 10.3　The continuum of high- and low-context cultures

**LOW-CONTEXT CULTURES**　　　　　　　　　　　　　　　　　　　　**HIGH-CONTEXT CULTURES**

Swiss　German　Scandinavian　North American　English　French　Italian　Spanish　Latin American　African　Arab　Asian

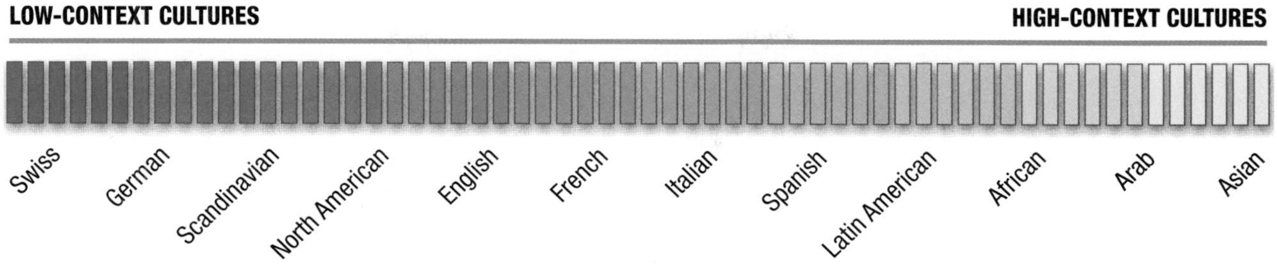

ing with someone from a different culture. Being attuned to culture-based communication differences will help you interact comfortably with people who come from different parts of the world.

Language barriers may also arise when communicating cross-culturally. When speaking with someone who is struggling with your language, make the conversation easier by choosing words the person is likely to know, avoiding slang expressions, being patient, and using body language to fill in what words can't say. Also, invite questions—and ask them yourself—so you both can be as clear as possible.

## FIGURE 10.4　Some ways communication differs in high- and low-context cultures

| FACTORS AFFECTING COMMUNICATION | LOW-CONTEXT CULTURES | HIGH-CONTEXT CULTURES |
|---|---|---|
| Personal Relationships | The specific details of the conversation are more important than what people know about each other. | Personal trust is the basis for communication, so sharing personal information forms a basis for strong, long-lasting relationships. |
| Time | People expect others to be punctual and to meet schedules. | Time is seen as a force beyond the person's control. Therefore lateness is common, and not considered rude. |
| Formality | A certain degree of civility is expected when people meet, including hand-shakes and introductions. | People often require formal introductions that emphasize status differences. As a result, a student will speak with great respect to an instructor. |
| Eye Contact | Expect little direct eye contact. | • Arab natives may use prolonged, direct eye contact. <br> • Students from Japan and other Far Eastern countries are likely to turn their eyes away from instructors as a sign of respect. |
| Personal Space | In the United States, people converse while remaining between 4 and 12 feet apart. | People from Latin America and the Middle East may sit or stand between 18 inches and 4 feet away from you. |

*Source*: Adapted from Louis E. Boone, David L. Kurtz, and Judy R. Block, *Contemporary Business Communication,* 2nd ed. (Upper Saddle River, NJ: Prentice Hall, 1997), p. 72.

One of the biggest barriers to successful communication is conflict, which can result in anger and even violence. With effort, you can manage conflict successfully and stay away from those who cannot.

## Manage Conflict

Conflicts, both large and small, arise when ideas or interests clash. You may have small conflicts with a housemate over a door left unlocked. You may have major conflicts with your partner about finances or with an instructor about a failing grade. Conflict, as unpleasant as it can be, is a natural element in the dynamic of getting along with others. Prevent it when you can—and when you can't, use problem-solving strategies to resolve it.

### Conflict Prevention Strategies

These two strategies can help you to prevent conflict from starting in the first place.

**Being Assertive.** No matter what your dominant learning styles, you tend to express yourself in one of three ways—aggressively, assertively, or passively. Aggressive communicators focus primarily on their own needs and can become impatient when needs are not satisfied. **Assertive** communicators are likely both to get their message across and to give listeners the opportunity to speak, without attacking others or sacrificing their own needs. Passive communicators focus primarily on the needs of others and often deny themselves power, causing frustration.

Figure 10.5 contrasts the characteristics of these three. Assertive behavior strikes a balance between aggression and passivity and promotes the most productive communication. Aggressive and passive communicators can use practical strategies to move toward a more assertive style of communication.

- Aggressive communicators might take time before speaking, use "I" statements, listen to others, and avoid giving orders.

ASSERTIVE
Able to declare and affirm one's own opinions while respecting the rights of others to do the same.

---

**FIGURE 10.5**   Assertiveness fosters successful communication

| AGGRESSIVE | ASSERTIVE | PASSIVE |
|---|---|---|
| Loud, heated arguing | Expressing feelings without being nasty or overbearing | Concealing one's own feelings |
| Blaming, name-calling, and verbal insults | Expressing oneself and giving others the chance to express themselves | Feeling that one has no right to express anger |
| Walking out of arguments before they are resolved | Using "I" statements to defuse arguments | Avoiding arguments |
| Being demanding: "Do this" | Asking and giving reasons: "I would appreciate it if you would do this, and here's why . . ." | Being noncommittal: "You don't have to do this unless you really want to . . ." |

- Passive communicators might acknowledge anger, express opinions, exercise the right to make requests, and know that their ideas and feelings are important.

**Send "I" Messages.** "I" messages help you communicate your needs rather than attacking someone else. Creating these messages involves some simple rephrasing: "You didn't lock the door!" becomes "I felt uneasy when I came to work and the door was unlocked." Similarly, "You never called last night" becomes "I was worried when I didn't hear from you last night."

"I" statements soften the conflict by highlighting the effects that the other person's actions have on you, rather than focusing on the person or the actions themselves. These statements help the receiver feel freer to respond, perhaps offering help and even acknowledging mistakes.

## Conflict Resolution

All too often, people deal with conflict through avoidance (a passive tactic that shuts down communication) or escalation (an aggressive tactic that often leads to fighting). Conflict resolution demands calm communication, motivation, and careful thinking. Use your analytical, creative, and practical thinking skills to apply the problem-solving plan (Chapter 5):

- Define and analyze the problem.
- Brainstorm possible solutions.
- Analyze potential solutions.
- Choose a solution and make it happen with practical action.

Trying to calm anger is an important part of resolving conflict. All people get angry at times—at people, events, and themselves. However, excessive anger can contaminate relationships, stifle communication, and turn friends and family away.

## Manage Anger

Strong emotions can get in the way of happiness and success. It is hard to concentrate on American history when you are raging over being cut off in traffic or can't let go of your anger with a friend. Psychologists report that angry outbursts may actually make things worse. When you feel yourself losing control, try some of these practical anger-management techniques.

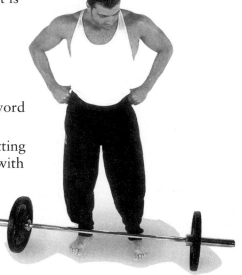

- **Relax.** Breathe deeply. Slowly repeat a calming phrase or word like "Take it easy" or "Relax."
- **Change your environment.** Take a break from what's upsetting you. Go for a walk, go to the gym, see a movie. Come up with some creative ideas about what might calm you down.
- **Think before you speak.** When angry, most people tend to say the first thing that comes to mind, even if it's hurtful. Inevitably, this escalates the hard feelings and the intensity of the argument. Instead, wait to say something until you are in control.

- **Do your best to solve a problem, but remember that not all problems can be solved.** Instead of blowing up, think about how you can handle what's happening. Analyze a challenging situation, make a plan, resolve to do your best, and begin. If you fall short, you will know you made an effort and be less likely to turn your frustration into anger.
- **Get help if you can't keep your anger in check.** If you consistently lash out, you may need the help of a counselor. Many schools have mental health professionals available to students.

Your ability to communicate and manage conflict has a major impact on your relationships with friends and family. Successful relationships are built on self-knowledge, good communication, and hard work.

# How Do You Make the Most of *Personal Relationships?*

Personal relationships with friends, classmates, spouses and partners, and parents can be sources of great satisfaction and inner peace. Good relationships can motivate you to do your best in school, on the job, and in life. When relationships fall apart, however, nothing may seem right. You may be unable to eat, sleep, or concentrate. Relationships have enormous power.

## Use Positive Relationship Strategies

Here are some strategies for improving personal relationships.

### Make Personal Relationships a High Priority

Life is meant to be shared. In some marriage ceremonies, the bride and groom share a cup of wine, symbolizing that the sweetness of life is doubled by tasting it together and the bitterness is cut in half when shared by two.

### Invest Time

You devote time to education, work, and sports. Relationships benefit from the same investment. In addition, spending time with people you like can relieve stress.

### Spend Time with People You Respect and Admire

Life is too short to hang out with people who bring you down or encourage you to ignore your values. "Try to nurture at least one friendship in each class," advises a Palo Alto College student. "If you know negative people who will try to discourage you and crush your spirit, avoid them. . . . You need nurturing and positivity."[13]

### If You Want a Friend, Be a Friend

If you treat others with the kind of loyalty and support that you appreciate yourself, you are likely to receive the same in return.

## Work Through Tensions

Negative feelings can fester when left unspoken. Get to the root of a problem by discussing it, compromising, forgiving, and moving on.

## Take Risks

It can be frightening to reveal your deepest dreams and frustrations, to devote yourself to a friend, or to fall in love. However, if you open yourself up, you stand to gain the incredible benefits of companionship, which for most people outweigh the risks.

## Find a Pattern That Suits You

Some students date exclusively and commit early. Some students prefer to socialize in groups. Some students date casually. Be honest with yourself—and others—about what you want in a relationship.

## If a Relationship Fails, Find Ways to Cope

When an important relationship becomes strained or breaks up, analyze the situation and choose practical strategies to help you move on. Some people need time alone; others need to be with friends and family. Some seek counseling. Some throw their energy into school or exercise. Some cry. Whatever you do, believe that in time you will emerge from the experience stronger.

# Avoid Destructive Relationships

On the far end of the spectrum are relationships that turn destructive. College campuses see their share of violent incidents. The more informed you are, the less likely you are to add to the sobering statistics.

## Sexual Harassment

Both men and women can be victims, although the most common targets are women. Sexual harassment basically consists of these two types:

- *Quid pro quo harassment* refers to a request for a sexual favor or activity in exchange for something else. "If you don't do X for me, I will fail you/fire you/make your life miserable."

- *Hostile environment harassment* indicates any situation where sexually charged remarks, behavior, or items cause discomfort. Examples include lewd jokes and pornography.

**How to Cope.** If you feel degraded by anything that goes on at school or work, address the person whom you believe is harassing you, or speak to a dean or supervisor.

## Violence in Relationships

Statistics indicate that violent relationships among students are increasing.[14]

- One in five college students has experienced and reported at least one violent incident while dating, from being slapped to more serious violence.

- In three of four violent relationships, problems surface after the couple has dated for a while.
- In six of ten cases, drinking and drugs are associated with the violence.

Women in their teens and 20s are more likely to be victims of domestic violence than older women. Here's why: First, when trouble occurs, students are likely to turn to friends rather than counselors or the law. Second, peer pressure makes them uneasy about leaving the relationship. And finally, some inexperienced women may believe that the violence is normal.[15]

**How to Cope.** Analyze your situation and use problem-solving skills to come up with options. If you see warning signs such as controlling behavior, unpredictable mood swings, personality changes associated with alcohol and drugs, and outbursts of anger, consider ending the relationship. If you are being abused, call a shelter or abuse hotline or seek counseling at school or at a community center. If you need medical attention, go to a clinic or hospital emergency room. If you believe your life is in danger, get out and obtain a restraining order that requires your abuser to stay away from you.

## Rape and Date Rape

Any intercourse or anal or oral penetration by a person against another person's will is defined as rape. Rape is primarily an act of rage and control, not a sexual act. Acquaintance rape, or **date rape,** refers to sexual activity during a date that is against one partner's will, including situations where one partner is too drunk or drugged to give consent. A drug called Rohypnol, known as roofies, is sometimes used by date rapists to sedate victims and is difficult to detect in a drink.

Campus Advocates for Rape Education (CARE), an organization at Wheaton College in Massachusetts, describes date rape's particular damage. "One's trust in a friend, date, or acquaintance is violated . . . fear, self-blame, guilt, and shame are magnified because the assailant is known."[16]

**How to Cope.** Communicate—clearly and early—what you want and don't want to do. When on a date with someone who seems unstable or angry, stick to safe, public places. Keep a cell phone handy. Avoid alcohol or drugs that might make it difficult for you to stay in control.

If you are raped, whether by an acquaintance or a stranger, seek medical attention immediately. Next, talk to a close friend or counselor. Consider reporting the incident to the police or to campus officials. Whether or not you take legal action, continue to get help through counseling, a rape survivor group, or a hotline.

## Choose Communities That Enhance Your Life

Personal relationships often take place within communities, or groups, that include people who share your interests—for example, sororities and fraternities, athletic clubs, and political groups. So much of what you accomplish in life is linked to your network of personal contacts.

If you affiliate with communities that are involved in positive activities, you are more likely to surround yourself with responsible and character-rich people who may become your friends and colleagues. You may find among them your future spouse or partner, your best friend, a person who helps you land a job, your doctor, accountant, real estate agent, and so on.

DATE RAPE
Sexual assault perpetrated by the victim's escort during an arranged social encounter.

Finding and working with a community of people with similar interests can have positive effects in personal relationships and in workplace readiness, as Eastern Kentucky University student Kasey Doyle explains:

> During my sophomore year, a friend persuaded me to join a service sorority on campus. I was hesitant at first, but once I began to get involved, I realized that I had missed out on many opportunities. Not only have I made many friends, I have also become more outgoing and personable. . . . I found a place where I fit in.
>
> Joining this organization also prepared me for my major and my job at [the campus newspaper] *The Progress*.
>
> As a reporter, you are expected to be outgoing and personable, and before joining an organization, I was extremely shy. I'm definitely not timid anymore, and I have matured and become more self-confident.[17]

If you find yourself drawn toward communities that encourage negative and even harmful behavior, such as gangs or groups that haze pledges, stop and think. Analyze why you are drawn to these groups. Resist the temptation to join. If you are already involved and want out, stand up for yourself and be determined.

# PERSONAL TRIUMPH CASE STUDY

GUSTAVO MINAYA
Student at Essex Community College, Baltimore, Maryland

*Connecting with others can be difficult, especially if you start out feeling exceptionally different. Gustavo Minaya spoke no English when he came to the United States as a child. Through learning and getting involved in activities, he has found his niche. Read the account; then use a separate piece of paper to answer the questions on page 330.*

I am a native of Peru. When I was six years old, my mother told me that we were going to America for a better life. My father was already living in the United States so my mother went to the embassy to apply for a visa, but our visa was denied. In desperation, she decided to hire "coyotes." These are people who know secret routes to the United States. Their job was to help us cross the border.

Our journey began at night with cold train rides. At different points, we stopped to eat or to get on a different train. Along the way other families joined us. At the Mexico-Texas border, the coyotes instructed us to walk under a highway. Once we were out again in the open, everyone began running for the U.S. border. Helicopters were circling overhead with their search lights on, and people were shouting. It was pandemonium.

Exhausted, we made it across the border and into a van, where people were stacked on top of each other. At another border check, my mother and I were arrested and taken into custody by immigration officers who took our fingerprints. They arranged to have us transported to an emergency shelter run by the American Red Cross. Meanwhile, my dad completed the paperwork for legal immigration, and we joined him a few months later.

Of course, I didn't know English. When I started school in the second grade I looked different from the other kids, and I sounded different because of my accent. Some of the kids picked on me. I cried a lot back then. The next year I took English as a Second Language (ESL) classes. Gradually, I learned English and began to feel like I fit in.

When I look back over my experiences, I believe the one thing that has helped me adjust to the changes is friendliness. I like to make people laugh, and I go into things with a positive attitude. Being friendly with other students, and people in general, has helped me gain a sense of belonging.

My main advice to international students who want to make the most of their education is to participate in campus activities. You can join a club or work on campus, maybe at the school store or library. This way you meet new people, and you'll learn English faster. You can't fit in if you isolate yourself.

Participation is also important for developing leadership skills. I look at clubs and other campus activities as opportunities to enhance my education. For example, I joined the International Student Association (ISA) and am now the president. During the meetings, I give my ideas and show my support by volunteering for projects. I've discovered that one of my strengths is bringing people together for a good cause.

I'm very proud of my parents for how hard they worked to make a better life for me and my brothers and sisters. In my native country of Peru, you can work as hard as you want, but it gets you nowhere. Some of the smartest people there are taxicab drivers because they can't find jobs doing anything else. Here, if you are willing to work, you can have a profession and achieve what you want. I plan to achieve as much as I can.

# Kente

The African word *kente* means "that which will not tear under any condition." Kente cloth is worn by men and women in African countries such as Ghana, Ivory Coast, and Togo. There are many brightly colored patterns of kente, each beautiful and special.

Think of how this concept applies to people. Like the cloth, all people are unique, with brilliant and subdued aspects. Despite mistreatment or misunderstanding by others, you need to remain strong so that you don't tear, allowing the weaker fibers of your character to show through. The *kente* of your character can help you endure, stand up against injustice, and fight peacefully, but relentlessly, for the rights of all people.

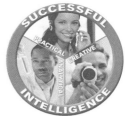

# Building World-Class Skills
## for College, Career, and Life Success

### Create Your Future

## DEVELOPING SUCCESSFUL INTELLIGENCE
### *Putting It All Together*

**Learn from the Experiences of Others.** Look back to Gustavo Minaya's Personal Triumph on page 328. After you've read his story, relate his experience to your own life by completing the following:

**Step 1. Think it through:** *Analyze your experience and compare it to Gustavo's.* When in your life have you felt like an outsider, and how does this relate to Gustavo's experience? What was his key to finding his place in his new world? What was yours?

**Step 2. Think out of the box:** *Create a challenge.* Think about the activities and organizations at your school with which you would most feel at home. Then imagine that none of those are available—and that you are required to get involved with three organizations or activities that you would never naturally choose. How would you challenge yourself? Name the three choices and describe what you think you could gain from your experiences. Consider trying one—for real!

**Step 3. Make it happen:** *Use practical strategies to connect with others.* Choose one of those organizations or activities that feel natural to you. Then choose one from your list of those that would be your challenges. Now try them both. Contact a person involved with each organization or activity and ask them for details: when the group meets, what they do, what the time commitment would likely be, what the benefit would be. Then join both in the coming semester, making an effort to get to know others who are involved.

**Definition of a Term Important to Culture and Health.** Ethnocentrism: The belief that ones own cultural view is the only view or is superior. Occurs when we use our own cultural biases to interpret another's beliefs. Ethnocentrism is a threat to a patient's health because of miscommunication. These are the three main consequences:

1. Lack of information means we use our own beliefs, ideas and experiences to interpret situations. We may not see an important part of a patient situation. Why does this matter?

2. If we don't have much experience with people from a certain cultural group we are likely to prejudge based on stereotypes, emotions, hearsay. Why does this matter?

3. With a lack of awareness of the ways we are treated due to our race, or age, or gender (our experiences differ from those of others), there is the tendency to see others as we see ourselves. Why does this matter?

# WRITING

## *Discovery Through Journaling*

*Record your thoughts on a separate piece of paper or in a journal.*

**Opening Your Mind.** On what topic is it most difficult for you to be accepting? Describe your difficulty with race, culture, ethnic origin, weight, gender, sexual orientation, or any other human characteristic. What do you think is the source of your uneasiness—parents, peers, experience, any other source? Describe what you can do now to think more openly, and think about why it may help you to combat your prejudices.

# TEAM BUILDING

## *Collaborative Solutions*

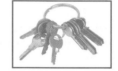

**Understanding Your Own Culture.** Divide into groups of two to five students. Assign one group member to take notes. Discuss the following questions, one at a time:
    Definition of Culture: Shared knowledge, beliefs, values, language, attitudes, experiences among a population group
    Think about and discuss your answers to these questions:

1. What racial, ethnic, or cultural groups do you belong to (socioeconomic, religion, profession, age group, gender, community)?

2. What experiences have you had with people from groups that are different from yours?

3. What personal qualities do you have that will help you, as a nurse, establish relationships with persons from other groups? What qualities might be detrimental?

**Problem Solving Close to Home.** Divide into groups of two to five students. Assign one group member to take notes. Discuss the following questions, one at a time:

1. What are the three largest problems the world faces with regard to how people get along with and accept others?

2. What could we do to deal with these three problems?

3. What can each individual student do to make improvements? (Talk about what you specifically feel that you can do.)

When all groups have finished, gather as a class and hear each group's responses. Observe the variety of problems and solutions. Notice whether more than one group came up with one or more of the same problems. If there is time, one person in the class, together with your instructor, could gather the responses to question 3 into an organized document that you can send to your school or local paper.

# CAREER PORTFOLIO

## *Plan for Success*

*Complete the following in your electronic portfolio or on separate sheets of paper.*

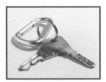

**Compiling a Résumé.** What you have accomplished in various work and school situations will be important for you to emphasize as you strive to land a job that is right for you. Your roles—on the job, in school, at home, or in the community—help you gain knowledge and experience.

On one electronic page or a sheet of paper, list your education and skills information. On another, list job experience. For each job, record job title, the dates of employment, and the tasks that this job entailed (if the job had no particular title, come up with one yourself). Be as detailed as possible: It's best to write down everything you remember. When you compile your résumé, you can make this material more concise. Keep this list current by adding experiences and accomplishments as you go along.

Using the information you have gathered and Figure 10.6 as your guide, draft a résumé for yourself. Remember there are many ways to construct a résumé; consult other resources, such as those listed in the bibliography, for different styles. You may want to reformat your résumé according to a style that your career counselor or instructor recommends, that best suits the career area you plan to enter, or that you like best.

Keep your résumé draft on hand—and on a computer disk. When you need to submit a résumé with a job application, update the draft and print it out on high-quality paper.

Here are some general tips for writing a résumé:

- Always put your name and contact information at the top. Make it stand out.

- State an objective if it is appropriate—if your focus is specific or you are designing this résumé for a particular interview or career area.

- List your postsecondary education, starting from the latest and working backward. This may include summer school, night school, seminars, and accreditations.

- List jobs in reverse chronological order (most recent job first). Include all types of work experience (full time, part time, volunteer, internship, and so on).

- When you describe your work experience, use action verbs and focus on what you have accomplished, rather than on the description of assigned tasks.

# Désirée Williams

237 Custer Street, San Francisco, CA 94101  •  650/555-5252 (w) or 415/555-7865 (h)  •  fax: 707/555-2735  •  e-mail: desiree@example.com

**EDUCATION**

| 2004 to present | San Francisco State University, San Francisco, CA |
|---|---|
| | Pursuing a B.A. in the Spanish BCLAD (Bilingual, Cross-Cultural Language Acquisition Development) Education and Multiple Subject Credential Program. Expected graduation: June 2008 |

**PROFESSIONAL EMPLOYMENT**

| 10/04–present | **Research Assistant, Knowledge Media Lab** |
|---|---|
| | Developing ways for teachers to exhibit their inquiry into their practice of teaching in an on-line, collaborative, multimedia environment. |
| 5/03–present | **Webmaster/Web Designer** |
| | Work in various capacities at QuakeNet, an Internet Service Provider and Web Commerce Specialist in San Mateo, CA. Designed several sites for the University of California, Berkeley, Graduate School of Education, as well as private clients such as A Body of Work and Yoga Forever. |
| 9/03–6/04 | **Literacy Coordinator** |
| | Coordinated, advised, and created literacy curriculum for an America Reads literacy project at Prescott School in West Oakland. Worked with non-reader 4th graders on writing and publishing, incorporating digital photography, Internet resources, and graphic design. |
| 8/03 | **Bilingual Educational Consultant** |
| | Consulted for Children's Television Workshop, field-testing bilingual materials. With a research team, designed bilingual educational materials for an ecotourism project run by an indigenous rain forest community in Ecuador. |
| 1/03–6/03 | **Technology Consultant** |
| | Worked with 24 Hours in Cyberspace, an online worldwide photojournalism event. Coordinated participation of schools, translated documents, and facilitated public relations. |

**SKILLS**

| Languages: | Fluent in Spanish. |
|---|---|
| | Proficient in Italian and Shona (majority language of Zimbabwe). |
| Computer: | Programming ability in HTML, Javascript, Pascal, and Lisp. Multimedia design expertise in Adobe Photoshop, Netobjects Fusion, Adobe Premiere, Macromedia Flash, and many other visual design programs. |
| Personal: | Perform professionally in Mary Schmary, a women's a cappella quartet. Have climbed Mt. Kilimanjaro. |

**FIGURE 10.6**    Set yourself apart with an attractive, clear résumé

- Include keywords that are linked to the description of the jobs for which you will be applying (see page 270 for more on keywords).
- List references on a separate sheet. You may want to put "References upon request" at the bottom of your résumé.
- Use formatting (larger font sizes, different fonts, italics, bold, and so on) and indents selectively to help the important information stand out.
- Get several people to look at your résumé before you send it out. Other readers will have ideas that you haven't thought of and may find errors you have missed.

## Suggested Readings

Dublin, Thomas, ed. *Becoming American, Becoming Ethnic: College Students Explore Their Roots.* Philadelphia: Temple University Press, 1996.

Feagin, Joe R., Hernan Vera, and Nikitah O. Imani. *The Agony of Education: Black Students at White Colleges and Universities.* New York: Routledge, 1996.

Gonzales, Juan L., Jr. *The Lives of Ethnic Americans,* 2nd ed. Dubuque, IA: Kendall/Hunt, 1994.

Hockenberry, John. *Moving Violations.* New York: Hyperion, 1996.

Levey, Marc, Michael Blanco, and W. Terrell Jones. *How to Succeed on a Majority Campus: A Guide for Minority Students.* Belmont, CA: Wadsworth, 1997.

Qubein, Nido R. *How to Be a Great Communicator: In Person, on Paper, and at the Podium.* New York: John Wiley, 1996.

Schuman, David. *Diversity on Campus.* Dubuque, IA: Kendall/Hunt, 2001.

Suskind, Ron. *A Hope in the Unseen: An American Odyssey from the Inner City to the Ivy League.* New York: Broadway Books, 1999.

Takaki, Ronald. *A Different Mirror: A History of Multicultural America.* Boston: Little, Brown, 1994.

Tannen, Deborah. *You Just Don't Understand: Women and Men in Conversation.* New York: Perennial Currents, 2001.

Tatum, Beverly Daniel. *"Why Are All the Black Kids Sitting Together in the Cafeteria?" and Other Conversations About Race: A Psychologist Explains the Development of Racial Identity.* Philadelphia: Basic Books, 2003.

Terkel, Studs. *Race: How Blacks and Whites Think and Feel About the American Obsession.* New York: Free Press, 1995.

Trotter, Tamera, and Joycelyn Allen. *Talking Justice: 602 Ways to Build and Promote Racial Harmony.* Saratoga, FL: R & E Publishers, 1993.

## Internet Resources

Prentice Hall Student Success Supersite (success stories from students from a diversity of backgrounds): **www.prenhall.com/success**

Asian American Resources: **www.ar.mit.edu/people/irie/aar/**

Britannica Guide to Black History: **http://blackhistory.eb.com**

Latino USA: **www.latinousa.org**

The Sociology of Race and Ethnicity (with multiple links to other resources): **www.trinity.edu/~mkear/race.html**

# Endnotes

[1]"For 7 Million, One Census Race Category Wasn't Enough," *New York Times*, March 13, 2001, pp. A1 and A14.

[2]T. L. Cross, B. J. Bazron, and K. Dennis, *Toward a Culturally Competent System of Care*. (Washington, DC: Georgetown University Child Development Center, 1989).

[3]Robert T. Trotter, *National Health Service Corps Educational Program for Clinical and Community Issues in Primary Care: Cross-Cultural Issues in Primary Care Module* (revised in 1999 for U.S. Department of Health and Human Services) (Reston, VA: AMA Student Association, 1994).

[4]Information in the sections on the five stages of building competency is based on Mark A. King, Anthony Sims, and David Osher, "How Is Cultural Competence Integrated in Education?" Cultural Competence. Retrieved May 2004, from: www.air.org/cecp/cultural/Q_integrated. htm#def.

[5]FBI Hate Crime statistics, from a grid created by the Anti-Defamation League (2001). Retrieved May 2004, from: www.adl.org/combating_hate/.

[6]Jen Lin-Liu, "China's 'Harvard Girl:' A College Student Has Become an Example for a New Style of Raising Children," *The Chronicle of Higher Education*, May 30, 2003. Retrieved March 2004, from: http://chronicle.com/weekly/v49/i38/ 38a04001.htm.

[7]Martin Luther King Jr., from his sermon "A Tough Mind and a Tender Heart," *Strength in Love* (Philadelphia: Fortress Press, 1986), p. 14.

[8]Sheryl McCarthy, *Why Are the Heroes Always White?* (Kansas City, MO: Andrews and McMeel, 1995), p. 137.

[9]Doug Gavel, "Students Speak Out at Hate Crime Forum," *Harvard University Gazette*, www. news.harvard.edu/gazette/2001/02.15/01- hatecrime.html.

[10]Paul Barrett Jr., "Solutions Offered to Address Racism on Campus," *Earlham Word Online* 13, no. 11 (November 20, 1998). Retrieved November 2004, from: http://word.cs.earlham. edu/issues/XIII/112098/opin91.html.

[11]Media Watch, *Diversity Web* (Fall 1997). Retrieved November 2004, from: www.diversityweb.org/ Digest/F97/mediawatch.html#top.

[12]Information for this section from Philip R. Harris and Robert T. Moran, *Managing Cultural Differences*, 3rd ed. (Houston, TX: Gulf Publishing Company, 1991), and Lennie Copeland and Lewis Griggs, *Going International: How to Make Friends and Deal Effectively in the Global Marketplace* (New York: Random House, 1985).

[13]Student essay submitted by the First Year Experience students of Patry Parma, Palo Alto College, San Antonio, Texas, January 2004.

[14]Tina Kelley, "On Campuses, Warnings About Violence in Relationships," *New York Times*, February 13, 2000, p. 40.

[15]Ibid.

[16]U.S. Department of Justice, Bureau of Justice Statistics, "Sex Offenses and Offenders," 1997, and "Criminal Victimization," 1994.

[17]Kasey Doyle, "Getting Involved on Campus Important," *The Eastern Progress* (November 4, 2004). Available: www.easternprogress.com/ news/2004/11/04/Perspective/Getting.Involved. On.Campus.Important-792180.shtml.

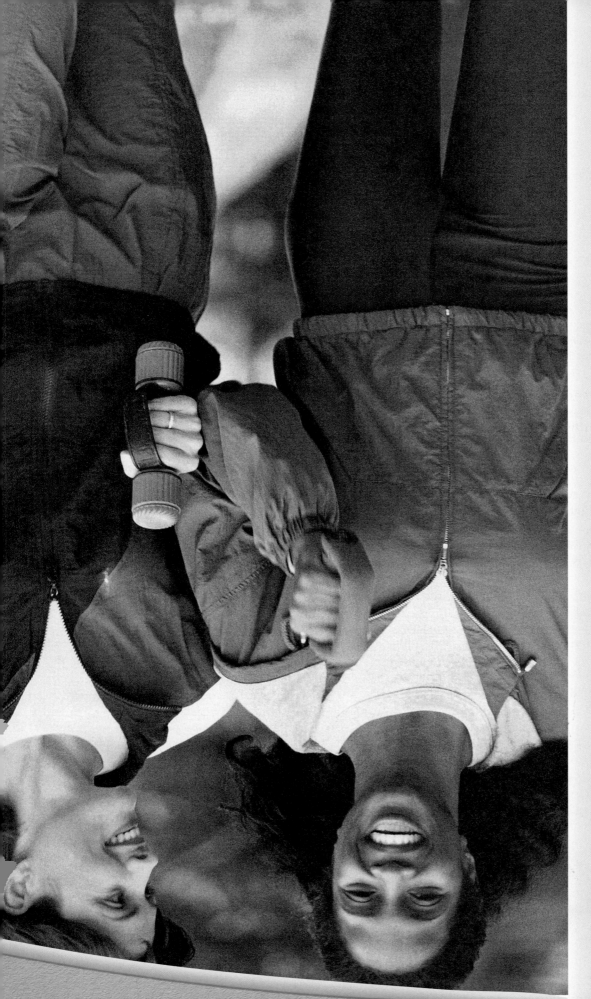

# INVEST: PERSONAL WELLNESS

*TAKING CARE OF YOURSELF*

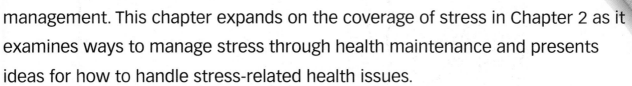

ocusing on personal wellness means targeting preventive actions you can take to stay healthy. Most likely, you have learned from personal experience that how well you do in school is directly related to your physical and mental health. Among the most important wellness strategies are those that deal with stress management. This chapter expands on the coverage of stress in Chapter 2 as it examines ways to manage stress through health maintenance and presents ideas for how to handle stress-related health issues.

Your personal wellness also depends on your decisions about drugs, alcohol, tobacco, and sex. Nearly every college student faces important choices on these issues. Your goal is to make decisions that are in your best interest and keep you healthy.

Approach all the topics in this chapter with successful intelligence. Analyze your situations and choices, brainstorm creative options, and take practical actions that work for you.

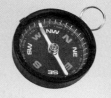

# Q & A BLUE SKY QUESTIONS DOWN-TO-EARTH ANSWERS

## *How can I secure my future?*

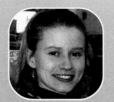

I'm a single mother with a special needs child. Recently I graduated from Central Michigan University with a BSN and entered graduate school at the University of Pennsylvania. I worked as a cake decorator at a bakery to pay for the moving costs, and all along I've borrowed money through school loans so that I could afford an education. It's been difficult to work, attend school, and be a mom, but I know nursing is what I want to do with my life.

Erika Sellekaerts
Senior, University of Pennsylvania, Philadelphia, Pennsylvania

I knew the University of Pennsylvania was a private school, but I still wasn't prepared for the shock or receiving my first bill. Instead of panicking, I sat down and wrote a letter to the administrative office and explained that my success as a student was already fragile because of being a single parent. I also explained how much I wanted to become an advanced practice nurse and that I plan to specialize in pediatric oncology. Thankfully, this effort paid off because I was awarded a grant. But that's only half the battle because I have to pay for housing. I qualified for a work-study program, which paid $7.00 an hour, but I had to pay $5.00 an hour for child care. You can't live on $2.00 an hour.

My graduate program requires that students work for nine months as a staff nurse before they can start clinicals. I would look for a staff nurse job right away; my daughter must have hip surgery. I'll be her personal nurse for six weeks, so I can't start work until she's well enough to go back to school. In the meantime, I'm working part time as a research assistant in an outpatient oncology clinic where I study the late effects of cancer. Needless to say, I'm on a very tight budget.

In spite of the grant, the job, and my determination to succeed, I continue to feel burdened about managing my finances. Even if I get a job right out of graduate school, I'll probably have to work nights, because often nurses must earn the day shifts. Working nights means I'll have to pay someone to take care of my daughter. Of course, I can try to get a job at an outpatient clinic with daytime hours, but I've heard those don't pay as well as hospital nursing positions. On top of all this, I'll have student loans to pay off. Sometimes I wonder if I'll ever get out of debt.

## PRACTICAL ANSWERS

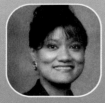

Dr. Roy Ann Sherrod
Assistant to the President, Professor of Nursing, The University of Alabama, Tuscaloosa, Alabama

### *There are many scholarships for nursing students.*

First let me congratulate you for achieving so much already. At my campus, we frequently see college students in terribly stressful predicaments like yours. The good news is you have many options. Networking is one of these options. I suggest that you intentionally network to help provide for your various needs; assistance with child care; emotional and spiritual support; and financial backing.

With so much going on in your life, you need the support of caring relationships. Cultivating adult companionship, so that you are interacting with people other than your child, can help you feel more connected to your new residence. Furthermore, we all need nurturing and replenishing, and close relationships can provide that.

There are many areas of funding and support for you to consider. One that is often overlooked by students is the local church. Churches often have scholarship programs for members and nonmembers of their congregations. Some churches also provide ministries for single parents, as well as other spiritually enriching outlets.

Professional nursing associations, such as the national association of nurse practitioners, usually offer scholarships and loans. The American Nurses Association is a good place to start your search because they offer several programs, especially for nurses who are seeking advanced degrees. Check with local associations first because they can provide information and contact for support, both locally and nationally.

Another potential funding source is health care institutions, such as hospitals and clinics. They may present conditional scholarship programs that pay your tuition and some expenses, if you agree to work for them for a period of time upon graduation. Of course, if you decide you don't want to work for them, you must pay the money back.

There are also local women's groups that offer scholarships, and they do not limit themselves to one professional area.

I applaud the letter you wrote to the administrator at your school. Now, make an appointment with a counselor in the student services office within your graduate program. These people are aware of sources of funding that are specific to nurses. Whereas your financial aid counselor might not be.

To help make end meet, you might want to consider a roommate. You can arrange for this person to share housing expenses and/or barter some of the rent in exchange for child care. A roommate might also help you feel more supported than living alone. Obviously, you would want to be very careful about whom you choose, especially since you have a daughter.

With regard to your graduate program requirement of working nine months, investigate what is meant by that time frame. How many hours per week does that translate into? Their definition of "nine months" may not be as unmanageable as it sounds. In addition, many universities have student counseling centers to help you cope with the stress you're feeling. Perhaps you would find that useful as well.

# How Can You Maintain a Healthy *Body and Mind?*

The healthier you are, the more you'll be able to reach your potential. Make your physical health a priority by eating right, exercising, getting enough sleep, reviewing your vaccinations, and taking steps to stay safe. Make your mental health a priority by recognizing mental health problems, related to stress or other causes, and understanding ways to get help.

## Eat Right

Making healthier choices about what you eat can lead to more energy, better general health, and an improved quality of life. Medical and nutritional experts in the federal government publish *Dietary Guidelines for Americans*, which lists seven practical, basic rules of healthy eating:

1. Eat a variety of foods.
2. Maintain a healthy weight.
3. Choose a diet low in fat and cholesterol.

4. Choose a diet with plenty of vegetables, fruits, and grain products.

5. Use sugars in moderation.

6. Use salt and sodium only in moderation.

7. If you drink alcoholic beverages, do so in moderation.

You can sum up this list with two words: *balance* and *moderation*. For balance, try to vary your diet by targeting different food groups: meats, fish, poultry, and other protein sources; dairy; breads and grains; and fruits and vegetables. For moderation, eat reasonable amounts. Just because you are served a supersized portion doesn't mean you have to eat it all. Decide how much food is enough and stop when you are full.

## Take Steps to Avoid Obesity

Obesity is a serious problem in the United States.[1] Government statistics indicate how widespread obesity is:[2]

- The **overweight** and the **obese** make up the majority of the population, with 61% of women and 67% of men currently falling into these two groups.[3]

- Between 1960 and 2000, the number of obese people in the United States more than doubled, to 30% of Americans now considered obese.

Obesity is a major risk factor in the development of adult-onset diabetes, coronary heart disease, high blood pressure, stroke, cancer, and other illnesses. In fact, after smoking, obesity is the second leading cause of preventable death. In addition, obese people often suffer social and employment discrimination and may find daily life difficult.

College life can make it tough to eat right. Students spend hours sitting in class or studying and tend to eat on the run, build social events around food, and eat as a reaction to stress. Many new students find that the "freshman 15"—referring to 15 pounds that people say freshmen tend to gain in the first year of school—is much more than a myth.

These practical tips will help you pay attention to how you eat and to make changes when you need, so you can lose weight or avoid gaining.

**Target Your Ideal Weight.** Your college health clinic has charts of ideal weight ranges for men and women with different body builds and heights. You can also find this information on Internet sites such as the Centers for Disease Control and Prevention, which has a calculator for body mass index (BMI) at www.cdc.gov/nccdphp/dnpa/bmi/calc-bmi.htm.

**Make Small But Effective Changes.** Pledge to stop drinking sugar-filled soda and to give up fried foods. Record your goals on paper so they become real.

**Reduce Portion Size.** A serving of cooked pasta is about one-half cup, for example, and cheese about 1.2 ounces. At restaurants, ask for a half portion or take home what you don't finish.

**Make Smart Choices.** Avoid high-fat, high-sugar foods. If you eat out, order a low-fat and balanced meal and limit your portions. Choose snacks with fewer than 200 calories such as a frozen fruit juice bar or a container of low-fat fruit yogurt.

**Plan Your Meals.** Try to eat at regular times and in a regular location. Attempt to minimize late-night eating sprees during study sessions. Avoid skipping meals because it may make you more likely to overeat later.

**Identify "Emotional Triggers" for Your Eating.** If you eat to relieve stress or handle disappointment, try substituting a positive activity. If you are upset about a course, spend more time studying, talk with your instructor, or write in your journal.

**Get Help.** If you need to lose weight, find a support group, such as Weight Watchers or an on-campus organization, that can help you stay on target.

**Set Reasonable Goals.** Losing weight and keeping it off take time and patience. Start by aiming to lose 5% to 10% of your current weight; for example, if you weigh 200 pounds, your weight-loss goal is 10 to 20 pounds. Work toward your goal at a pace of approximately 1 to 2 pounds a week. When you reach it, set a new goal if you need to lose more, or begin a maintenance program.

## Exercise

Being physically fit enhances your general health, increases your energy, and helps you cope with stress. During physical activity, the brain releases endorphins, chemical compounds that have a positive and calming effect on the body.

College athletes use daily exercise as a stress reliever. Larisa Kindell, a senior and co-captain of Wesleyan University's swimming team, credits her athletic routine with helping her balance her life. "If I didn't have swimming, a place to release my academic stress, I don't think I'd be as effective in the classroom or studying at night," she said. Swimming has taught her "discipline, time management, and motivation" and has contributed to her academic success.[4]

Always check with a physician before beginning an exercise program, and adjust your program to your physical needs and fitness level. If you don't currently exercise, walking daily is a good way to begin. If you exercise frequently and are already in good shape, you may prefer an intense workout.

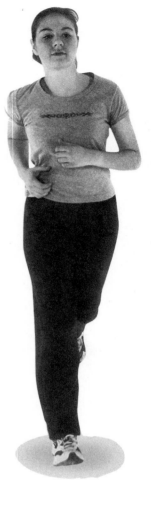

## Types of Exercise

There are three general categories of exercises. The type you choose depends on your exercise goals, available equipment, your time and fitness level, and other factors.

- *Cardiovascular training* strengthens your heart and lung capacity. Examples include running, swimming, inline skating, aerobic dancing, and biking.

- *Strength training* strengthens different muscle groups. Examples include using weight machines and free weights and doing push-ups and abdominal crunches.

- *Flexibility training* increases muscle flexibility. Examples include stretching and yoga.

Some exercises, such as lifting weights or biking, fall primarily into one category. Others, like power yoga, combine elements of two or all three. For maximum benefit, try alternating exercise methods through **cross-training**. For example, if you lift weights, use a stationary bike for cardiovascular work and build stretching into your workout.

CROSS-TRAINING
Alternating types of exercise and combining elements from different types of exercise.

## Making Exercise a Priority

Busy students often have trouble getting to the gym, even when there is a fully equipped athletic center on campus. Use these ideas to help make exercise a priority, even in the busiest weeks:

- Walk to classes and meetings. When you reach your building, use the stairs.
- Use your school's fitness facilities.
- Play team recreational sports at school or in your community.
- Use home exercise equipment such as weights, a treadmill, or an elliptical trainer.
- Find activities you can do outside of a club, such as running or pickup basketball.
- Work out with friends or family to combine socializing and exercise.

## Get Enough Sleep

College students are infamous for being sleep deprived. Research indicates that students need eight to nine hours of sleep a night to function well, but recent studies show that students average six to seven hours—and often get much less.[5]

During sleep your body repairs itself while your mind sorts through problems and questions. Inadequate sleep hinders your ability to concentrate, raises stress levels, increases irritability, and makes you more susceptible to illness. It can also have more serious effects such as an increased risk of auto accidents. According to Tracy Kuo, a clinical psychologist at the Stanford Sleep Disorders Clinic, "A sleepy driver is just as dangerous as a drunk driver."[6]

Students, overwhelmed with responsibilities, often feel that they have no choice but to prioritize schoolwork over sleep. Michelle Feldman, a sophomore at Syracuse University, stays up regularly until 4 A.M. getting her reading and studying done. Fellow Syracuse student Brian Nelson, a junior aiming to complete a triple major, only manages two hours a night as he works to keep up with the 24 credits he's taking in one semester.[7]

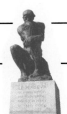

## The groundwork of all happiness is health.

LEIGH HUNT

For the sake of both your health and your GPA, find a way to get the sleep you need. Gauge your needs by first analyzing how you feel. If you are groggy in the morning, doze off during the day, or regularly need caffeine to make it through your classes, you may be sleep deprived. Sleep expert Gregg D. Jacobs, recommends the following practical suggestions for improving sleep habits:[8]

- **Reduce consumption of alcohol and caffeine.** Caffeine may keep you awake, especially if you drink it late in the day. Alcohol causes you to sleep lightly, making you feel less rested when you awaken.
- **Exercise regularly.** Regular exercise, especially in the afternoon or early evening, promotes sleep.
- **Take naps.** Studies have shown that taking short afternoon naps can reduce the effects of sleep deprivation.

- **Be consistent.** Try to establish somewhat regular times to wake up and go to bed.

- **Complete tasks an hour or so before sleep.** Give yourself a chance to wind down.

- **Establish a comfortable sleeping environment.** Wear something comfortable, turn down the lights and noise, find a blanket and pillow that you like, and keep the room cool. Use earplugs, soft music, or a white noise machine if you're dealing with outside distractions.

## Review Your Immunizations

Immunizations are not just for kids. Adults often need them to prevent diseases in particular circumstances or because they didn't receive a full course of shots as children. Following is immunization information from the Centers for Disease Control and Prevention (CDC) that may prevent major illness or literally save your life (check the "Recommended Adult Immunization Schedule" at www.cdc.gov for more detailed information). If you think you need these vaccines, check with your doctor or the college health service:

- The CDC recommends that college freshmen living in dormitories receive the *meningococcal meningitis* vaccine. This vaccine prevents the spread of a bacterial infection that can quickly kill even healthy young adults and often leaves survivors with permanent, serious disabilities. Meningococcal bacteria are spread through direct contact (such as sharing a glass) or indirect contact (such as sneezing) with infected individuals. Outbreaks are linked to close living situations, such as those common in college dormitories and military barracks.

- For women younger than age 26, the new *human papillomavirus* (HPV) vaccine is recommended. Three doses are required within a six-month period. The vaccine prevents HPV infections, which have been linked to cervical cancer, and they are most effective when the woman has never been exposed to HPV. The vaccine is *not* recommended during pregnancy.

- A *tetanus* booster is recommended every 10 years to protect you from bacterial infections related to certain wounds. When untreated, the toxin in tetanus is lethal.

- Three shots to prevent *hepatitis B* and two shots to prevent *hepatitis A* (both blood diseases) are recommended in college if you have not been immunized. Homosexuals, intravenous drug users, and some healthcare professionals are at increased risk.

- The *chicken pox* vaccine is recommended for any adult who did not have this illness as a child and who risks exposure. Chicken pox in adults can be severe and painful. Adults who have had chicken pox can also get shingles, a second outbreak of the virus.

- Although it used to be given only to adults who are over 65 or who have weak immune systems, the *influenza* vaccine is now recommended for many adults and children. It is available each year for a few months, starting around mid-October.

- Adults over 65 years of age and younger adults with chronic illnesses like diabetes, chronic pulmonary disease, or compromised immune systems should get the *pneumococcal polysaccharide* vaccine. This vaccine prevents a serious, often fatal, bacterial cause of pneumonia, bloodstream infections, and meningitis.

- The *measles-mumps-rubella (MMR)* vaccine is recommended for unvaccinated adults born after 1956 as well as adults who received vaccinations between 1963 and 1967.

A common illness, not protected by immunization, is *mononucleosis.* "Mono" is caused by a virus passed in saliva and is related to kissing and sharing drinking cups. Major symptoms, which can last for a few days or a few months, are fever, sore throat, swollen lymph glands, and fatigue. The only treatment is rest, fluids, and a balanced diet. Protect yourself by being careful in your relationships with friends, family, and roommates.[9]

## Stay Safe

Staying safe is another part of staying well. Take these practical measures to prevent incidents that jeopardize your well-being.

### Avoid Situations That Present Clear Dangers

Don't walk or exercise alone at night, especially in isolated areas. Don't work or study alone in a building. If a person looks suspicious, contact someone who can help.

### Avoid Drugs or Overuse of Alcohol

Anything that impairs judgment makes you vulnerable to assault. Avoid driving while impaired or riding with someone who has taken drugs or alcohol.

### Avoid People Who Make You Uneasy

If a fellow student gives you bad feelings, avoid situations that place you alone together. Speak to an instructor if you feel threatened.

It is not enough to have a healthy body. Your well-being also depends on a healthy mind.

## Recognize Mental Health Problems

With life's ups and downs, no one is happy all the time. However, you can target positive mental health by finding ways to feel good about who you are and what you are doing right now, to have hope for the future, and to build the resilience to cope with life's setbacks.

College students who feel overwhelmed by stress are susceptible to developing mental health problems or to having existing problems grow worse. Use the following information to analyze your situation and, if necessary, to take practical steps to improve your health.

### Depression

Almost everyone has experienced sadness after the death of a friend or relative, the end of a relationship, or a setback such as failing a course. However, as many as 10% of Americans experience a major depression, going beyond temporary blues, at some point in their lives. A depressive disorder is an illness, not a sign of weakness or a mental state that can be

# Improve Your Physical Health

*Make a change in how you eat, exercise, or sleep.*

First, decide what you most need to change. What's most important to your health right now—to eat better, exercise more, or get more sleep? Name it:

Now, considering your individual situation and looking at the strategies in this chapter, list five practical actions you can take right away to improve in this area. Word them as action statements. *Examples:* "I will leave earlier so that I can walk to my first class." "I will stop keeping candy bars in my room." "I will take a nap whenever I'm dragging in the afternoon."

1.
2.
3.
4.
5.

The final step: Just do it!

escaped by trying to "snap out of it." This illness requires a medical evaluation and is treatable.

A depressive disorder is "a "whole-body" illness, involving your body, mood, and thoughts."[10] Among the symptoms of depression are the following:

- Feeling constantly sad, worried, or anxious
- Difficulty with decisions or concentration
- No interest in classes, people, or activities
- Frequent crying
- Hopeless feelings and thoughts of suicide
- Constant fatigue
- Sleeping too much or too little
- Low self-esteem
- Eating too much or too little
- Physical aches and pains
- Low motivation

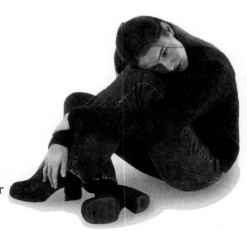

Depression can have a genetic, psychological, physiological, or environmental cause, or a combination. Figure 11.1 describes these causes along with strategies for fighting depression.

If you recognize any of these feelings in yourself, seek help. Start with your school's counseling office or student health service, which may also post information on the school website. You may be referred to a specialist who will help you sort through your symptoms and determine treatment. For some people, adequate sleep, a regular exercise program, a healthy diet, and the passage of time are enough to lessen stress and ease the disorder. For others, medication is important. If you are diagnosed with depression, know that your condition is common, even among college students. Be proud that you have taken a step toward recovery.

At its worst, depression can lead to suicide. SAVE (Suicide Awareness\ Voices of Education) lists these suicide warning signs:[11]

- Statements about hopelessness or worthlessness: "The world would be better off without me."
- Loss of interest in people, things, or activities.
- Preoccupation with suicide or death.
- Making final arrangements such as visiting or calling family and friends and giving things away.
- Sudden sense of happiness or calm. (A decision to commit suicide often brings a sense of relief that convinces others that the person "seemed to be on an upswing.")

If you recognize these symptoms in someone you know, begin talking with the person about his or her feelings. Then do everything you can to convince the individual to see a doctor or mental health professional. Don't keep your concerns a secret; sound an alarm that may save a life. If you recognize these symptoms in yourself, know that you can find help if you reach out.

## Eating Disorders

Millions of people develop serious and sometimes life-threatening eating disorders every year, including anorexia nervosa, bulimia, and binge eating.

**FIGURE 11.1**   What causes depression and what can help

| POSSIBLE CAUSES OF DEPRESSION | HELPFUL STRATEGIES IF YOU FEEL DEPRESSED |
|---|---|
| A genetic trait that makes depression more likely | Do the best you can and don't have unreasonable expectations of yourself. |
| A chemical imbalance in the brain | Try to be with others rather than alone. |
| Seasonal affective disorder, which occurs when a person becomes depressed in reaction to reduced daylight during autumn and winter | Don't expect your mood to change right away; feeling better takes time. |
| Highly stressful situations such as financial trouble, school failure, a death in the family | Try to avoid making major life decisions until your condition improves. |
| Illnesses, injuries, lack of exercise, poor diet, reaction to medication | Remember not to blame yourself for your condition. |

*Source:* National Institutes of Health Publication No. 94-3561, National Institutes of Health, 1994.

Because these disorders are common on college campuses, student health and counseling centers generally offer medical and psychological help, including referrals to trained specialists.

> One ceases to recognize the significance of mountain peaks if they are not viewed occasionally from the deepest valleys.

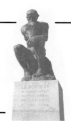

DR. AL LORIN

**Anorexia Nervosa.** People with anorexia become dangerously thin through restricted food intake, constant exercise, and use of laxatives, all the time believing they are overweight. An estimated 5% to 7% of college undergraduates, most of whom are women, suffer from anorexia.[12] The desire to emulate an "ideal" body type is one cause of the disease. In addition, eating disorders tend to run in families. Effects of anorexia-induced starvation include loss of menstrual periods in women, impotence in men, organ and bone damage, heart failure, and death.

**Bulimia.** People who binge on excessive amounts of food, usually sweets and fattening foods, and then purge through self-induced vomiting have bulimia. They may also use laxatives or exercise obsessively. Bulimia can be hard to notice because bulimics are often able to maintain a normal appearance. The causes of bulimia, like those of anorexia, can be rooted in a desire to fulfill a body-type ideal or can come from a chemical imbalance. Bulimics often suffer from depression or other psychiatric illnesses. Effects of bulimia include damage to the digestive tract and even heart failure due to the loss of important minerals.

**Binge Eating.** Like bulimics, people with binge eating disorder eat large amounts of food and have a hard time stopping. However, they do not purge afterward. Binge eaters are often overweight and feel they cannot control their eating. As with bulimia, depression and other psychiatric illnesses may contribute to the problem. Binge eaters may suffer from all of the health problems associated with obesity.

The stresses of college lead some students to experiment with alcohol, tobacco, and other potentially addictive substances. Although these substances may be quick, temporary fixes that alleviate stress, they have potentially serious consequences that can do long-term damage.

## How Can You Make Successfully *Intelligent Decisions* About Alcohol, Tobacco, and Drugs?

Abusing alcohol, tobacco, and drugs can cause financial struggles, emotional traumas, family and financial upheaval, health problems, and even death. As you read, think about the effects of your actions on yourself and others, and consider how to make positive, life-affirming choices.

## Alcohol

Alcohol, a depressant that slows vital body functions, is the most frequently abused drug on campus. Even a few drinks affect thinking and muscle coordination. Heavy drinking can damage the liver, the digestive system, and brain cells and can impair the central nervous system. Prolonged use also leads to **addiction**, making it seem impossible to quit. In addition, alcohol contributes to the deaths of 100,000 people every year through both alcohol-related illnesses and accidents involving drunk drivers.[13]

The National Institute on Alcohol Abuse and Alcoholism (NIAAA) offers these statistics about college students and alcohol:[14]

- Nearly 9 out of 10 students have used alcohol.
- Among heavy drinkers, there is an increased incidence of sexual assault and unwanted sexual advances as a result of drinking.
- Drinking with a group and serving one's own drinks may contribute to greater alcohol consumption. Both situations are common at large gatherings such as fraternity parties.

Of all alcohol consumption, **binge drinking** is associated with the greatest problems. Here are statistics from a recent survey:[15]

- Forty-three percent of the students surveyed labeled themselves as binge drinkers, and 21% said they binge-drink frequently.
- Eight out of 10 of the students who do not binge-drink reported experiencing such "secondhand effects" as vandalism, sexual assault or unwanted sexual advances, or interrupted sleep or study.[16]
- Students who binge-drink are more likely to miss classes, be less able to work, have hangovers, become depressed, and engage in unplanned or unsafe sexual activity.[17]

From what Darra Clark, a freshman at a large university in the Southwest, has seen, it is not possible to be a successful student if you drink too much. You can't do well in school and have friends if you "get drunk and stoned out of your gourd every night," she explains. "I think that the whole drinking scene is probably the thing I've found most appalling about college (our student handbook specifically outlaws beer funnels, for example). The problem, of course, is that drinking becomes a really hard behavior to regulate. . . . Drinking and drugs have done some awful things to some of the kids I've seen around here."[18]

The Get Analytical exercise on page 349, a self-test, will help you analyze your drinking habits. If you think you have a problem, use your creative and practical thinking skills to come up with a viable solution. The information on addiction on pages 352 and 353 introduces possible options.

## Tobacco

The National Institute on Drug Abuse (NIDA) found that nearly 40% of college students reported smoking at least once in the year before they were surveyed, and 25% had smoked once within the previous month. Nationally, about 60 million people are habitual smokers.[19]

When people smoke they inhale nicotine, a highly addictive drug found in all tobacco products. Nicotine's immediate effects may include an increase in blood pressure and heart rate, sweating, and throat irritation. Long-term effects may include high blood pressure, bronchitis, emphysema, stomach ulcers, and heart disease. Pregnant women who smoke increase their risk of having infants with low birth weight, premature births, or stillbirths.

---

**ADDICTION**
Compulsive physiological need for a habit-forming substance.

**BINGE DRINKING**
Having five or more drinks at one sitting.

# Evaluate Your Substance Use

Even one "yes" answer may indicate a need to look carefully at your habits. Three or more "yes" answers indicates that you may benefit from discussing your use with a counselor.

## Within the Last Year:

Y  N  1. Have you tried to stop drinking or taking drugs but found that you couldn't do so for long?

Y  N  2. Do you get tired of people telling you they're concerned about your drinking or drug use?

Y  N  3. Have you felt guilty about your drinking or drug use?

Y  N  4. Have you felt that you needed a drink or drugs in the morning—as an "eye-opener"—in order to cope with a hangover?

Y  N  5. Do you drink or use drugs alone?

Y  N  6. Do you drink or use drugs every day?

Y  N  7. Have you found yourself regularly thinking or saying, "I need" a drink or any type of drug?

Y  N  8. Have you lied about or concealed your drinking or drug use?

Y  N  9. Do you drink or use drugs to escape worries, problems, mistakes, or shyness?

Y  N  10. Do you find you need increasingly larger amounts of drugs or alcohol in order to achieve a desired effect?

Y  N  11. Have you forgotten what happened while drinking or using drugs because you had a blackout?

Y  N  12. Have you been surprised by how much you were using alcohol or drugs?

Y  N  13. Have you spent a lot of time, energy, and/or money getting alcohol or drugs?

Y  N  14. Has your drinking or drug use caused you to neglect friends, your partner, your children, or other family members, or caused other problems at home?

Y  N  15. Have you gotten into an argument or a fight that was alcohol- or drug-related?

Y  N  16. Has your drinking or drug use caused you to miss class, fail a test, or ignore schoolwork?

Y  N  17. Have you rejected planned social events in favor of drinking or using drugs?

Y  N  18. Have you been choosing to drink or use drugs instead of performing other activities or hobbies you used to enjoy?

Y  N  19. Has your drinking or drug use affected your efficiency on the job or caused you to fail to show up at work?

Y  N  20. Have you continued to drink or use drugs despite any physical problems or health risks that your use has caused or made worse?

Y  N  21. Have you driven a car or performed any other potentially dangerous tasks while under the influence of alcohol or drugs?

Y  N  22. Have you had a drug- or alcohol-related legal problem or arrest (possession, use, disorderly conduct, driving while intoxicated, etc.)?

*Source:* Adapted from the Criteria for Substance Dependence and Criteria for Substance Abuse in the *Diagnositc and Statistical Manual of Mental Disorders,* Fourth Edition, published by the American Psychiatric Association, Washington, DC, and from materials entitled "Are You an Alcoholic?" developed by Johns Hopkins University.

Inhaling tobacco smoke damages the cells that line the air sacs of the lungs and can cause lung cancer. Lung cancer causes more deaths in the United States than any other type of cancer. Smoking also increases the risk of mouth, throat, and other cancers.[20] Over time, smoking will wrinkle your skin, cause chronic coughing, and even change the sound of your voice.

In recent years, the health dangers of secondhand smoke have been recognized. Simply being around smokers regularly causes about 3,000 lung cancer deaths per year in nonsmokers.[21] This awareness has led many colleges (and local jurisdictions) to ban smoking in classrooms and other public spaces and even in many dorm rooms. If you smoke regularly, you can quit by being motivated, persevering, and seeking help. Practical suggestions for quitting include:[22]

- Try a nicotine patch or nicotine gum, and be sure to use them consistently.
- Get support and encouragement from a health care provider, a "quit smoking" program, a support group, and friends and family.
- Avoid situations that increase your desire to smoke, such as being around other smokers and drinking heavily.
- Find other ways to lower stress, such as exercise or other activities you enjoy.
- Set goals. Set a quit date and tell friends and family. Make and keep medical appointments.

The positive effects of quitting—increased life expectancy, greater lung capacity, and more energy—may inspire any smoker to consider making a lifestyle change.

To assess the level of your potential addiction, you may want to take the self-test in the exercise on page 349, replacing the words "alcohol" or "drugs" with "cigarettes" or "smoking." Think about your results, weigh your options, and make a responsible choice.

## Drugs

The NIDA reports that nearly 32% of college students have used illicit drugs at least once in the year prior to being surveyed, and 16% in the month before.[23] College students may use drugs to relieve stress, be accepted by peers, or just to try something new.

In most cases, the negative consequences of drug use outweigh any temporary high. Drug use violates federal, state, and local laws, and you may be arrested, tried, and imprisoned for possessing even a small amount of drugs. You can jeopardize your reputation, your student status, and your ability to get a job if you are caught using drugs or if drug use impairs your performance. Finally, long-term drug use can damage your body and mind. Figure 11.2 shows commonly used drugs and their potential effects.

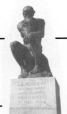

A habit is no damn private hell. . . . A habit is hell for those you love.

BILLIE HOLIDAY

One drug that doesn't fit cleanly into a particular category is methylenedioxymethamphetamine (MDMA), better known as Ecstasy. The use of this drug, a combination stimulant and hallucinogen, is on the rise at college

FIGURE 11.2 Drugs have potent effects on the user

| DRUG | DRUG CATEGORY | USERS MAY FEEL ... | POTENTIAL PHYSICAL EFFECTS | DANGER OF DEPENDENCE |
|---|---|---|---|---|
| **Cocaine** (also called *coke, blow, snow*) and **crack cocaine** (also called *crack* or *rock*) | Stimulant | Alert, stimulated, excited, energetic, confident | Nervousness, mood swings, sexual problems, stroke or convulsions, psychoses, paranoia, coma at large doses | Strong |
| **Alcohol** | Depressant | Sedated, relaxed, loose | Impaired brain function, impaired reflexes and judgment, cirrhosis, impaired blood production, greater risk of cancer, heart attack, and stroke | Strong with regular, heavy use |
| **Marijuana and hashish** (also called *pot, weed, herb*) | Cannabinol | Euphoric, mellow, little sensation of time, paranoid | Impaired judgment and coordination, bronchitis and asthma, lung and throat cancers, anxiety, lack of energy and motivation | Moderate |
| **Heroin** (also called *smack, dope, horse*) and **codeine** | Opiate | Warm, relaxed, without pain, without anxiety | Abscesses, risk of needle-transmitted diseases such as hepatitis and HIV | Strong, with heavy use |
| **Lysergic acid diethylamide (LSD)** (also called *acid, blotter, trips*) | Hallucinogen | Heightened sensual perception, hallucinations, distortions of sight and sound, little sense of time | Impaired brain function, paranoia, agitation and confusion, flashbacks | Insubstantial |
| **Hallucinogenic mushrooms** (also called *shrooms, magic mushrooms*) | Hallucinogen | Strong emotions, hallucinations, distortions of sight and sound, "out of body" experience | Paranoia, agitation, poisoning | Insubstantial |
| **Glue, aerosols** (also called *whippets, poppers, rush*) | Inhalants | Giddy, lightheaded, dizzy, excited | Damage to brain, liver, lungs, and kidneys; suffocation | Insubstantial |
| **Ecstasy** (also called *X, XTC, vitamin E*) | Stimulant | Heightened sensual perception, relaxed, clear, fearless | Fatigue, anxiety, depression, heart arrhythmia, hyperthermia from lack of fluid intake during use | Insubstantial |
| **Ephedrine** (also called *chi powder, zest*) | Stimulant | Energetic | Anxiety, elevated blood pressure, heart palpitations, memory loss, stroke, psychosis, insomnia | Moderate |

*(continued)*

| DRUG | DRUG CATEGORY | USERS MAY FEEL ... | POTENTIAL PHYSICAL EFFECTS | DANGER OF DEPENDENCE |
|---|---|---|---|---|
| **Gamma hydroxybutyrate (GHB)** (also called *G, liquid ecstasy, goop*) | Depressant | Uninhibited, relaxed, euphoric | Anxiety, vertigo, increased heart rate, delirium, agitation | Moderate |
| **Ketamine** (also called *K, Special K, vitamin K*) | Anesthetic | Dreamy, floating, having an "out of body" sensation, numb | Neuroses, disruptions in consciousness, reduced ability to move | Moderate |
| **OxyContin** (also called *Oxy, OC, legal heroin*) | Analgesic (containing opiate) | Relaxed, detached without pain or anxiety | Overdose death can result when users ingest or inhale crushed time-release pills, or take them in conjunction with alcohol or narcotics | Moderate, with long-term use |
| **Anabolic steroids** (also called *roids, juice, hype*) | Steroid | Increased muscle strength and physical performance, energetic | Stunted growth, mood swings, male-pattern baldness, breast development (in men) or body hair development (in women), mood swings, liver damage, insomnia, aggression, irritability | Insubstantial |
| **Methamphetamine** (also called *meth, speed, crank*) | Stimulant | Euphoric, confident, alert, energetic | Seizures, heart attack, strokes, vein damage (if injected), sleeplessness, hallucinations, high blood pressure, paranoia, psychoses, depression, anxiety, loss of appetite | Strong, especially if taken by smoking |

Source: "Drug Facts," n.d., Safety First, Drug Policy Alliance (www.safety1st.org/drugfacts.html).

parties, raves, and concerts. Its immediate effects include diminished anxiety and relaxation. When the drug wears off, nausea, hallucinations, shaking, vision problems, anxiety, and depression replace these highs. Long-term users risk permanent brain damage in the form of memory loss, chronic depression, and other disorders.[24]

You are responsible for analyzing the potential consequences of what you introduce into your body. Ask questions like the following: Why do I want to do this? What positive and negative effects might my behavior have? Why do others want me to take drugs? What do I really think of these people? How would my drug use affect the people in my life?

Use the self-test to assess your relationship with drugs. If you believe you have a problem, read the following section on steps that can help you get your life back on track.

## Identifying and Overcoming Addiction

People with addictions have lost control. Many addicts hide their addictions well and continue to function, but their lives are severely impaired. If you think you may be addicted, take the initiative to change. Those suffering from addiction have to help themselves for others to help them.

## Facing Addiction

Because substances often cause physical and chemical changes and psychological dependence, habits are tough to break and quitting may involve a painful withdrawal. Asking for help isn't an admission of failure but a courageous move to reclaim your life.

Even one "yes" answer on the self-test on page 349 may indicate that you need to evaluate your alcohol or drug use and to monitor it more carefully. If you answered yes to three or more questions, you may benefit from talking to a professional about your use and the problems it may be causing you.

## Working Through Addiction

The following resources can help you generate options and develop practical plans for recovery.

**Counseling and Medical Care.** You can find help from school-based, private, government-sponsored, or workplace-sponsored resources. Ask your school's counseling or health center, your personal physician, or a local hospital for a referral.

**Detoxification ("Detox") Centers.** If you have a severe addiction, you may need a controlled environment where you can separate yourself completely from drugs or alcohol. Some are outpatient facilities. Other programs provide a 24-hour environment through the withdrawal period.

**Support Groups.** Alcoholics Anonymous (AA) is the premier support group for alcoholics. Based on a 12-step recovery program, AA membership costs little or nothing. AA has led to other support groups for addicts such as Overeaters Anonymous (OA) and Narcotics Anonymous (NA). Many schools have AA, NA, or other group sessions on campus. Al-Anon is a 12-step program for families and friends of alcoholics.

When people address their problems directly instead of avoiding them through substance abuse, they can begin to grow and improve. Working through substance-abuse problems can lead to a restoration of health and self-respect.

Another important aspect of both physical and mental health involves being comfortable with your sexuality and making wise sexual decisions. Choosing birth control and knowing how to avoid sexually transmitted infections have short- and long-term consequences for the rest of your life.

# How Can You Make Successfully Intelligent Decisions *About Sex?*

What sexuality means to you and the role it plays in your life are your own business. However, the physical act of sex goes beyond the private realm. Individual sexual conduct can result in an unexpected pregnancy and in contracting or passing a sexually transmitted infection (STI). These consequences affect everyone involved in the sexual act and, often, their families.

Your self-respect depends on making choices that maintain health and safety—yours as well as those of the person with whom you are involved.

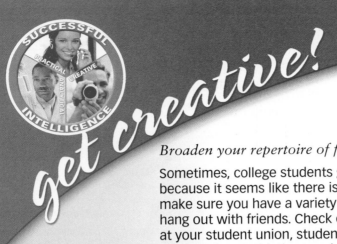

# Find More Fun

*Broaden your repertoire of fun things to do.*

Sometimes, college students get involved in potentially unsafe activities because it seems like there isn't anything else to do. Use your creativity to make sure you have a variety of enjoyable activities to choose from when you hang out with friends. Check out your resources: What possibilities can you find at your student union, student activities center, college or local arts organizations, athletic organizations, various clubs, nature groups? Could you go hiking? Paint pottery? Check out a baseball game? Run a 5K? Try a new kind of cuisine? Volunteer at a children's hospital ward? See a play?

Expand your horizons. List here 10 specific activities available to you.

1. _____
2. _____
3. _____
4. _____
5. _____
6. _____
7. _____
8. _____
9. _____
10. _____

Analyze sexual issues carefully, weighing the positive and negative effects of your choices. Ask questions like the following:

- Is this what I really want? Does it fit with my values?
- Do I feel ready or do I feel pressured?
- Is this the right person/moment/situation? Does my partner truly care for me and not just for what we might be doing? Will this enhance or damage our emotional relationship?
- Do I have what I need to prevent pregnancy and exposure to STIs? If not, is having unprotected sex worth the risk?

## Birth Control

Using birth control is a choice, and it is not for everyone. For some, using any kind of birth control goes against religious or personal beliefs. Others may want to have children. Many sexually active people, however, choose one or more methods of birth control.

In addition to preventing pregnancy, some birth control methods also protect against STIs. Figure 11.3 describes established methods, with effectiveness percentages and STI prevention based on proper and regular use.

Evaluate the pros and cons of each option for yourself as well as for your partner. Consider cost, ease of use, reliability, comfort, and protection against STIs. Communicate with your partner and together make a choice that is comfortable for both of you. For more information, check your library, the Internet, or a bookstore; talk to your doctor; or ask a counselor at the student health center.

**FIGURE 11.3**  Make an educated decision about birth control

| METHOD | APPROXIMATE EFFECTIVENESS | PREVENTS SEXUALLY TRANSMITTED INFECTIONS (STIs)? | DESCRIPTION |
| --- | --- | --- | --- |
| Abstinence | 100% | Only if no sexual activity occurs | Just saying no. No intercourse means no risk of pregnancy. However, alternative modes of sexual activity can still spread STIs. |
| Condom | 85% (95% with spermicide) | Yes, if made of latex | A sheath that fits over the penis and prevents sperm from entering the vagina. |
| Diaphragm, cervical cap, or shield | 85% | No | A bendable rubber cap that fits over the cervix and pelvic bone inside the vagina (the cervical cap and shield are smaller and fit over the cervix only). The diaphragm and cervical cap must be fitted initially by a gynecologist. All must be used with a spermicide. |
| Oral contraceptives (the Pill) | 99% with perfect use; 92% for typical users | No | A dosage of hormones taken daily by a woman, preventing the ovaries from releasing eggs. Side effects can include headaches, weight gain, and increased chances of blood clotting. Various brands and dosages; must be prescribed by a gynecologist. |
| Injectable contraceptives (Depo-Provera) | 97% | No | An injection that a woman must receive from a doctor every few months. Possible side effects may resemble those of oral contraceptives. |
| Vaginal ring (NuvaRing) | 92% | No | A ring inserted into the vagina that releases hormones. Must be replaced monthly. Possible side effects may resemble those of oral contraceptives. |
| Spermicidal foams, jellies, inserts | 71% if used alone | No | Usually used with diaphragms or condoms to enhance effectiveness, they have an ingredient that kills sperm cells (but not STIs). They stay effective for a limited period of time after insertion. |
| Intrauterine device (IUD) | 99% | No | A small coil of wire inserted into the uterus by a gynecologist (who must also remove it). Prevents fertilized eggs from implanting in the uterine wall. May or may not have a hormone component. Possible side effects include increased or abnormal bleeding. |

*(continued)*

**FIGURE 11.3** Continued.

| METHOD | APPROXIMATE EFFECTIVENESS | PREVENTS SEXUALLY TRANSMITTED INFECTIONS (STIs)? | DESCRIPTION |
|---|---|---|---|
| Tubal ligation | Nearly 100% | No | Surgery for women that cuts and ties the fallopian tubes, preventing eggs from traveling to the uterus. Difficult and expensive to reverse. Recommended for those who do not want any, or any more, children. |
| Vasectomy | Nearly 100% | No | Surgery for men that blocks the tube that delivers sperm to the penis. Like tubal ligation, difficult to reverse and only recommended for those who do not want any, or any more, children. |
| Rhythm method | Variable | No | Abstaining from intercourse during the ovulation segment of the woman's menstrual cycle. Can be difficult to time and may not account for cycle irregularities. |
| Withdrawal | Variable | No | Pulling the penis out of the vagina before ejaculation. Unreliable because some sperm can escape in the fluid released prior to ejaculation. Dependent on a controlled partner. |

Source: Adapted from MayoClinic.com, http://www.mayoclinic.com/health/birth-control/BI99999/PAGE=BI00020.

## Sexually Transmitted Infections

STIs spread through sexual contact (intercourse or other sexual activity that involves contact with the genitals). All are highly contagious. The only birth control methods that offer protection are the male and female condoms (latex or polyurethane only), which prevent skin-to-skin contact. Most STIs can also spread to infants of infected mothers during birth. Have a doctor examine any irregularity or discomfort as soon as you detect it. Figure 11.4 describes common STIs.

### AIDS and HIV

The most serious of the STIs is AIDS (acquired immune deficiency syndrome), which is caused by the human immunodeficiency virus (HIV). Not everyone who tests positive for HIV will develop AIDS, but AIDS has no cure and results in eventual death. Figure 11.5 shows some alarming statistics on AIDS.

HIV can lie undetected in the body for up to 10 years before surfacing, and a carrier can spread it during that time. Medical science continues to develop drugs to combat AIDS and its related illnesses. The drugs can cause severe side effects, however, and none are cures.

HIV is transmitted through two types of bodily fluids: fluids associated with sex (semen and vaginal fluids) and blood. People have acquired HIV through sexual relations, by sharing hypodermic needles for drug use, and by receiving infected blood transfusions. You cannot become infected unless one of those fluids is involved. Therefore, it is unlikely you can contract HIV from toilet seats, hugging, kissing, or sharing a glass.

FIGURE 11.4
To stay safe, know these facts about sexually transmitted infections

| DISEASE | SYMPTOMS | HEALTH PROBLEMS IF UNTREATED | TREATMENTS |
|---|---|---|---|
| Chlamydia | Discharge, painful urination, swollen or painful joints, change in menstrual periods for women | Can cause pelvic inflammatory disease (PID) in women, which can lead to sterility or ectopic pregnancies; infection; miscarriage or premature birth. | Curable with full course of antibiotics; avoid sex until treatment is complete. |
| Gonorrhea | Discharge, burning while urinating | Can cause PID, swelling of testicles and penis, arthritis, skin problems, infections. | Usually curable with antibiotics; however, certain strains are becoming resistant to medication. |
| Genital herpes | Blisterlike itchy sores in the genital area, headache, fever, chills | Symptoms may subside and then recur, often in response to high stress levels; carriers can transmit the virus even when it is dormant. | No cure; some medications, such as acyclovir, reduce and help heal the sores and may shorten recurring outbreaks. |
| Syphilis | A genital sore lasting one to five weeks, followed by a rash, fatigue, fever, sore throat, headaches, swollen glands | If it lasts more than four years, it can cause blindness, destruction of bone, insanity, or heart failure; can cause death or deformity of a child born to an infected woman. | Curable with full course of antibiotics. |
| Human papilloma virus (HPV, or genital warts) | Genital itching and irritation, small clusters of warts | Can increase risk of cervical cancer in women; virus may remain in body and cause recurrences even when warts are removed. | Treatable with drugs applied to warts or various kinds of wart removal surgery. Vaccine (Gardasil) newly available; most effective when given to women before exposure to HPV. |
| Hepatitis B | Fatigue, poor appetite, vomiting, jaundice, hives | Some carriers have few symptoms; others may develop chronic liver disease that may lead to other diseases of the liver. | No cure; some recover, some do not. Bed rest may help ease symptoms. Vaccine is available. |

## Protecting Yourself

The best defense against AIDS is not having sex or being in a long-term monogamous relationship. Condoms are the next best choice. The U.S. Department of Health and Human Services reports, "*There's absolutely no guarantee even when you use a condom.* But most experts believe that the risk of getting AIDS and other sexually transmitted diseases can be greatly reduced if a condom is used properly. . . . Sex with condoms ISN'T totally 'safe sex,' but it IS 'less risky' sex."[25] Always use a latex condom because natural skin condoms may let the virus pass through. Avoid petroleum jelly, which can destroy the latex in condoms.

## FIGURE 11.5 — AIDS and HIV continue to spread in the United States

- Since the AIDS epidemic began in the United States, an estimated 886,575 people have been diagnosed, and approximately 501,669 have died of AIDS.

- Since the epidemic began, well over one million Americans have been infected with HIV.

- It is estimated that between 850,000 and 950,000 people in the United States are currently HIV-positive.

- The year 2002 brought over 40,000 newly diagnosed AIDS patients. Over half of these were people under the age of 25.

- As of the end of 2002, 384,906 Americans were living with AIDS.

- Approximately 60 percent of newly infected men contracted HIV from homosexual sex, 25 percent through injection drug use, and 15 percent through heterosexual sex.

- Approximately 75 percent of newly infected women contracted HIV through heterosexual sex and 25 percent through injection drug use.

*Source:* National Institute of Allergy and Infectious Diseases, "HIV/AIDS Statistics" (January 2004). Retrieved May 2004, from: www.niaid.nih.gov/factsheets/aidsstat.htm#2.

Keep in mind that your emotional defenses can cloud your thinking about safe sex. If you are young and healthy, you may believe, incorrectly, that nothing bad can happen to you. This sense of invulnerability is leading an increasing number of gay students to engage in unprotected sex. For example, John, a gay student at Tufts University, tries to be safe but often rationalizes his failure to use condoms during all sexual encounters. When Benjamin, a student at Hunter College of the City University of New York, complains of "safe sex fatigue," he is also admitting that he isn't always willing to assess his risks.[26]

To be safe, have an HIV test done at your doctor's office or at a government-sponsored clinic. Your school's health department may also administer HIV tests, and home HIV tests are available over the counter. If you are infected, first inform all sexual partners and seek medical assistance. Then, contact support organizations in your area or call the National AIDS Hotline at 1-800-342-AIDS.

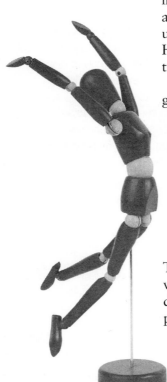

# *Joie de vivre*

The French have a phrase that is commonly used in the English language as well: *joie de vivre*, which literally means "joy of living." A person with joie de vivre finds joy and optimism in all parts of life, is able to enjoy life's pleasures, and can find something positive in its struggles. Without experiencing challenges, people might have a hard time recognizing and appreciating happiness and satisfaction.

Think of this concept as you examine your personal wellness. If you focus on the positive, your attitude can enhance all areas of your life.

# Building World-Class Skills
## for College, Career, and Life Success

## Create Your Future

## DEVELOPING SUCCESSFUL INTELLIGENCE
### *Putting It All Together*

**Take Steps Toward Better Health**. Put your successful intelligence to work in improving your physical health.

**Step 1. Think it through:** *Analyze your habits*. Pick a topic—eating, drinking, sleeping, sexual activity—that is an issue for you. To examine why it is a problem, identify behaviors and attitudes and note their positive and negative effects.

**Example:**   *Issue:* binge drinking

*Behavior:* I binge-drink probably three times a week.

*Attitude:* I don't think it's any big deal. I like using it to escape.

*Positive effects:* I have fun with my friends. I feel confident, accepted, social.

*Negative effects:* I feel hung over and foggy the next day. I miss class. I'm irritable.

**Your turn:**   *Issue:*

*Behavior:*

*Attitude:*

*Positive effects:*

*Negative effects:*

Question to think about: Is it worth it?

**Step 2. Think out of the box:** *Brainstorm ways to change*. First think about what you want to be different, and why. Then come up with changes you could make. Be creative!

*How you might change your behavior:*

*How you might change your attitude:*

*Positive effects you think these changes would have:*

**Step 3. Make it happen:** *Put a practical health improvement plan into action.* Choose two actions to take—one that would improve your attitude and one that would improve your behavior—that you think would have the most positive effect for you. Commit to these actions with specific plans and watch the positive change happen.

*Attitude improvement plan:*

*Behavior improvement plan:*

# TEAM BUILDING
## Collaborative Solutions

**Actively Dealing with Stress.** By yourself, make a list of stressors—whatever events or factors cause you stress. As a class, discuss the stressors you have listed. Choose the five most common. Divide into five groups according to who would choose what stressor as his or her most important (redistribute some people if the group sizes are unbalanced). Each group should discuss its assigned stressor, brainstorming solutions, and strategies. List your best coping strategies and present them to the class. Groups may want to make extra copies of the lists so every member of the class has five, one for each stressor.

# WRITING
## Discovery Through Journaling

*Record your thoughts on a separate piece of paper or in a journal.*

**Addiction.** Many people have, at one time or another, had to cope with some kind of addiction. Describe how you feel about addiction in any form—to alcohol, drugs, food, sex, the Internet, gambling. How has addiction ensnared you, if at all? How did you deal with it? If you have never faced an addiction or been close to someone who did, describe how you think you would work through the problem it if it ever happened to you.

# CAREER PORTFOLIO
## Plan for Success

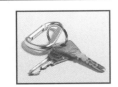

*Complete the following in your electronic portfolio or on separate sheets of paper.*

**Setting Effective Boundaries at Work.** In the current working world, many companies are putting pressure on their employees to do more in less time. The result is an environment that places workers under a great deal of stress. If you work in this environment, you may be asked to step up your efforts in different ways—do more work, add tasks to your job description, work late nights, keep your cell phone on for work calls on weekends, and so on.

However, there is a boundary—a limit—to what you can do successfully. If you hit that limit and don't overstep it, you may indeed keep your job and earn promotions. If you cross that boundary, your health and the quality of your work can suffer. If you don't work hard enough to approach it, you may lose your job or not advance.

Your challenge is to determine your limit and then monitor yourself to make sure that you work up to potential but don't overdo it. Answer the following questions in the effort to identify the most effective boundary for yourself as an employee:

- Are you willing to take on any job-related task, or do you get upset when people pile work on your desk that is not part of your job description?

- Are you willing to work late to meet a deadline, or do you get upset if you don't leave on time?

- Do you try to do your best work on everything or to get by with doing as little as possible?

- Are you likely to initiate different ideas that will improve your work product and then find ways to make them happen?

- Do you take a leadership position in your work team or try to stay in the background?

- When given a work request, do you tend to say "yes" right away, "no" right away, or take time to think about it thoroughly?

- Do you bring work into your personal life—socialize with coworkers, take work calls on personal time—or do you leave your job behind when you leave the workplace?

Analyze your answers as honestly as possible. Then, answer these questions: How do you think your attitudes will help or hurt you as a team member in your relationships with peers, managers, and others, and how do you think they will affect your career advancement? Check your personal attitude assessment against someone in a field you are interested in to see if you are on target or off base.

If you realize that your attitudes may stand in the way of success in a particular job or career area, consider what specific steps you are willing to take to change them. You might also consider whether you want to rethink your career or company choice to find a position or area that suits you better. Finally, think about how your ability to set effective boundaries may affect your success in school. Working up to your limits, but not too far beyond, will help you become the person you want to be both at school and in the world of work.

# Suggested Readings

Duyff, Roberta Larson. *The American Dietetic Association's Complete Food and Nutrition Guide*. Hoboken, NJ: Wiley, 2003.

Grayson, Paul A., Phil Meilman, and Philip W. Meilman. *Beating the College Blues*. New York: Checkmark Books, 1999.

Kadison, Richard D., and Theresa Foy DiGeronimo. *College of the Overwhelmed: The Campus Mental Health Crisis and What to Do About It*. San Francisco: Jossey-Bass, 2004.

Kuhn, Cynthia, et al. *Buzzed: The Straight Facts About the Most Used and Abused Drugs from Alcohol to Ecstasy*, 2nd ed. New York: W. W. Norton, 2003.

*Mayo Clinic Family Health Book: The Ultimate Home Medical Reference*, 3rd ed. New York: HarperResource, 2003.

The Physician's Desk Reference. *The Physician's Desk Reference Family Guide Encyclopedia of Medical Care*. New York: Ballantine Books, 1999.

Schuckit, Marc Alan. *Educating Yourself About Alcohol and Drugs: A People's Primer*. New York: HarperCollins, 1998.

Selkowitz, Ann. *The College Student's Guide to Eating Well on Campus*. Bethesda, MD: Tulip Hill Press, 2000.

Ward, Darrell. *The Amfar AIDS Handbook: The Complete Guide to Understanding HIV and AIDS*. New York: W. W. Norton, 1998.

# Internet Resources

Prentice Hall Student Success Supersite (fitness and well-being information): **www.prenhall.com/success**

American Cancer Society (general information, prevention, and early detection tips): **www.cancer.org**

Centers for Disease Control and Prevention (disease prevention and health information): **www.cdc.gov**

Columbia University's Health Education Program: **www.alice.columbia.edu**

It's Your (Sex) Life: **www.itsyoursexlife.com**

MayoClinic.com (medical information from this world-renowned medical center): **www.mayohealth.org**

HIV Prevention: **www.thebody.com/safesex.html**

# Endnotes

[1] The sources used in this section include Jane E. Brody, "Added Sugars Are Taking a Toll on Health," *New York Times*, September 12, 2000, p. F8; "Diabetes as Looming Epidemic," *New York Times*, January 30, 2001, p. F8; "Extra Soft Drink Is Cited as Major Factor in Obesity," *New York Times*, February 16, 2001, p. A12; Josh Stroud, "No More Fast Forward," *Dallas Business Journal*, January 21, 2000, p. 10C; "U.S. Favors Traditional Weight-Loss Plans," *New York Times*, January 16, 2001, p. F12.

[2] Statistics in these bullets taken from K. M. Flegal, M. D. Carroll, C. L. Ogden, and C. L. Johnson, "Prevalence and Trends in Obesity Among US Adults, 1999–2000," *Journal of the American Medical Association*, 288(2002): 1723–27.

[3] Definitions from "Defining Overweight and Obesity," Centers for Disease Control and Prevention. Retrieved May 2004, from: www.cdc.gov/nccdphp/dnpa/obesity/defining.htm.

[4] Jennifer Jacobson, "How Much Sports Is Too Much? Athletes Dislike Conferences' Efforts to Give Players More Time to Be Students," *The Chronicle of Higher Education* (December 6, 2002). Retrieved March 2004, from: http://chronicle.com/weekly/v49/i15a03801.htm.

[5] CBS News, "Help for Sleep-Deprived Students," Durham, NC (April 19, 2004). Retrieved May 2004, from: www.cbsnews.com/stories/2004/04/19/health/main612476.shtml.

[6] "College Students Sleep Habits Harmful to Health, Study Finds," *The Daily Orange—Feature Issue*

(September 25, 2002). Retrieved May 2004, from: www.dailyorange.com/news/2002/09/25/Feature/College.Students.Sleep.Habits.Harmful.To.Health.Study.Finds-280340.shtml.

[7]Ibid.

[8]Herbert Benson, M.D., and Eileen M. Stuart, R.N., C.M.S., et al., *The Wellness Book* (New York: Simon & Schuster, 1992), p. 292; and Gregg Jacobs, Ph.D., "Insomnia Corner," *Talk About Sleep* (2004) Retrieved May 2004, from: www.talkaboutsleep.com/sleepdisorders/insomnia_corner.htm.

[9]Information in this section based on materials from the Centers from Disease Control and Prevention (table at http://www.cdc.gov/hip/recs/adult/schedule.htm) and on advice from Dr. Orin Levine, associate professor of epidemiology at Johns Hopkins University.

[10]National Institutes of Health Publication No. 94-3561, National Institutes of Health, 1994.

[11]Retrieved May 9, 2004, from: www.save.org/depressed/symptoms.html (SA/VE website).

[12]Kim Hubbard, Anne-Marie O'Neill, and Christina Cheakalos, "Out of Control," *People*, April 12, 1999, p. 54.

[13]J. McGinnis and W. Foege, "Actual Causes of Death in the United States," *Journal of the American Medical Association* 270, no. 18 (1993): 2208.

[14]National Institute on Alcohol Abuse and Alcoholism, No. 29 PH 357, July 1995.

[15]H. Wechsler et al., "Changes in Binge Drinking and Related Problems Among American College Students Between 1993 and 1997," *Journal of American College Health* 47 (September 1998): 57.

[16]Ibid., pp. 63–64.

[17]National Institute on Alcohol Abuse and Alcoholism, No. 29 PH 357, July 1995.

[18]Darra Clark, Arizona State Freshman's Comments on EssayEdge.com. Retrieved March 2004, from: www.essayedge.com/college/admissions/speakout/arizona.shtml.

[19]National Institute on Drug Abuse, Capsule Series C-83-08, "Cigarette Smoking" (Bethesda, MD: National Institutes of Health, 1994).

[20]David Stout, "Direct Link Found Between Smoking and Lung Cancer," *New York Times*, October 18, 1996, pp. A1, A19.

[21]*Chicago Tribune*, "Secondhand Smoke Blamed in 3,000 Yearly Cancer Deaths" (February 26, 1997). [on-line]. Retrieved April 1997, from: http://archives.chicago.tribune.com.

[22]National Institutes of Health, Agency for Health Care Policy and Research, "Nicotine: A Powerful Addiction."

[23]National Institute on Drug Abuse, *National Survey Results on Drug Abuse from Monitoring the Future Study* (Bethesda, MD: National Institutes of Health, 1994).

[24]Drug Enforcement Administration, U.S. Department of Justice. Retrieved February 2003, from: www.usdoj.gov/dea/concern/mdma/mdmaindex.htm.

[25]U.S Department of Health and Human Services, "A Condom Could Save Your Life," Publication no. 90-4239.

[26]Alex P. Kellogg, "'Safe Sex Fatigue' Grows Among Gay Students: Health Officials Change Their HIV-Education Strategies as Condom Use Declines," *The Chronicle of Higher Education* (January 18, 2002). Retrieved March 2004, from: http://chronicle.com/weekly/v38/i19/19a03701.htm.

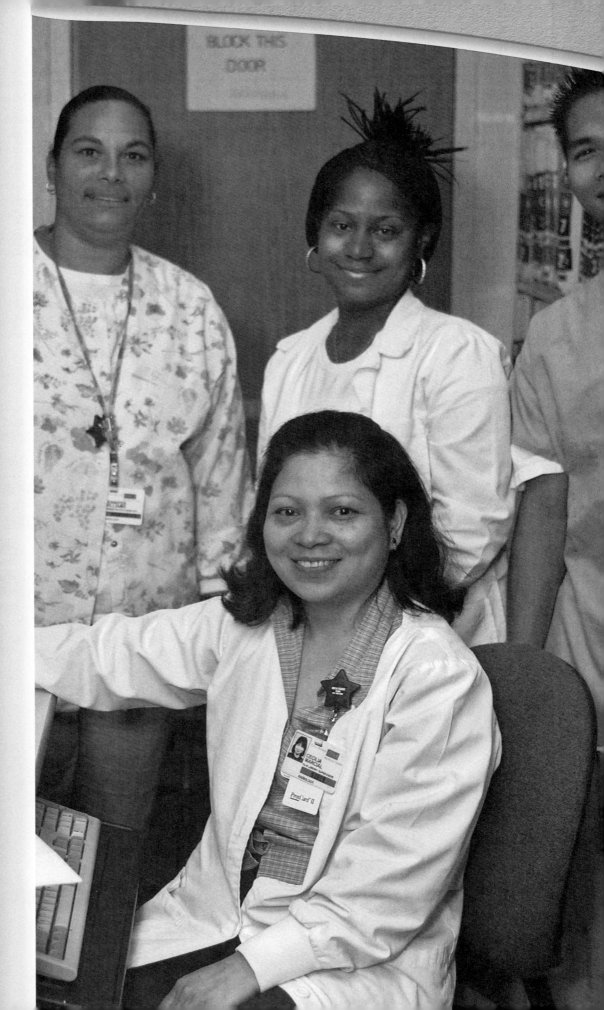

**PROSPER: MANAGING CAREER AND MONEY**

*REALITY RESOURCES*

**A**ll of the ways that you grow and learn in college will help you in your future career. Beginning to explore careers now, while you are a student, will help you find a career that suits you, whether it is being a teacher in Minnesota, an attorney in Manhattan, an archaeologist in Egypt, or anything else you dream of.

Money issues are another important concern—now, as you figure out how to finance school costs and manage credit cards, and later, when you are earning money in the working world. This chapter will show you how your successful intelligence can help you explore careers, hunt for jobs effectively, balance work and school, and manage your money so you can make the most of what you earn.

### *I'm deeply concerned about some of the ethical situations that affect a nurse, specifically quality of life.*

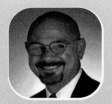

I'm a former police officer who served on the force for eight years in a suburb of Kansas City. One of my responsibilities at that time was to investigate car accidents. This meant some of my work hours were spent at the local hospital. I've also given CPR while on duty. Of course, I got great satisfaction from knowing I helped save someone's life. After I got hurt on the job, I began to think about pursuing a new career, and nursing became the obvious choice for me.

**Robert Dary**
*Senior, University of Kansas, Kansas City, Kansas*

What drives me to be a nurse is that I'm making a difference in the life of a patient. I feel very comfortable working in ICU because I can get to know the patients and their families. Having someone you love in ICU can be a very traumatic experience. I find it gratifying to interact with the patient's family. By explaining the purpose of medical procedures and how different hospital equipment works, I help them understand what's going on with the patient.

Working toward a bachelor's degree is a real stretch for me. I've been forced to think in more creative ways. Back when I was in high school, learning seemed less complicated. I memorized the facts and regurgitated what I knew. In nursing, learning requires more than memorization. There's so much material to absorb that I've needed to understand how each component relates to the whole. I know I'll need to continue learning long after graduation. Advances in technology cause procedures to change, and I'm also interested in learning more about pathophysiological processes. The idea of continuing to reeducate myself excites me.

Thinking about my future also raises another core issue of nursing. I'm deeply concerned about some of the ethical situations that affect a nurse, specifically quality of life. I've seen patients come out of ICU who were on feeding tubes, and they are still ventilator dependent. Their survival depends on the machine. Sometimes I think technology takes away the natural process of dying, and I wonder if in my future career I'll be setting up some of my patients for poorer quality of life. Other than my brief exposure to Hospice, I've seen very little educational material that addresses death and dying. Can you offer suggestions for helping me come to terms with these tough issues as they relate to my future career?

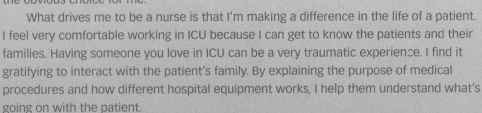

# PRACTICAL ANSWERS

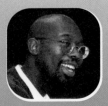

**Dr. Courtney H. Lyder**
*Yale School of Nursing, New Haven, Connecticut*

### *One of the most difficult challenges for critical care nurses is patients who are facing the end of life.*

You raised very thoughtful issues about the profession of nursing. With regard to continuing education, I think we have an inherent accountability both to our patients and to their families to expand our knowledge and clinical skills. Given the advances in health care technology, the methods by which we deliver nursing care could radically change; therefore, it is imperative that you keep up to date with the latest technology and effective care modalities based on nursing research.

One of the best things I ever did to continue my education was a brief study abroad program in England. In this course we compared the British system of psychiatric nursing care of the American model. This course gave me a different perspective and I changed some of my nursing practices because of this experience. Sometimes the best learning isn't confined to the classroom; it happens experientially. Perhaps you can volunteer in a cultural setting different from what you are accustomed to or take a nontraditional course.

One of the most difficult challenges for critical care nurses is patients who are facing the end of life. You will definitely confront this issue again and again as a critical care nurse. Historically, the nursing profession has focused on maintaining or enhancing the quality of life for patients, as well as helping the families adjust to the changes that chronic and acute illnesses bring. I can't point you to any one seminal piece of literature or strategy for grappling with this complex issue. However, I can tell you that coming to terms with dying patients is a process, as you move from being a novice to an expert. Several years ago I was a nurse in the medical intensive care unit (MICU) and it became clear to me that I had to depend on the expertise of the senior nurses. I tapped their brains for help in dealing with my thoughts and feelings related to caring for patients with poor prognostic outcomes.

Palliative care is a type of nursing that deals with end-of-life issues, and the goal of nursing care may change depending on whether the patient's condition is chronic or acute. There are courses you can take in palliative care that address death and dying. As you know, the goal of hospice isn't cure but to provide the best comfort for the patient. Nevertheless, you can have palliative care in the critical care area as well.

I have never felt more like a nurse than when I am helping a patient die peacefully. Nurses, unlike physicians, are with the patient around the clock. Being able to tell patients that you are there for them and that they will not die alone can help make death less frightening for them. My earlier experience as a MICU nurse taught me that death and dying were mechanical and technical processes. When I chose geriatric nursing, which is my current specialty, I began to see death as a more natural, even beautiful process. One of the wonderful things I've learned from caring for our elders is that they can teach us how to live.

# How Can You Prepare for *Workplace Success?*

Now is the time to take steps toward a fulfilling nursing career. You are already preparing for career success with your work in this course, because every skill in this book—thinking, teamwork, writing skills, and goal setting, among others—prepares you to thrive in your chosen profession. Use the following strategies to get more specific in your preparation.

## Investigate Paths in Nursing

Look back at Chapters 1 and 2 for ideas of paths to take within nursing. The working world changes all the time. You can get an idea of what's out there—and what you think of it all—by exploring potential careers and building knowledge and experience.

**FIGURE 12.1** Ask questions like these to analyze how a workplace may fit you

| | |
|---|---|
| What can I do in this area that I like and do well? | Do I respect the company or organization? |
| What are the educational or degree requirements? | Does this organization accommodate special needs (child care, sick days, flex time)? |
| What are workplace requirements? | Do I need to belong to a professional union? What does union membership involve? |
| What wage or salary and benefits can I expect? | Are there opportunities near where I live (or want to live)? Are they on par nationally? |
| What are the people like? | What are the people like at the organization? |
| What are the prospects for moving up to higher-level positions? | Do I prefer the service or production end of this industry? |
| What is the orientation, residency, or internship? | Does the organization provide for on the job learning? |

## Explore Potential Paths

Possibilities extend far beyond what you can imagine. Ask instructors, relatives, mentors, and fellow students. Check your library for books on nursing or biographies of people who worked areas that interest you. Explore through job shadowing or interviewing

Use your analytical thinking skills to broaden your investigation. Look at Figure 12.1 for the kinds of questions that will aid your search when you are ready to look for a job. You may discover that:

**A Wide Array of Job Possibilities Exists.** For example, nurses are also administrators who run hospitals, researchers who test new drugs, and so on.

**Within Each Job, There Is Variety of Tasks and Skills.** You may know that an instructor teaches, but you may not see that instructors also often write, research, study, design courses, give presentations, and counsel. Take your exploration beyond your first impression of a career.

**Common Assumptions About Salaries Don't Always Hold.** Finance, medicine, law, and computer science aren't the only high-paying careers. According to data from the U.S. Labor Department, nurses are gaining high earnings.[1] Remember to place earnings in perspective: Even if you earn a high salary, you may not be happy unless you enjoy your work.

Your school's career center may offer job listings, assessments of skills and personality types, questionnaires to help you pinpoint areas that may suit you, and information about different organizations and companies. Visit the center early and work with a counselor to develop a solid career game plan.

## Build Knowledge and Experience

Having knowledge and experience specific to the career you wish to pursue is valuable on the job hunt. Courses, internships, jobs, and volunteering are four great ways to build both.

**Internships and Residencies.** When you become a nurse your first job should offer a orientation period of up to one year. Look for this!

**Jobs.** You may discover opportunities while earning money during a part-time job. Some nursing students work at an organization part time while attending nursing school. This can lead to opportunities after graduation. Jobs in the health field can help you get into nursing school too.

**Volunteering.** Helping others in need can introduce you to careers and increase your experience. Some schools have programs that link you to volunteering opportunities. Include volunteer activities on your résumé. Many employers and nursing schools look favorably on volunteering.

Even after you've completed college, the key is to continually build on what you know. With the work world changing so quickly, today's employers value those who are always improving in their skills and knowledge.

## Know What Employers Want

In the jobs you seek after you graduate, employers will look for specific technical skills, work experience, and academic credentials. They will also look for other skills and qualities that indicate that you are a promising candidate.

### Important Skills

Figure 12.2 describes the particular skills and qualities that tell an employer you are likely to be an efficient and effective employee.

These skills, which you have built throughout this book, are as much a part of your school success as they are of your work success. The more you develop them now, the more employable and promotable you will be.

### Emotional Intelligence

Another quality employers seek is *emotional intelligence*. In his book *Working with Emotional Intelligence*, psychologist Daniel Goleman states that emotional intelligence can be even more important than IQ and knowledge. He defines emotional intelligence as a combination of these factors:[2]

- *Personal competence* refers to how you manage yourself—your self-awareness, self-regulation, and motivation.

- *Social competence* refers to how you handle relationships with others, including awareness of the needs and feelings of others and ability to encourage others to do things.

| FIGURE 12.2 | Employers look for candidates with these important skills |

| SKILLS | WHY IS IT USEFUL? |
|---|---|
| Communication | Good listening, speaking, and writing skills are keys to working with others, as is being able to adjust to different communication styles. |
| Analytical thinking | An employee who can analyze choices and challenges, as well as assess the value of new ideas, stands out. |
| Creativity | The ability to come up with new concepts, plans, and products helps companies improve and innovate. |
| Practical thinking | No job gets done without employees who can think through a plan for achieving a goal, put it into action, and complete it successfully. |
| Teamwork | All workers interact with others on the job. Working well with others is essential for achieving workplace goals. |
| Goal setting | Teams fail if goals are unclear or unreasonable. Employees and company benefit from setting realistic, specific goals and achieving them reliably. |
| Cultural competence | The workplace is increasingly diverse. An employee who can work with, adjust to, and respect people from different backgrounds and cultures is valuable. |
| Leadership | The ability to influence and motivate others in a positive way earns respect and career advancement. |
| Positive attitude | Other employees will gladly work with, and often advance, someone who completes tasks with positive, upbeat energy. |
| Integrity | Acting with integrity at work—communicating promptly, being truthful and honest, following rules, giving proper notice—enhances value. |
| Flexibility | The most valuable employees understand the constancy of change and have developed the skills to adapt to its challenge. |
| Continual learning | The most valuable employees take personal responsibility to stay current in their fields. |

Look at Figure 12.3 for specific skills that are part of these two factors.

An important part of personal competence is knowledge of your values. Think back to how you explored your values in Chapter 3. These values give you a framework from which to make all kinds of important decisions, including those about your career goals. Because you usually enjoy, excel at, and are most motivated by what is important to you, pursuing a career that incorporates your values increases your chances of fulfillment and success.

The current emphasis on teamwork has made emotional intelligence very important in the workplace. The more adept you are at working comfortably and productively with others (i.e., the more emotionally intelligent you are and the more you use this intelligence), the more likely you are to succeed.

## FIGURE 12.3 — Being emotionally intelligent means developing these key qualities

### PERSONAL COMPETENCE

**Self-Awareness**

- I know my emotions and how they affect me.
- I understand my strengths and my limits.
- I am confident in my abilities.
- I am open to improvement.

**Self-Management**

- I can control my emotions and impulses.
- I can delay gratification when there is something more important to be gained.
- I am trustworthy.
- I can adapt to change and new ideas.
- I persist toward my goals despite obstacles.

### SOCIAL COMPETENCE

**Social Awareness**

- I sense the feelings and perspectives of others.
- I help others improve themselves.
- I know how to relate to people from different cultures.
- I can sense how to serve the needs of others.

**Social Skills**

- I know how to work in a team.
- I can inspire people to act.
- I understand how to lead a group.
- I know how to persuade people.
- I can make positive change happen.

## Expect Change

The working world is always in flux, responding to technological developments, global competition, and other factors. Reading newspapers and magazines, scanning business sites on the Internet, and watching television news all help you keep abreast of what you face as you make career decisions. Think about the following as you prepare to adjust to change.

### Growing and Declining Career Areas

Rapid workplace change means that a growth area today may be declining tomorrow—witness the sudden drop in Internet company jobs and fortunes in 2001. The U.S. Bureau of Labor keeps updated statistics on the status of various career areas. For example, for the period 1998 to 2008, of the 10 fastest growing occupations identified by the bureau, five are computer-related occupations.

### Workplace Trends

What's happening now? Companies, to save money, are hiring more temporary employees (temps) and fewer full-time employees. Temporary jobs offer flexibility, few obligations, and often more take-home pay, but they have limited benefits. Also, in response to the changing needs of the modern workforce, companies are offering more "quality of life" benefits such as telecommuting, job sharing, and on-site child care.

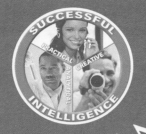

# GET ANALYTICAL!

## Connect Values to Career

*Use your values as a career exploration guide.*

First, look at the following list of "value words." Put a check mark by those qualities that are most important to you as a working person. Circle your top five.

- Accepting
- Adventurous
- Ambitious
- Calm
- Caring
- Conscientious
- Cooperative
- Creative
- Decisive
- Demonstrating leadership
- Efficient
- Enthusiastic
- Focused on learning
- Honest/fair
- Independent
- Kind
- Loyal
- Organized
- Powerful
- Prompt
- Serious
- Trustworthy
- Wealthy

Keeping your top values in mind, answer the following questions:

The kind of work I enjoy most is
I can't see myself working as a
Self-fulfillment at work consists of
Being in charge of others makes me feel
Being responsible makes me feel
Working independently makes me feel
Working in a team makes me feel
Imagining that I'm being promoted after two years on a job, I think my employer would say it is because of these exemplary characteristics:

*Source:* Adapted from Gary Izumo et al., *Keys to Career Success* (Upper Saddle River, NJ: Prentice Hall, 2002), pp. 67–69.

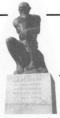

Standing still is the fastest way of moving backwards in a rapidly changing world.

LAUREN BACALL

## Personal Change

Even difficult personal changes can open doors that you never imagined were there. For example, Susan Davenny Wyner, a successful classical singer, was hit by a car while biking. The accident damaged her vocal cords beyond repair. She later discovered that conducting held an opportunity for her to express herself musically in a way she didn't think she could ever do again.[3]

As this story demonstrates, if you think creatively about your marketable skills and job possibilities, you will be able to find new ways to achieve. What you know about your learning style should play an important role in your thinking.

# What Does Your *Learning Style* Mean for Your Career?

If you think you want to go into nursing or some health care field but are not sure, you are not alone. Many students who have not been in the workplace—and even some who have—aren't sure what career to pursue. Start with what you know about yourself. Ask yourself questions like the following:

- What do I know best, do best, and enjoy best?
- Out of the jobs I have had, what did I like and not like to do?
- What kinds of careers could make the most of everything I am?

What you know about your learning style from Chapter 3 will give you important clues in the search for the right career. The Multiple Intelligences assessment points to information about your innate learning strengths and challenges, which, in turn, can lead you to careers that involve these strengths. Your Personality Spectrum assessment results are perhaps even more significant to career success because they provide insight on how you work best with others. Career success depends, in large part, on your ability to function in a team.

Figure 12.4 focuses the four dimensions of the Personality Spectrum on career ideas and strategies. Look for your strengths and decide what you may want to keep in mind as you search. Look also at the skills that challenge you because even the most ideal job involves some tasks that may not be in your area of comfort. Identifying ways to boost your abilities in those areas will help you succeed.

Keep in mind a few important points as you consider the information in this table:

## Use Information as a Guide, Not a Label

You may not necessarily have all the strengths and challenges that your dominant areas indicate. Chances are, though, that thinking through them will help you narrow your focus and clarify your abilities and interests.

## Avoid Thinking That Challenges Are Weaknesses

Work challenges describe qualities that may cause issues in particular work situations. They aren't necessarily weaknesses in and of themselves. For example, not many people would say that a need for structure and stability

FIGURE 12.4

## Personality Spectrum dimensions indicate strengths and challenges

| DIMENSION | STRENGTHS ON THE JOB | CHALLENGES ON THE JOB | LOOK FOR JOBS/CAREERS THAT FEATURE . . . |
|---|---|---|---|
| Thinker | • Problem solving<br>• Development of ideas<br>• Keen analysis of situations<br>• Fairness to others<br>• Efficiency in working through tasks<br>• Innovation of plans and systems<br>• Ability to look strategically at the future | • A need for private time to think and work<br>• A need, at times, to move away from established rules<br>• A dislike of sameness—systems that don't change, repetitive tasks<br>• Not always being open to expressing thoughts and feelings to others | • Some level of solo work/think time<br>• Problem solving<br>• Opportunity for innovation<br>• Freedom to think creatively and to bend the rules<br>• Technical work<br>• Big-picture strategic planning |
| Organizer | • High level of responsibility<br>• Enthusiastic support of social structures<br>• Order and reliability<br>• Loyalty<br>• Ability to follow through on tasks according to requirements<br>• Detailed planning skills with competent follow-through<br>• Neatness and efficiency | • A need for tasks to be clearly, concretely defined<br>• A need for structure and stability<br>• A preference for less rapid change<br>• A need for frequent feedback<br>• A need for tangible appreciation<br>• Low tolerance for people who don't conform to rules and regulations | • Clear, well-laid-out tasks and plans<br>• Stable environment with consistent, repeated tasks<br>• Organized supervisors<br>• Clear structure of how employees interact and report to one another<br>• Value of, and reward for, loyalty |
| Giver | • Honesty and integrity<br>• Commitment to putting energy toward close relationships with others<br>• Finding ways to bring out the best in self and others<br>• Peacemaker and mediator<br>• Ability to listen well, respect opinions, and prioritize the needs of coworkers | • Difficulty in handling conflict, either personal or between others in the work environment<br>• Strong need for appreciation and praise<br>• Low tolerance for perceived dishonesty or deception<br>• Avoidance of people perceived as hostile, cold, or indifferent | • Emphasis on teamwork and relationship building<br>• Indications of strong and open lines of communication among workers<br>• Encouragement of personal expression in the workplace (arrangement of personal space, tolerance of personal celebrations, and so on) |
| Adventurer | • Skillfulness in many different areas<br>• Willingness to try new things<br>• Ability to take action<br>• Hands-on problem-solving skills<br>• Initiative and energy<br>• Ability to negotiate<br>• Spontaneity and creativity | • Intolerance of being kept waiting<br>• Lack of detail focus<br>• Impulsiveness<br>• Dislike of sameness and authority<br>• Need for freedom, constant change, and constant action<br>• Tendency not to consider consequences of actions | • A spontaneous atmosphere<br>• Less structure, more freedom<br>• Adventuresome tasks<br>• Situations involving change<br>• Encouragement of hands-on problem solving<br>• Travel and physical activity<br>• Support of creative ideas and endeavors |

(a challenge of the Giver) is a weakness. However, it can be a challenge in a workplace that operates in an unstructured manner.

### Know That You Are Capable of Change

Use ideas about strengths and challenges as a starting point and make some decisions about how you would like to grow.

Now that you've done your homework, it's time to get to the search. What you know, along with the strategies that follow, will help you along the path to a career that works for you.

# How Can You Explore Career Options in Nursing?

To have a clearer sense of your goals in nursing, reflect on Chapter 2's discussion of career options beginning on page 57. To be certain, maximize your nursing career opportunities by using the resources available to you, making a strategic search plan, and knowing some basics about résumés and interviews.

## Use Available Resources

Use your school's nursing advisers and career planning office, your **networking** skills and online services to help you explore postgraduation job opportunities.

NETWORKING
The exchange of information or services among individuals, groups, or institutions.

### Your School's Nursing Advisers

Generally, the nursing advisers deal with postgraduation job opportunities along with financial aid information.

The advisers can help you understand the prerequisites needed to get into nursing school. They can help you with the application process. Ask them about what GPA you should have and how to find tutors.

If your school has a **cooperative education** or career office, it can help you land a job before graduation. Jason Roach, a nursing student at New Mexico State University, used the co-op office as a job-referral source. He explains, "The Cooperative Education office works very hard to notify students when health care organizations will be on campus interviewing. I receive at least ten e-mails a week telling me who would be on campus and a quick background on the each."[4]

COOPERATIVE EDUCATION
A program offered by some colleges that combines credit-earning course work with paid work experience in a field that relates to the course.

### Networking

The most basic type of networking—talking to nurses about specialties that interest you—is one of the most important strategies. Networking **contacts** can answer questions regarding job responsibilities and challenges. You can network with friends and family members, instructors, administrators, counselors, alumni, employers, coworkers, and others. Go job-shadow with a nurse—this is *the* best way to see what the career is like.

CONTACT
A person who serves as a carrier or source of information.

You can also network with people you meet through your extracurricular activities. Christine Muñoz, a student at New Mexico State University, chose a prenursing club that she knew could help her prepare for nursing school and a career. "I am currently the president of SNA—the Hispanic Student Nurse

Association," said Muñoz. "This semester we did several fund-raisers and community service projects. We have biweekly meetings, and we also have socials where we all just get together and hang out. Professional speakers come and speak about résumé and interview skills, and nursing specialty practice areas, something that is beneficial to everyone."[5]

### Online Services

The Internet has exploded into one of the most fruitful sources of nursing opportunities. There are many sites to learn more about nursing. Try www.nursingworld.org.

## Make a Strategic Job Search Plan

After gathering information, make a practical plan to achieve your career goals by mapping out your long-term timeline and keeping track of specific actions.

### Make a Big-Picture Timeline

Make a career timeline that illustrates the steps toward your goal, as shown in Figure 12.5. Write in the steps when you think they should happen. If

**FIGURE 12.5** A career timeline helps you plan ahead

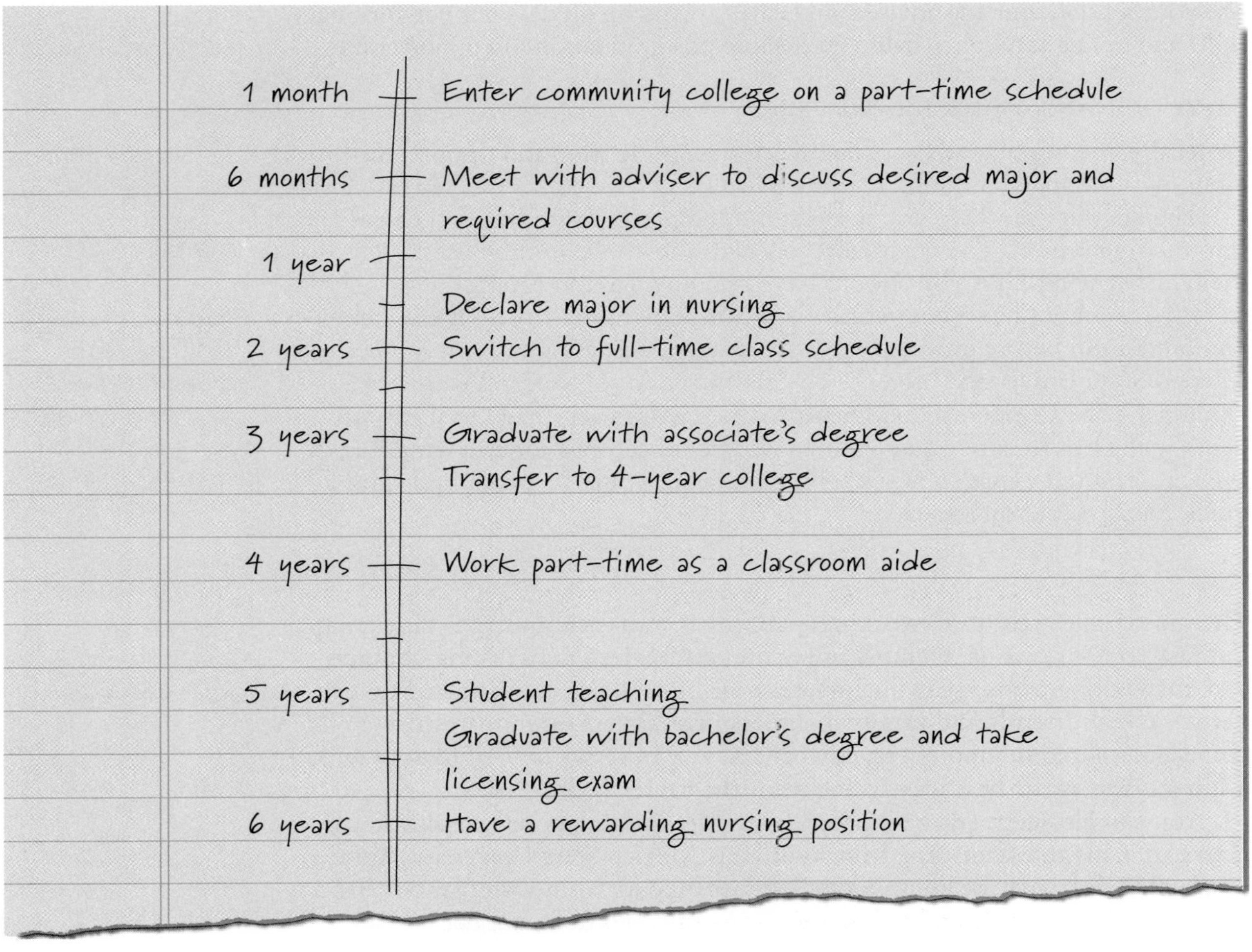

|  |  |
|------|------|
| 1 month | Enter community college on a part-time schedule |
| 6 months | Meet with adviser to discuss desired major and required courses |
| 1 year | |
| | Declare major in nursing |
| 2 years | Switch to full-time class schedule |
| 3 years | Graduate with associate's degree |
| | Transfer to 4-year college |
| 4 years | Work part-time as a classroom aide |
| 5 years | Student teaching |
| | Graduate with bachelor's degree and take licensing exam |
| 6 years | Have a rewarding nursing position |

your plan is five years long, indicate what you plan to do by the fourth, third, and second years, and then the first year, including a six-month goal and a one-month goal for that first year. Your path may change, of course; use your timeline as a guide rather than as an inflexible plan.

On road to a truly satisfying nursing career, seek support as you work toward goals. Confide in supportive people, talk positively to yourself, and read books about nursing such as those listed at the end of this chapter.

# Your Résumé, Cover Letter, and Interview

Information on résumés, cover letters, and interviews fills entire books. You'll find specific sources listed at the end of the chapter. To get you started, here are a few basic tips on giving yourself the best possible chance at a job.

## Résumé and Cover Letter

Your résumé should always be typed or printed on high-quality paper. Design your résumé neatly, using an acceptable format (books or your career office can show you some standard formats).

Proofread it for errors and have someone else proofread it as well. Type or print it on a heavier bond paper than is used for ordinary copies. Include a cover letter along with your résumé that tells the employer what job you are interested in and why he or she should hire you.

Prospective employers often use a computer to scan résumés. The computer program will select résumés if they contain enough *keywords*—words relating to the job opening or industry. Résumés without enough keywords probably won't even make it to the human resources desk. When you construct your résumé, make sure to include as many keywords as you can. For example, if you are seeking a computer-related job, list computer programs you use and other specific technical proficiencies. To figure out what keywords you need, check out job descriptions, job postings, and other current résumés.[6]

## Interview

Be clean, neat, and appropriately dressed. Choose a nice pair of shoes—people notice. Bring an extra copy of your résumé and any other materials that you want to show the interviewer, even if you have already sent a copy ahead of time. Avoid chewing gum or smoking. Offer a confident handshake. Make eye contact. Show your integrity by speaking honestly about yourself. After the interview, no matter what the outcome, follow up right away with a formal but pleasant thank-you note.

Being on time to your interview makes a positive impression—and being late will almost certainly be held against you. If you are from a culture that does not consider being late a sign of disrespect, remember that your interviewer may not agree.

Having a job may not only be a thought for the future; it may be something you are concerned about right now. Many students need to work and take classes at the same time to fund their education. Although you may not necessarily work in an area that interests you, you can hold a job that helps you pay the bills and still make the most of your school time.

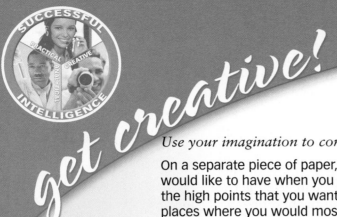

## Make a Dream Résumé

*Use your imagination to conjure up an ideal work history.*

On a separate piece of paper, write your "dream résumé," the résumé that you would like to have when you graduate college, the résumé that would hit all the high points that you want to achieve and that would open the door at the places where you would most like to work. Use questions like these to brainstorm:

- What would be your academic record?
- What awards and honors would you have?
- What internship or work experience would you have?
- What special skills would you have?

The person who can hand out this résumé is the person you are committed to becoming.

# What Will Help You *Juggle* Work and School?

What you are studying today can prepare you to find a job when you graduate. In the meantime, though, you can make work a part of your student life to make money, explore a career, and increase your future employability through contacts or résumé building.

As the cost of education continues to rise, more and more students are working and taking classes at the same time. Figure 12.6 shows statistics related to working for both part-time and full-time college students.

Many people want to work and many need to work to pay for school. Gather information about what you need, analyze the potential positive and negative effects of working, generate options, and make practical choices that are right for you.

## Establish Your Needs

Think about what you need from a job before you begin your job hunt. Ask questions like these:

- How much money do I need to make—weekly, per semester, for the year?
- What time of day is best for me? Should I consider night or weekend work?

FIGURE 12.6    Many students are working while in school

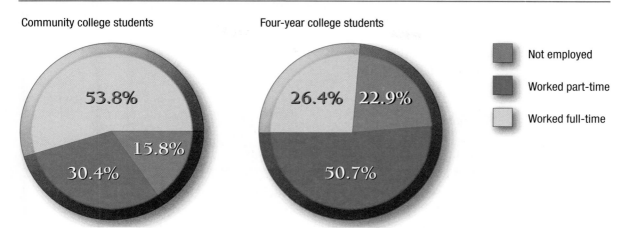

Community college students          Four-year college students

53.8%
15.8%
30.4%

26.4%  22.9%
50.7%

Not employed
Worked part-time
Worked full-time

*Source:* U.S. Department of Education, National Center for Educational Statistics. *Profile of Undergraduates in U.S. Postsecondary Education Institutions:* 1999–2000. (NCES 98-084), July 2002, Table 12.5.1.

- Can my schedule handle a full-time job or should I look for part-time work?
- Do I want hands-on experience in a particular field? What do I like and dislike doing?
- Does location matter? Where do I want to work and how far am I willing to commute?
- How flexible a job do I need?
- Can I, or should I, find work at my school or as part of a work-study?

## Analyze Effects of Working While in School

Evaluate any job opportunity by looking at these effects. Potential positive effects include:

- Money earned.
- General and career-specific experience.
- Enhanced school and work performance (working up to 15 hours a week may encourage students to manage time more effectively and build confidence).

Potential negative effects include:

- Demanding time commitment.
- Reduced opportunity for social and extracurricular activities.
- Having to shift gears mentally from work to classroom.

The right part-time job can help you develop skills that you can use after graduation. For example, "techies" on the University of Denver's Technology Services help desk learn to solve hardware, software, and Internet problems as they polish their customer-service etiquette. On an average day, each staffer handles nearly 100 calls and visits, many of which involve angry, frustrated people. "We're on the front line, so if something goes wrong, we're the first to know, and we get blamed for everything," said technician Andrew Chan. Because Chan solves problems quickly and efficiently while treating people with respect, he will receive positive recommendations from his supervisors.[7]

No matter where your money comes from—financial aid or one or more jobs—budgeting skills will help you cover your expenses and have some cash left over for savings and fun.

# How Can You *Create a Budget* That Works?

For the vast majority of college students, money is tight. You may have to rely on loans or money from a job to cover tuition, textbooks, and the products and services you need every day. Even if your family pays for your education, you will almost certainly need to monitor your monthly personal expenses. Effective **budgeting** relieves money-related stress and helps you feel more in control.

Your biggest expense right now is probably the cost of your education, including tuition and room and board. However, that expense may not hit you fully until after you graduate and begin to pay back your student loans. For now, include in your budget only the part of the cost of your education you are paying while you are in school.

Budgeting demands analytical, creative, and practical thinking. You gather information about your resources (money flowing in) and expenditures (money flowing out) and analyze the difference. Next, you come up with ideas about how you can make changes. Finally, you take practical action to adjust spending or earning so that you come out even or ahead. Most people budget on a month-by-month basis.

BUDGETING
Making a plan for the coordination of resources and expenditures; setting goals regarding money.

## Figure Out What You Earn

Add up all of the money you receive during the year—the actual after-tax money you have to pay your bills. Common sources of income include:

- Take-home pay from a regular full-time or part-time job during the school year
- Take-home pay from summer and holiday employment
- Money you earn as part of a work-study program
- Money you receive from your parents or other relatives for your college expenses
- Scholarships or grants that provide spending money

Money can't buy you happiness. It just helps you look for it in more places.

MILTON BERLE

If you have savings specifically earmarked for your education, decide how much you will withdraw every month for your school-related expenses.

## Figure Out What You Spend

Start by recording every check you write for fixed expenses like rent and telephone. Then, over the next month, record personal expenditures in a small notebook. Indicate any expenditure over five dollars, making sure to count smaller expenditures if they are frequent (for example, a bus pass for a month, soda or newspaper purchases per week).

Some expenses, like automobile and health insurance, may be billed only a few times a year. In these cases, convert the expense to monthly by dividing the yearly cost by 12. Be sure to count only current expenses, not expenses that you will pay after you graduate. Among these are the following:

- Rent or mortgage
- Tuition that you are paying right now (the portion remaining after all forms of financial aid, including loans, scholarships and grants, are taken into account)
- Books, lab fees, and other educational expenses
- Regular bills (electric, gas, oil, phone, water)
- Food, clothing, toiletries, and household supplies
- Child care
- Transportation and auto expenses (gas, maintenance)
- Credit cards and other payments on credit (car payments)
- Insurance (health, auto, homeowner's or renter's, life)
- Entertainment and related items (cable TV, movies, eating out, books and magazines)
- Computer-related expenses, including the cost of your online service
- Miscellaneous unplanned expenses

Use the total of all your monthly expenses as a baseline for other months, realizing that your expenditures will vary depending on what is happening in your life.

## Evaluate the Difference

Focusing again on your current situation, subtract your monthly expenses from your monthly income. Ideally, you have money left over—to save or to spend. However, if you are spending more than you take in, your first job is to analyze the problem by looking carefully at your budget, your spending patterns, and priorities. Use your analytical thinking skills to ask some focused questions.

### Question Your Budget

Did you forget to budget for recurring expenses such as the cost for semiannual dental visits? Or was your budget derailed by an emergency expense that you did not foresee, such as the cost of a new transmission for your car? Is your budget realistic? Is your income sufficient for your needs?

## Question Your Spending Patterns and Priorities

Did you spend money wisely during the month? Did you go to too many restaurants or movies? Can you afford the luxury of your own car? Are you putting too many purchases on your credit card and being hit by high interest payments? When you are spending more than you are taking in during a "typical month," you may have to adjust your budget over the long term.

## Adjust Spending or Earning

Look carefully at what may cause you to overspend and brainstorm possible solutions that address those causes. Solutions can involve either increasing resources or decreasing spending. To deal with spending, prioritize your expenditures and trim the ones you really don't need to make. Cut out unaffordable extras.

As for resources, investigate ways to take in more money. Start your summer job search early. Taking a part-time job, hunting down scholarships or grants, increasing hours at a current job, or looking for a higher-paying job may also help.

### A Sample Budget

Figure 12.7 shows a sample budget of an unmarried student living with two other students in off-campus housing with no meal plan. Included are all regular and out-of-pocket expenses with the exception of tuition expenses, which the student will pay back after graduation in student loan payments. In this case, the student is $164 over budget. How would you make up the shortfall?

Not everyone likes the work involved in keeping a budget. For example, whereas logical-mathematical learners may take to it easily, visual learners may resist the structure and detail of the budgeting process (see Chapter 3). Visual learners may want to create a budget chart such as the one in the example or use strategies that make budgeting more tangible, such as dumping receipts into a big jar and tallying them at the end of the month. Even if you have to force yourself to use a budget, you will realize that the process can reduce stress and help you take control of your finances and your life.

## Make Successfully Intelligent Financial Decisions

Every budgetary decision you make has particular effects, often involving a trade-off among options. When you spend $80 for that new pair of sneakers, for example, you may not have enough for movie tickets and dinner with friends that weekend. That is, there is an opportunity cost in addition to money. In this case, the new sneakers deprive you of the chance to attend the movie and go to dinner.

FIGURE 12.7 How one student mapped out a monthly budget

**A STUDENT'S SAMPLE MONTHLY BUDGET**

- Wages: $10 an hour (after taxes) × 20 hours a week = $200 a week × 4 1/3 weeks (one month) = $866.
- Withdrawals from savings (from summer earnings) = $200
- Total income per month: $1,066

**MONTHLY EXPENDITURES**

| | |
|---|---|
| School-related expenses (not covered by student loans, grants, scholarships—including books and supplies) | $ 150 |
| Public transportation | $ 90 |
| Phone | $ 40 |
| Food | $ 450 |
| Credit card payments | $ 100 |
| Rent (including utilities) | $ 200 |
| Entertainment | $ 100 |
| Miscellaneous expenses, including clothes and toiletries | $ 100 |
| **Total monthly spending** | **$1,230** |

$1,066 (income) − $1,230 (spending) = $−164 ($164 over budget)

## Use Decision-Making Strategies

Being a successfully intelligent money manager means using what you know about decision making (Chapter 4) to think through financial decisions carefully.

1. *Define the decision.* Be honest about what you need and what you just want. Do you really need a new bike? Or can the old one suffice while you pay off some credit card debt?
2. *Generate available options.* Imagine what you can do with your money.
3. *Evaluate options.* Look closely at the positive and negative effects of each option and make a choice.
4. *Take practical action.* Spend it—save it—invest it—whatever you decided to do.
5. *Evaluate the result.* Build knowledge that you can use in the future. What were the positive and negative effects of what you chose? Would you make that choice again?

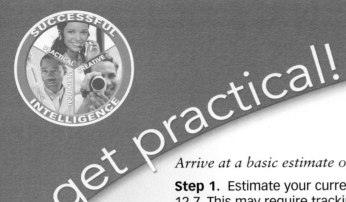

# Map Out Your Budget

*Arrive at a basic estimate of whether you are operating at a gain or a loss.*

**Step 1.** Estimate your current expenses in dollars per month, using Figure 12.7. This may require tracking expenses for a month, if you don't already keep a record of your spending. The grand total is your total monthly expenses.

**Step 2.** Calculate your average monthly income. If it's easiest to come up with a yearly figure, divide by 12 to derive the monthly figure. For example, if you have a $6,000 scholarship for the year, your monthly income would be $500 ($6,000 divided by 12).

**Step 3.** Subtract the grand total of your monthly expenses from the grand total of your monthly income:

**Step 4.** If you have a negative cash flow, you can increase your income, decrease your spending, or both. Think about what's possible for you to accomplish. List here your two most workable ideas about how you can get your cash flow back in the black.

1. _____

2. _____

## Balance Short-Term Satisfaction and Long-Term Money Growth

Making some short-term sacrifices to save money often can help you tremendously in the long run. However, this doesn't mean you should never spend money on things that bring you immediate satisfaction. The goal is to make choices that provide both short-term satisfaction and long-term money growth. Here are three ways to do just that:

- **Live beneath your means.** Spend less than you make. This helps you create savings. Saved money gives you a buffer that can help with emergencies or bigger expenditures.

- **Pay yourself.** After you pay your monthly bills, put whatever you can save in an account. Paying yourself helps you store money in your savings where it can grow. Make your payment to yourself a high priority so you honor it as you do your other bills.

- **Use banks to your advantage.** Choose a bank that has reasonable account fees and convenient ATMs—and, if you use it, online access for banking and bill payment. Know how much you can maintain in a checking account, and find one that can handle your minimum with the lowest fees.

## Use Savings Strategies

You can save money and still enjoy life. Think carefully about where your money goes and save your splurges for special items or events. Here are some savings suggestions for cutting corners. Small amounts can eventually add up to big savings and may keep you out of debt.

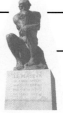

It is thrifty to prepare today for the wants of tomorrow.

AESOP

- Share living space.
- Rent or borrow movies.
- Eat at home more often than at restaurants.
- Use coupons, take advantage of sales, buy store brands, and buy in bulk.
- Find discounted play and concert tickets (students often receive discounts).
- Walk or use public transport.
- Bring your lunch from home.
- Shop in secondhand stores.
- Use e-mail or write letters.
- Ask a relative to help with child care.

# How Can You Manage Your *Credit Cards?*

College students often receive dozens of credit card offers from financial institutions issuing Visa and MasterCard. These offers—and the cards that go along with them—are a double-edged sword: They have the power to help you manage your money, but they also can plunge you into a hole of debt that may take you years to dig out of. Some statistics from a Nellie May survey of undergraduates illustrate the challenging situation:[8]

- Average number of credit cards per student—3.2
- Average credit card debt per student—$1,843
- Average available credit card limit—$3,683
- Percentage of students with debt between $3,000 and $7,000—9%
- Percentage of students with more than $7,000 in credit card debt—5%

When used properly, credit cards are a handy alternative to cash. They give you the peace of mind of knowing you always have money for emergencies and you have a record of all your purchases. In addition, if you pay your bills on time, you will be building a strong credit history that will affect your ability to take out future loans including auto loans and mortgages.

However, it takes self-control to avoid overspending, especially because it is so easy to hand over your credit card when you see something you like. To avoid excessive debt, ask yourself questions before charging: Would I buy it if I had to pay cash? Can I pay off the balance in full at the end of the first billing cycle? If I buy this, what purchases will I have to forgo? If I buy this, do I have enough to cover emergencies?

## How Credit Cards Work

Every time you charge a textbook, a present, or a pair of pants, you are creating a debt that must be repaid. The credit card issuer earns money by charging interest on your unpaid balance. With rates often higher than 20%, you may soon find yourself wishing you had paid cash.

Here's an example of how quickly credit card debt can mount. Say you have a $3,000 unpaid balance on your credit card at an annual interest rate of 18%. If you make the $60 minimum monthly payment every month, it will take you eight long years to pay off your debt, assuming that you make no other purchases. The math—and the effect on your wallet—is staggering:

- Original debt—$3,000
- Cost to repay credit card loan at an annual interest rate of 18% for 8 years—$5,760
- Cost of credit—$2,760

By the time you finish, you will repay nearly twice your original debt.

To avoid unmanageable debt that can lead to a personal financial crisis, learn as much as you can about credit cards, starting with the important concepts in Figure 12.8. Learn to use credit wisely while you are still in school. The habits you learn today can make a difference to your financial future.

## Managing Debt

The majority of American citizens have some level of debt, and many people go through periods when they have a hard time paying bills. Falling behind on payments, however, could result in a poor credit rating that makes it difficult for you to make large purchases or take out loans. Particular resources can help you solve credit problems; see Figure 12.9 for some ideas.

Avoiding the pitfalls of credit card debt means educating yourself about interest rates, late charges, credit ratings, bankruptcy, and more. Debbie Alford, a student at the University of Central Oklahoma, realized too late how poor financial decisions would affect her future. As a freshman, Debbie charged only necessities, such as books and tuition, and paid her credit card debt in full when her financial aid check arrived every semester. But her debt began to escalate when she started using her cards to cover expenses, like car repairs, food, and clothes. At age 23,

**FIGURE 12.8**   Learn to be a smart credit consumer

| **WHAT TO KNOW ABOUT . . .** | **. . . AND HOW TO USE WHAT YOU KNOW** |
|---|---|
| *Account balance*—a dollar amount that includes any unpaid balance, new purchases and cash advances, finance charges, and fees. Updated monthly on your card statement. | Charge only what you can afford to pay at the end of the month. Keep track of your balance. Hold on to receipts and call customer service if you have questions about recent purchases. |
| *Annual fee*—the yearly cost some companies charge for having a card. | Look for cards without an annual fee or, if you've paid your bills on time, ask your current company to waive the fee. |
| *Annual percentage rate (APR)*—the amount of interest charged on your unpaid balance, meaning the cost of credit if you carry a balance in any given month. The higher the APR, the more you pay in finance charges. | Credit card companies compete by charging different APRs. Shop around, especially on the Web. Two sites with competitive APR information are www.studentcredit.com and www.bankrate.com. Also, watch out for low, but temporary, introductory rates that skyrocket to over 20% after a few months. Look for *fixed* rates (guaranteed not to change). |
| *Available credit*—the unused portion of your credit line. Determine available credit by deducting your current card balance from your credit limit. | It is important to have credit available for emergencies, so avoid charging to the limit. |
| *Billing cycle*—the number of days between the last statement date and the current statement date. | Knowledge of your billing cycle can help you juggle funds. For example, if your cycle ends on the 3rd of the month, holding off on a large purchase until the 4th gives you an extra month to pay without incurring finance charges. |
| *Cash advance*—an immediate loan, in the form of cash, from the credit card company. You are charged interest immediately and may also pay a separate transaction fee. | Use a cash advance only in emergencies because the finance charges start as soon as you complete the transaction. It is a very expensive way to borrow money. |
| *Credit limit*—the debt ceiling the card company places on your account (e.g., $1,500). The total owed, including purchases, cash advances, finance charges, and fees, cannot exceed this limit. | Credit card companies generally set low credit limits for college students. Many students get around this limit by owning more than one card, which increases the credit available but most likely increases problems as well. |
| *Credit line*—a revolving amount of credit that can be used, paid back, then used again for future purchases or cash advances. | Work with the credit line of one card, paying the money you borrow back at the end of each month so you can borrow again. |
| *Delinquent account*—an account that is not paid on time or for which the minimum payment has not been met. | Avoid having a delinquent account at all costs. Not only will you be charged substantial late fees, but you also risk losing your good credit rating, affecting your ability to borrow in the future. Delinquent accounts remain part of your credit record for many years. |
| *Due date*—the date your payment must be received and after which you will be charged a late fee. | Avoid late fees and finance charges by mailing your payment a week in advance. |

**FIGURE 12.8** Continued

| WHAT TO KNOW ABOUT . . . | . . . AND HOW TO USE WHAT YOU KNOW |
|---|---|
| *Finance charges*—the total cost of credit, including interest and service and transaction fees. | Your goal is to incur no finance charges. The only way to do that is to pay your balance in full by the due date on your monthly statement. |
| *Grace period*—the interest-free time period between the date of purchase and the date your payment for that purchase is due once it appears on your statement. For example, a purchase on November 4 may first appear on your November 28 statement with payment due 25 days later. | It is important to know that interest-free grace periods only apply if you have no outstanding balance. If you carry a balance from month to month, all new purchases are immediately subject to interest charges. |
| *Minimum payment*—the smallest amount you can pay by the statement due date. The amount is set by the credit card company. | Making only the minimum payment each month can result in disaster if you continue to charge more than you can realistically afford. When you make a purchase, think in terms of total cost, not monthly payments. |
| *Outstanding balance*—the total amount you owe on your card. | If you carry a balance over several months, additional purchases are immediately hit with finance charges. Pay cash instead. |
| *Past due*—your account is considered "past due" when you fail to pay the minimum required payment on schedule. | Three credit bureaus note past due accounts on your credit history: Experian, TransUnion, and Equifax. You can contact each bureau for a copy of your credit report to make sure there are no errors. |

and only a junior in college, Debbie filed for bankruptcy. Looking back, she blames credit card companies for making it so easy to accumulate debt and herself for not understanding the financial hole she was digging until it was too late.[9]

The most basic way to stay in control is to pay bills regularly and on time. On credit card bills, pay at least the minimum amount due. If you get into trouble, deal with it in three steps. First, admit that you made a mistake, even though you may be embarrassed. Then, address the problem immediately to minimize damages. Call the **creditor** and see if you can pay your debt gradually using a payment plan. Finally, examine what got you into trouble and avoid it in the future if you can. Cut up a credit card or two if you have too many. If you clean up your act, your credit history will gradually clean up as well.

CREDITOR
A person or company to whom a debt is owed, usually money.

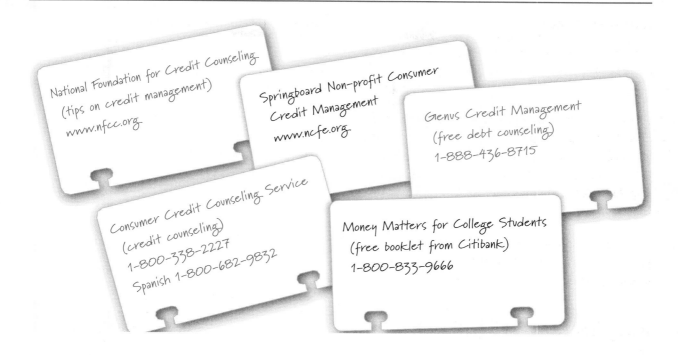

National Foundation for Credit Counseling (tips on credit management) www.nfcc.org

Springboard Non-profit Consumer Credit Management www.ncfe.org

Genus Credit Management (free debt counseling) 1-888-436-8715

Consumer Credit Counseling Service (credit counseling) 1-800-338-2227 Spanish 1-800-682-9832

Money Matters for College Students (free booklet from Citibank) 1-800-833-9666

# *Sacrifici*

In Italy, parents often use the term *sacrifici*, meaning "sacrifices," to refer to tough choices that they make to improve the lives of their children and family members. They may sacrifice a larger home so they can afford to pay for their children's sports and after-school activities. They may sacrifice a higher-paying job so they can live close to where they work. They give up something in exchange for something else that is more important to them.

Think of the concept of *sacrifici* as you analyze the sacrifices you can make to get out of debt, reach your savings goals, and prepare for a career that you find satisfying. Many of the short-term sacrifices you are making today will help you do and have what you want in the future.

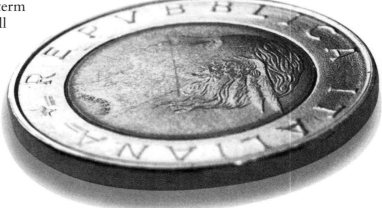

## Create Your Future

### DEVELOPING SUCCESSFUL INTELLIGENCE

#### *Putting It All Together*

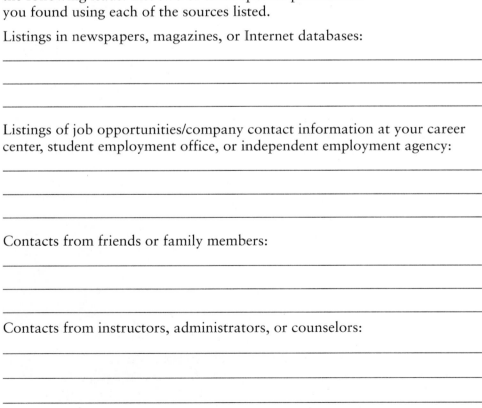

**Nursing Career Possibilities.** Choose one of the nursing career areas you have listed as an interest in any other exercise in this book. Follow up on it by using the following leads. List two or three specific possibilities you found using each of the sources listed.

Listings in newspapers, magazines, or Internet databases:

_____

_____

_____

Listings of job opportunities/company contact information at your career center, student employment office, or independent employment agency:

_____

_____

_____

Contacts from friends or family members:

_____

_____

_____

Contacts from instructors, administrators, or counselors:

_____

_____

_____

_____

Current or former employers or coworkers:

_____

_____

_____

_____

# TEAM BUILDING
## Collaborative Solutions

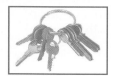

**Building Interview Skills.** Divide into pairs. Each student will have a turn interviewing the other about themselves and their career aspirations. Follow these steps.

1. Independently, take three minutes to brainstorm questions you'll ask the other person. Focus on learning style, interests, and initial career ideas. You might ask questions like these:
   - If you could have any job in the world, what would it be?
   - What do you think would be the toughest part of achieving success in that profession?
   - Who are you as a learner and worker—what is your learning style?
   - What sacrifices are you willing to make to realize your dreams?
   - What is your greatest failure, and what have you learned from it?
   - Who is a role model to you in terms of career success?

2. Person A interviews Person B for 5 to 10 minutes and takes notes.

3. Switch roles: Person B interviews Person A and takes notes. Remember that each person uses the questions he or she developed in Step 1.

4. Share with each other what interesting ideas stand out to you from the interviews. If you have any, offer constructive criticism to your interviewee about his or her interview skills.

5. Finally, submit your notes to your instructor for feedback.

This exercise will build your ability to glean information from others and to answer questions during an interview. You will use this skill throughout your professional life. Probe deeply when interviewing others so you develop the ability to draw out the best in someone. Be as interested—and interesting—as you can.

# WRITING
## Discovery Through Journaling

*Record your thoughts on a separate piece of paper or in a journal.*

**Money and You.** Describe your relationship with money. What do you buy? How much do you spend? Are you careful? Reckless? Unattentive? Focused on every detail? How much do you use credit cards, and do you pay credit card bills in full each month or run a balance? If you could change how you handle money, what would you do?

# CAREER PORTFOLIO

## Plan for Success

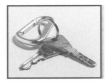

*Complete the following in your electronic portfolio or on separate sheets of paper.*

**Being Specific About Your Job Needs.** As you consider specific job directions and opportunities, you will have to begin thinking about a variety of job-related factors that different employers offer and that may affect your job experience and personal life. Among these factors are the following:

- Benefits, including health insurance, vacation, 401(k)
- Integrity of company (What is its reputation?)
- Integrity of organization in its dealings with employees
- Promotion prospects/your chances for advancement
- Job stability
- Training and educational opportunities (Does the company offer in-house training? Will it pay for job-related courses or degrees?)
- Starting salary
- Quality of employees
- Quality of management
- Nature of the work you will be doing (Will you be required to travel extensively? Will you be expected to work long hours? Will you be working in an office or in the field?)
- Your official relationship with the company (Will you be a full-time or part-time employee or an independent contractor?)
- Job title
- Location of your primary workplace
- Company size
- Company's financial performance over time

Think about how important each factor is in your job choice. Then rate each on a scale of 1 to 10, with 1 being the least important and 10 being the most important. As you consider each factor, keep in mind that even if you consider something very important, you may not get it right away if you are just beginning your career.

Finally, consider the results of a survey of college students conducted by the National Association of Colleges and Employers. When asked their top two reasons for choosing an employer, students named *integrity of organization in its dealings with employees* as number one and *job stability* as number two. How do these top choices compare to your own?[10]

## Suggested Readings

Adams, Robert Lang, et al. *The Complete Résumé and Job Search Book for College Students.* Holbrook, MA: Adams Publishing, 1999.

Beatty, Richard H. *The Resume Kit,* 5th ed. New York: John Wiley, 2003.

Boldt, Laurence G. *Zen and the Art of Making a Living: A Practical Guide to Creative Career Design.* New York: Arkana, 1999.

Bolles, Richard Nelson. *What Color Is Your Parachute? 2003: A Practical Manual for Job Hunters and Career Changers.* Berkeley, CA: Ten Speed Press, 2003.

Detweiler, Gerri. *The Ultimate Credit Handbook*, 3rd ed. New York: Plume, 2003.

Goleman, Daniel. *Emotional Intelligence.* New York: Bantam Books, 1997.

Goleman, Daniel. *Working with Emotional Intelligence.* New York: Bantam Books, 2000.

Kennedy, Joyce Lain. *Job Interviews for Dummies.* Foster City, CA: IDG Books Worldwide, 2000.

Tyson, Eric. *Personal Finance for Dummies.* Foster City, CA: IDG Books Worldwide, 2000.

## Internet Resources

U.S. Bureau of Labor—statistics: **www.bls.gov/oco/**

Student Advantage—information on discounts: **www.studentadvantage.com**

Monster.com (online job search): **www.monster.com**

The Motley Fool (money and investment advice): **www.fool.com**

1st Steps in the Hunt: Daily News for Online Job Hunters (advice on finding a job via an online search): **www.interbiznet.com/hunt/**

College Grad Job Hunter (advice on résumés, interviews, and a database of entry-level jobs): **www.collegegrad.com**

Women Working 2000 and Beyond (information for working women): **www.womenworking2000.com**

JobWeb (career information site for college students): **www.jobweb.com**

Prentice Hall Student Success Supersite—Money Matters: **www.prenhall.com/success/MoneyMat/index.html**

Career Path: **www.prenhall.com/success/CareerPath/index.html**

Résumé Edge (résumé advice): **www.resumeedge.com**

## Endnotes

[1] Peter Passell, "Royal Blue Collars," *New York Times*, March 22, 1998, p. 12.

[2] Daniel Goleman, *Working with Emotional Intelligence* (New York: Bantam Books, 1998), pp. 26–27.

[3] Women's Review of Books, "Rebuilding a Life: Susan Davenny Wyner Replays Her Transformation from Singer to Conductor," reprinted on the website for the New England String Ensemble (December 2000). Retrieved May 2004, from: www.newenglandstringensemble.org.

[4] New Mexico State University FAQ, "Does NMSU Do Anything to Help People Get Jobs After They Graduate?" (October 2000). Retrieved March 2004, from: www.nmsu.edu/aggieland/students/faq_jobs.html.

[5] New Mexico State University FAQ, "What Kind of Student Clubs and Organizations Are There?" (June 1999). Retrieved March 2004, from: www.nmsu.edu/aggieland/students/faq_orgs.html.

[6] ResumeEdge.com, "Resume Keyword Search" (2004). Retrieved May 2004, from: www.enetsc.com/ResumeTips23.htm.

[7] Scott Carlson, "Help-Desk Diary: Tech-Savvy Students Learn People Skills and Patience by Solving Campus Computer Problems," *The Chronicle of Higher Education* (June 20, 2003). Retrieved March 2004, from: http://chronicle.com/weekly/v49/i41a02701.htm.

[8] Laura A. Bruce, "College Kids' Credit Card Use Can Leave Them Drowning in High-Interest Debt," Bankrate.com (2001). Retrieved March 2001, from: www.bankrate.com/brm/news/cc/20000815.asp.

[9] Eric Hoover, "The Lure of Easy Credit Leaves More Students Struggling with Debt: Consumer Advocates Blame Lenders, Congress, and Some Colleges," *The Chronicle of Higher Education* (June 15, 2001). Retrieved March 2004, from: http://chronicle.com/weekly/v47/i40/40a03501.htm.

[10] Eduardo Porter and Greg Winter, "'04 Graduates Learned Lesson in Practicality," *New York Times*, May 30, 2004, pp. A1 and A24.

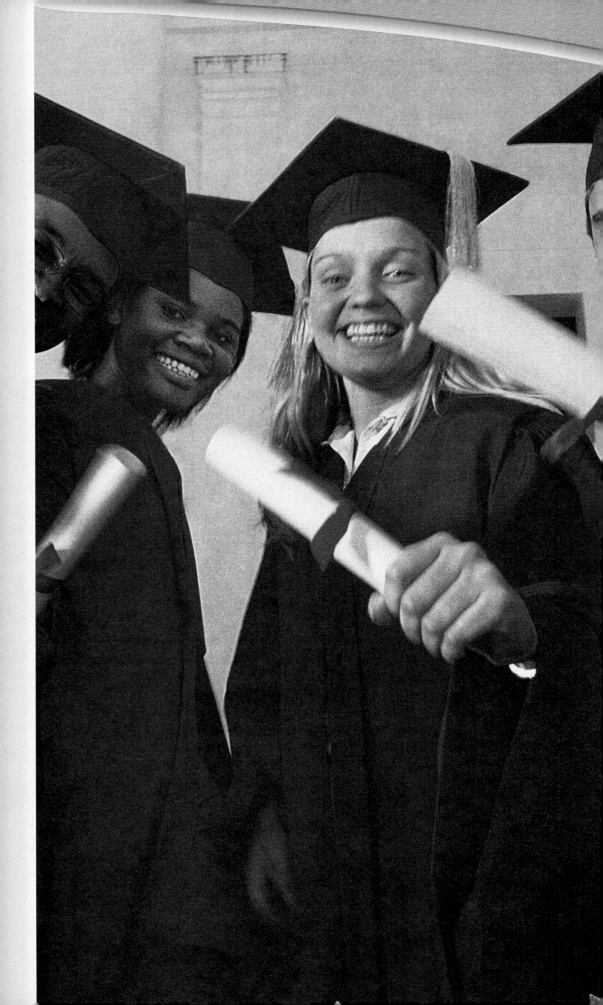

**THRIVE: CREATING YOUR LIFE**

*BUILDING A SUCCESSFUL FUTURE*

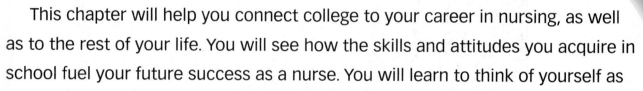

A s you come to the end of your work in this course, you have built up a wealth of knowledge. You will soon be analyzing how you fared in your first college semester. You are facing important decisions about what direction you want to go in your future nursing career—and starting to think about where the choices you make now will ultimately lead you.

This chapter will help you connect college to your career in nursing, as well as to the rest of your life. You will see how the skills and attitudes you acquire in school fuel your future success as a nurse. You will learn to think of yourself as a member of a broader community of health professionals and to take on the challenge of being an active participant in the health care system. You will gather 20 important tools that will help you transfer the power of successful intelligence into your nursing career. Finally, you will create your personal mission, exploring how to use it to guide your dreams.

**IN THIS CHAPTER ...**

*You will explore answers to the following questions:*

- How do ethical dilemmas affect nursing? 397
- What is the future of nursing? 398
- How will what you've learned bring success? 401
- How can you make a difference in your community? 405
- How can you continue to activate your successful intelligence? 410
- How can you create and live your personal mission? 412

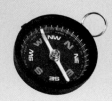

# Q & A BLUE SKY QUESTIONS DOWN-TO-EARTH ANSWERS

### How can I make decisions about my professional nursing career?

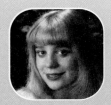

Wendy Casciato
Senior, University of Iowa,
Iowa City, Iowa

My area of interest is community health nursing. Upon graduation, I would like to pursue a career in parish or school nursing. One of the challenges I've faced as a college student is information overload. There's so much material to absorb, and sometimes my concerns aren't addressed in textbooks.

For example, I've been receiving quite a bit of advice from faculty and other nurses. They recommend that even though I know I want to be a community health nurse, I should work for a year or two at a hospital. They say floor work provides an opportunity to solidify a nurse's assessment skills. For me, this suggestion presents a real internal conflict. I'm eager to launch my career in community health, yet I also want to be fully prepared to assume the challenges of community health nursing.

This brings me to another related concern, which is the often subtle but very real insinuations I receive about community health nursing being a less respected position than that of a hospital nurse. I sense that this branch of the nursing profession isn't viewed with the same esteem as other nursing specialties. Of course, I don't believe that, but I'm not sure how to counter this stereotype. Their advice makes me wonder if my education has been enough.

As beneficial as my studies are, I realize there's more knowledge for me to tap. Today we have many written resources available at our fingertips, and I want to make the most of this opportunity. However, weeding through what's relevant, whether I'm on the Internet or in the library, can get overwhelming. If I could expand my understanding of how to set professional goals and what resources would best facilitate the fulfillment of these goals, I think I might have a better handle on making decisions that affect my nursing career. Can you offer suggestions for maximizing written resources?

## PRACTICAL ANSWERS

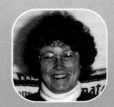

Kathryn H. Krauss,
RN, MSW
Parish Nurse, Central
United Methodist Church,
Spokane, Washington

### Explore all your options, and don't limit yourself!

My nursing career spans over 40 years of experience, when I began as a hospital nurse. I've also taught parenting classes for the American Red Cross, served as a Lamaze instructor, and developed a support group for women with breast cancer, as well as many other roles in between. But I've not found any area as personally fulfilling as community health nursing.

The advice you're receiving, in my opinion, is incorrect. Although hospital work is valuable in many ways, community health nursing offers such a wide range of experiences that you'll find yourself making assessments all the time. I work as a parish nurse for an inner-city church. Our church serves more than 25,000 meals per year to high school students, families, and the poor, homeless, and mentally ill. We provide health education, do assessments, and help connect folks to health care providers and agencies. We also promote health care among the residents of the low-income apartment buildings in our neighborhood. In one of the buildings, where many of the residents have mental illness, we offer art therapy classes and host an art exhibition of their work. In all of these activities, I'm constantly assessing people's needs.

Perhaps community health nursing isn't held in high esteem among the nurses you know because of the value they place on modern technology, which hospitals rely on. By contract, community health nursing emphasizes hospitality, which isn't usually a high-tech activity. However, building relationships is a key component to effective prevention of health problems. If you can't earn the trust and respect of the people in your community, they won't allow you to educate them about their health issues.

I suggest that you not try to change anyone else's stereotype of the specialty you've chosen. Instead, put your energy into enjoying what you do. Your intuition about the need to set professional goals is a keen observation. One goal you may want to set is to obtain certification through the ANA Credential Center. This requires rigorous and disciplined community health nursing education.

Information overload will continue to be an issue, even after you leave college. One of the most effective methods I've found for staying current is to join professional nurse organizations. I recommend the regional parish nurse organization, which publishes a monthly newsletter. The second organization worth checking out is your local parish nurse support group. The monthly meetings always contain an educational component, plus they have an e-mail bulletin board. From these resources, you can begin to develop your own library by collecting and filing inspiring articles. In the process, you will train your mind to notice interesting and pertinent information as it relates to your specialty.

Reading good literature, beyond what you were exposed to in the classroom, can also supplement your education. I have an extensive and diverse library that includes literature, philosophy, social work, nursing practice, psychology, and theology. I use these books and articles daily in many ways. For example, I crafted my personal mission statement based on the Bible, from Jesus' words: "I have come that they might have life and life in all its fullness" (John 10:10). My library also helps me serve the students under my supervision and is a useful resource when I write articles for nursing publications.

And take advantage of people resources. Enlisting the support of a spiritual director can help you define your call in life. I also suggest that you seek out a mentor who is a community health nurse. You can observe how this person handles snags in professional life, and what habits help them succeed. Studying another person might be the best book you'll ever read.

# How Do *Ethical Dilemmas* Affect Nursing?

As a nurse you will become familiar with ethical dilemmas. For instance, in genetics, the ability to be tested for your predisposition to diseases may pose a risk to your confidentiality and privacy. Would you want others to know this information? For that matter, would you want to know it? Discrimination based on genetic test results could be grounds for denial of employment or insurance, although the Americans with Disabilities Act may offer protection. People will need to be educated on test results and the possible consequences of releasing them.

The ability to perform gene therapy raises many ethical questions. Will we become legally or morally bound to fix everything with gene therapy?

Genetics, along with many other areas of research, offers great opportunities to learn more about human physiology, disease, and the world around us. But this new knowledge must be thought about critically. It is vitally important that you, as a nursing major, take at least one ethics course because nursing and health care are full of ethical problems.

Questions nurses deal with in everyday practice include the following:

*End-of-life care.* On a day-to-day, person-to-person basis, how are ethical decisions made that coincide with an individual's and society's values? Is it appropriate to keep a person alive at any cost? How are health care resources best used?

*Nursing shortage.* Will there be enough nurses? (See Chapter 1.)

*Emerging infectious diseases.* How will their spread be curtailed? How are they best treated?

*Bioterrorism and disaster response.* How can we create a national nursing response plan?

*Proposed cuts in Medicare and Medicaid.* Is it necessary to cut health benefits to the most vulnerable members of the population?

*Increasing health care costs.* Will patient care suffer?

*Safety issues such as gun control, protection of nurses from needle sticks, latex allergies, and workplace violence.* Nursing and safety, along with nursing and care, are synonymous. How can nurses use this expertise to promote important legislation and education?

*HIV/AIDS.* Is research funding utilized to its fullest to battle the HIV/AIDS epidemic? What biases may interfere with research funding and the care of HIV/AIDS patients? What is our responsibility on a global level?

## Nursing Is Complex

Thinking about tough questions will help you understand how nursing is also a philosophical, spiritual, social, and political pursuit. The more you understand these areas, along with science, the better off you'll be in planning and making decisions that affect you, your family, and your local and global communities. A thorough background in the sciences and in the liberal arts is a necessity in nursing and will help you in any career you choose. Big questions about truth and decisions based on values occur everywhere and they will occur throughout your lifetime.

# What Is the *Future* of Nursing?

The American Nurses Association's Health Care Agenda covers many issues that are involved in ethical dilemmas. Here is a sample of what the ANA thinks the future of health care should look like. The full text can be found on the American Nurses Association's website: www.nursingworld. org/naf. The main points that nurses are promoting include:

*Access to affordable, quality health care services is the right of all people.* "Nursing, as the pivotal health care profession, is well positioned to advocate on behalf of and in concert with individuals, families and communities who are in desperate need of a well financed, functional and coordinated health care system that provides safe, quality care." (from the ANA Health Care Agenda 2005)

*Health care should be both cost effective and high quality.* The main focus of health care should be on primary care, rather than more expensive care in emergency departments or hospitals. The emphasis is on disease prevention and health promotion.

*The American Nurses Association supports a single-payer health care system.* Nursing should be viewed as saving money through its focus on prevention and health promotion, rather than as a cost to the system. Nurses save money through access, quality care, and holistic perspectives on health.

## Present and Future Changes in Health Care

Biotechnology and genetics are examples of the rapid changes occurring in the health sciences today. The Human Genome Project, an international effort launched in 1989, has completed a basic map of the entire human genome. But genetic innovations have been used in health care for years; examples include the production of insulin, human hemoglobin produced in pigs, and Factor IX for hemophilia in sheep's milk. Newer innovations include genetic disease treatment, or gene therapy, which places a fully functioning gene into cells to replace, or augment, the function of a defective gene. At this time gene therapy is primarily experimental, but that will soon change as techniques are improved and tested.

Questions about the use of new technology and discoveries arise in all areas of the health sciences. Genetics is a good example of how questions concern not only researchers but citizens as well. For instance, gene therapy that affects only somatic cells, body cells that are not involved in reproduction, will not affect future generations. However, gene therapy performed on germ cells, the cells of reproduction, alters the genes so that these changes are passed on to future generations. This raises many important questions concerning the desirability of permanently altering the human gene pool. Most geneticists currently agree that germ cell therapy is not advisable.

More recently, the use of stem cells for research has been discussed. These cells have the possibility of regenerating human tissue. For example, experiments are being done with stem cells to see if they could be used in humans to grow arterial bypasses in the heart. If this works, many cardiac surgeries and invasive procedures would become unnecessary. This potential life- and cost-saving therapy raises ethical concerns for some people. Implications of research must be understood by researchers and nonresearchers or potentially breakthrough work may be overlooked and underfunded due to decisions based on uninformed reactions. Likewise, ethical issues must be equally considered.

## Nursing *Research*

When the answers in health care are not known, nursing research makes important contributions to the care of patients, as well as to public health, health policy, and all aspects of nursing. Inquiry is a part of nursing research and is just as it sounds—an inquiry, or exploration, into something you desire to know.

The *American Heritage College Dictionary* defines inquiry as follows:

1. The act of inquiring.
2. A question; a query.
3. A close examination of a matter in a search for information or truth.

As the definition states, inquiry is about asking questions and carefully examining evidence that helps you answer the questions. This is usually done by forming a hypothesis and then deciding how to test your hypothesis.

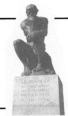

## *Wonder*

"Twinkle, twinkle, little star—I don't wonder what you are. For by spectroscopic ken, I know that you are hydrogen."

ANONYMOUS

A hypothesis is like an assumption or a likely explanation to your question. If you are wondering about the effect of alcohol consumption during pregnancy, you might ask the question, "Do women who drink alcohol during pregnancy give birth to infants who are small and poorly developed?" From this you develop a testable hypothesis:

Birth weight is lower among infants of women who drink alcohol than among infants of women who do not drink alcohol.

To test this directly you would have to have access to patient charts so you could look for women who drank during their pregnancy and women who didn't and then look for the weights of their infants and compare. Did the infants of women who drank weigh less than those of women who didn't drink? In the lab you could devise an experiment to see if alcohol affects individual cell development.

Often the answers to your questions are not known. This gives you an opportunity, in the lab or in the field, to take on the role of the researcher. You will learn how to

1. Ask questions.

2. Form ways to answer your questions, either experimentally or through observation.

3. Collect information and record it for later use or analysis.

## Nursing Theory

Any profession must have research-based theory to make itself distinct from other professions. Nursing must have its own theories to make it unique. Theories come from research. Research findings form a knowledge base that helps define what nursing is. At the end of this chapter you will read about nursing research on pain. Although many other professions, such as medicine, psychology, and physiology, do research on pain, nursing focuses on caring for patients in pain. Nursing shares many theories with other professions, but a growing body of knowledge is unique to nursing. This is important in giving nursing a unique identity.

The information gained from nursing research is added to what we already know or employed toward developing new information. As you plan for your future, consider nursing research as an option whether you eventually become a professor or work in a clinical situation, or both.

# How Will What You've Learned *Bring Success*?

You leave this course with far more than a final grade, a notebook full of work, and a credit hour or three on your transcript. You have gathered important attitudes and skills, developed flexibility, and opened the door to lifelong learning.

## New Attitudes and Skills Prepare You to Succeed

The attitudes and skills you gained this semester are your keys to success now and in the future (see Figure 13.1). As you move through your college years, keep motivation high by reminding yourself that you are creating tools that will benefit you in everything you do.

## Flexibility Helps You Adapt to Change

As a citizen of the twenty-first century, you are likely to move in and out of school, jobs, and careers in the years ahead. You are also likely to experience important personal changes. How you react to the changes you experience, especially if they are unexpected and difficult, is almost as important as the changes themselves in determining your future success. The ability to "make lemonade from lemons" is the hallmark of people who always land on their feet.

Successfully intelligent thinking will help you adapt to and benefit from both planned and unexpected changes. Your goal is flexibility as you analyze each change, generate and consider options, make decisions, and take practical actions. With flexibility and resourcefulness, you can adapt to the loss of a job or an exciting job offer, a personal health crisis or a happy change in family status, failing a course or winning an academic scholarship.

Although sudden changes may throw you off balance, the unpredictability of life can open new horizons. Margaret J. Wheatley and Myron Kellner-Rogers, leadership and community experts and founders of the Berkana Institute, explain: People "often look at this unpredictability with resentment, but . . . unpredictability gives us the freedom to experiment. It is this unpredictability that welcomes our creativity."[1] Here are some strategies they recommend for making the most of unpredictable changes:

- **Look for what happens when you meet someone or something new.** Be aware of new feelings or insights that arise. Observe where they lead you.

- **Be willing to be surprised.** Great creative energies can come from the force of a surprise. Instead of turning back to familiar patterns, explore new possibilities.

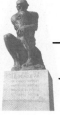

The word "impossible" is not in my dictionary.

NAPOLEON

FIGURE 13.1 Attitudes and skills acquired in college are tools for lifelong success

| ACQUIRED SKILL | IN COLLEGE, YOU'LL USE IT TO . . . | IN CAREER AND LIFE, YOU'LL USE IT TO . . . |
|---|---|---|
| Investigating resources | . . . find who and what can help you have the college experience you want | . . . get acclimated at a new job or in a new town—find the people, resources, and services that can help you succeed |
| Knowing and using your learning styles | . . . select study strategies that make the most of your learning styles | . . . select jobs, career areas, and other pursuits that suit what you do best |
| Setting goals and managing stress | . . . complete assignments and achieve educational goals, reduce stress by being in control | . . . accomplish tasks and reach career and personal goals, reduce stress by being in control |
| Managing time | . . . get to classes on time, juggle school and work, turn in assignments when they are due, plan study time | . . . finish work tasks on or before they are due, balance duties on the job and at home |
| Analytical, creative, and practical thinking | . . . think through writing assignments, solve math problems, analyze academic readings, brainstorm paper topics, work through academic issues, work effectively on team projects | . . . find ways to improve product design, increase market share, present ideas to customers; analyze life issues, come up with ideas, and take practical action |
| Reading | . . . read course texts and other materials | . . . read operating manuals, work guidebooks, media materials in your field; read for practical purposes, for learning, and for pleasure at home |
| Note taking | . . . take notes in class, in study groups, during studying, and during research | . . . take notes in work and community meetings and during important phone calls |
| Test taking | . . . take quizzes, tests, and final exams | . . . take tests for certification in particular work skills and for continuing education courses |
| Writing | . . . write essays and reports | . . . write work-related documents, including e-mails, reports, proposals, and speeches; write personal letters and journal entries |
| Building successful relationships | . . . get along with instructors, students, student groups | . . . get along with supervisors, coworkers, team members, friends, and family members |
| Staying healthy | . . . stay physically and mentally healthy so that you can make the most of school | . . . stay physically and mentally healthy so that you can be at your best at work and at home |
| Managing money | . . . stay on top of school costs and make decisions that earn and save you the money you need | . . . budget the money you earn so that you can pay your bills and save for the future |
| Establishing and maintaining a personal mission | . . . develop a big-picture idea of what you want from your education, and make choices that guide you toward those goals | . . . develop a big-picture idea of what you wish to accomplish in life, and make choices that guide you toward those goals |

- **Use your planning as a guide rather than a rule.** If you allow yourself to follow new paths when changes occur, you are able to grow from what life gives you.
- **Focus on what is rather than what is supposed to be.** Planning for the future works best as a guide when combined with an awareness of the realities of your situation.

## Lifelong Learning

As a student, your main focus is on learning—on acquiring knowledge and skills in the courses you take. Though you will graduate knowing much more than you did when you started college, you are not finished learning. On the contrary, with knowledge in many fields doubling every two to three years and with your personal interests and needs changing every day, what you learn in college is just the beginning of lifelong learning. With the *habit* of learning you will be able to achieve your career and personal goals—those that you set out for yourself today and those that you cannot anticipate but that will be part of your future.

You can make learning a habit through asking questions and being open to exploring new ideas and possibilities. Here are some ways to make that happen:

### Investigate New Interests

When information and events catch your attention, take your interest one step further and find out more. Instead of dreaming about it, just do it.

### Read, Read, Read

Reading expert Jim Trelease says that people who don't read "base their future decisions on what they used to know. If you don't read much, you really don't know much. You're dangerous."[2] Decrease the danger to yourself and others by opening a world of knowledge and perspectives through reading. Ask friends which books have changed their lives. Keep up with local, national, and world news through newspapers and magazines.

### Pursue Improvement in Your Studies and Career

When at school, take classes outside of your major if you have time. After graduation, continue your education both in nursing and in the realm of general knowledge. Stay on top of ideas, developments, and new technology in nursing by seeking out **continuing education** courses. Sign up for conferences in your area of interest. Make sure to work for an organization that offers additional education and pays for you to take courses and go to professional conferences. When you go for job interviews ask about this—make sure you are entering a learning and nurturing environment. With the nursing shortage you can be very selective about where you work. And go to graduate school!

CONTINUING EDUCATION
Courses that students can take without having to be part of a degree program.

### Spend Time with Interesting People

When you meet someone new who inspires you and makes you think, keep in touch. Form a study group, a film club, or a walking club. Host a potluck dinner party and invite people from different corners of your life—

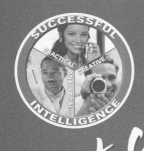

## get creative!

# Think 50 Positive Thoughts

*Appreciate yourself, and plan to expand your horizons.*

On a separate piece of paper, list 25 things you like about yourself. You can name anything—things you can do, things you think, things you've accomplished, things you like about your physical self, and so on.

Next, list 25 things you would like to do in your life. These can be anything from trying Vietnamese food to traveling to the Grand Canyon to working for Teach for America. They can be things you'd like to do tomorrow or things that you plan to do in 20 years. At least five items on each list should involve your current and future education.

Finally, come up with five things you can plan for the next year that combine what you like about yourself and what you want to do. If you like your strength as a mountain biker and you want to explore a state you've never seen, plan a mountain biking trip. If you like your writing and you want to be a published author, write an essay to submit to a magazine. Be creative. Let everything be possible.

1. _____
2. _____
3. _____
4. _____
5. _____

family, school, work, or neighborhood. Learn something new from everyone you meet.

## Talk to People from Different Generations

Younger people can learn from the experienced, broad perspective of those belonging to older generations; older people can learn from the fresh and often radical perspective of those younger than themselves. Communication builds mutual respect.

## Delve into Other Cultures

Talk with a friend who has grown up in a culture different from your own. Invite him or her to dinner. Eat food from a country you've never visited. Initiate conversations with people of different races, religions, values, and ethnic backgrounds. Travel internationally and locally. Take a course that deals with some aspect of cultural diversity. Try a semester or year abroad.

## Nurture a Spiritual Life

You don't have to attend a house of worship to be spiritual, although that may be part of your spiritual life. Wherever you find spirituality and soul—in music, organized religion, friendship, nature, cooking, sports, or anything else—they will help you find balance and meaning.

## Experience the Arts

Art is "an adventure of the mind" (Eugène Ionesco, playwright); "a means of knowing the world" (Angela Carter, author); something that "does not reproduce the visible; rather, it makes visible" (Paul Klee, painter); "a lie that makes us realize truth" (Pablo Picasso, painter); a revealer of "our most secret self" (Jean-Luc Godard, filmmaker). Through art forms you can discover new ideas and shed light on old ones. Seek out whatever moves you—music, visual arts, theater, photography, dance, domestic arts, performance art, film and television, poetry, prose, and more.

## Make Your Own Creations

Take a class in drawing, writing, or quilting. Learn to play an instrument. Write poems for your favorite people or stories to read to your children. Concoct a new recipe. Design and build a set of shelves for your home. Create a memoir of your life. Express yourself, and learn more about yourself, through art.

Lifelong learning is the master key that unlocks every door you encounter on your journey. If you keep it firmly in your hand, you will discover worlds of knowledge—and a place for yourself within them.

You are part of a world community of people who depend on one another. Giving what you can of your time, energy, and resources to those who need help makes you a valued community member.

COMMUNITY
(1) A group of people living in the same locality.
(2) A group of people having common interests.
(3) A group of people forming a distinct segment of society.

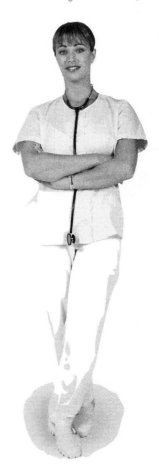

# How Can You *Make a Difference* in Your Community?

Everyday life is demanding. You can become so caught up in your own issues that you neglect to pay attention to anything else. However, you can make a difference in your **community**—by helping others; being an active, involved citizen; and doing your share for the environment.

## You Can Help Others

What you do for others has enormous impact. Giving others hope, comfort, or help can improve their ability to cope. Reaching out to others can also enhance your career. Being involved in causes and the community shows caring and community spirit, qualities companies look for in people they hire.

You can help others by volunteering, participating in service learning, and setting an example in how you live your life.

## Volunteering

Look for a volunteering activity that you can fit into your schedule. Figure 13.2 lists organizations that provide volunteer opportunities; you might also look into more local efforts or private clearinghouses that set up smaller projects.

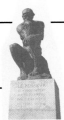

Never doubt that a small group of committed citizens can change the world; indeed, it's the only thing that ever has.

MARGARET MEAD

Many schools, realizing the importance of community involvement, sponsor volunteer groups or have committees that organize volunteering opportunities. For example, the University of Virginia has a student volunteer center called Madison House, which connects students to the surrounding community through projects such as youth mentoring, housing improvement, and a crisis hotline.

Volunteerism is also getting attention on the national level. AmeriCorps, a federal volunteer clearinghouse, offers financial awards for education in return for community service. If you work for AmeriCorps and you are enrolled in the National Service Trust, you will receive an award that you can use to pay current tuition expenses or repay student loans. You may work either before, during, or after your college education.

## Service Learning

In the past few years, looking for a way to help students become involved citizens as well as successful learners, many colleges have instituted *service learning* programs. The basic concept of service learning is to provide the community with service and the students with knowledge, creating positive

| **FIGURE 13.2** | Look into volunteering opportunities that these organizations offer |

- AIDS-related organizations
- American Red Cross
- Amnesty International
- Audubon Society
- Battered women shelters
- Big Brothers and Big Sisters
- Churches, synagogues, temples, mosques, and affiliated organizations such as the YM/WCA or YM/WHA
- Educational support organizations

- Environmental awareness/support organizations such as Greenpeace and Sierra Club
- Health-focused organizations such as the Avon Foundation for Breast Cancer or the Childhood Leukemia Foundation
- Hospitals
- Hotlines
- Kiwanis/Knights of Columbus/Lions Club/Rotary

- Libraries
- Meals on Wheels
- Nursing homes
- Planned Parenthood
- School districts
- Scouting organizations
- Share Our Strength/other food donation organizations
- Shelters and organizations supporting the homeless
- World Wildlife Fund

change for both and including specific opportunities for students to reflect on and analyze their experiences.[3]

In service learning, schools set up a system whereby students provide services in the context of a course for which they receive credit. The service and related assignments are required. The National Service Learning Clearinghouse presents this example of the difference between volunteering and service learning:

> If school students collect trash out of an urban streambed, they are providing a service to the community as volunteers; a service that is highly valued and important. When school students collect trash from an urban streambed, then analyze what they found and possible sources so they can share the results with residents of the neighborhood along with suggestions for reducing pollution, they are engaging in service-learning. In the service-learning example, the students are providing an important service to the community AND, at the same time, learning about water quality and laboratory analysis, developing an understanding of pollution issues, learning to interpret science issues to the public, and practicing communications skills by speaking to residents.[4]

Service learning builds a sense of civic responsibility, helps students learn useful skills through doing, and promotes values exploration and personal change. If you are interested in seeing these benefits firsthand, talk to your adviser about whether your school offers service learning programs. Service learning is a "win-win" situation: Everyone has something to gain.

## Setting an Example

The most basic—and perhaps the most important—way you can make a difference is to live your life in a way that sets an example for others. If you make life choices that show a value of learning and hard work, perseverance, commitment, responsibility, and love, you will inspire others to strive for their own personal best.

When you reach for the heights, you also leave an inspiring legacy to any children you have now or may one day have. A 31-year-old returning student and mother of four at Palo Alto College in San Antonio, Texas, is keenly aware of the relationship between what she is doing in school and her children's future. She explains,

> Having waited so long [to go to college] after high school and having a family has put a new perspective and priority on seeking a degree and my goals I want to accomplish in life. Throughout my high school years and even into my twenties, I didn't have any desire to pursue a degree or have any higher ambitions about work. I decided to go back to college after I realized that I could not get a job that paid more than minimum wage.
>
> Hopefully, I am setting a great example for my children. I want them to be confident in their talents and discover their skills. I know that I live in a very stressful environment and everything doesn't go the way I plan for it to go. That is why I try to stay open and flexible to the changes that occur. There is still a lot of spontaneity and it mostly feels like chaos around this house, but it is more of a controlled chaos. And there is always tomorrow.[5]

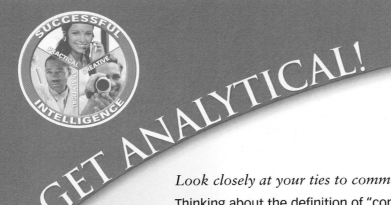

## GET ANALYTICAL!

# Evaluate Your Involvement in Communities[6]

*Look closely at your ties to communities important to you.*

Thinking about the definition of "community" that you read in the margin on page 405, come up with a list of communities to which you belong—professional, family, spiritual, academic, athletic, political, and so on. Write them here.

_____

_____

_____

Choose two of these communities that are especially important to you. On a separate sheet of paper, answer the following questions for each community. These questions will help you analyze your involvement and how you and your communities benefit.

- How do I help others in this community?
- How do others in this community help me?
- Do I get more than I give, or give more than I get, from this community?
- What about this community concerns me?
- What have I done, or can I do, to address my concerns?
- What is the extent of my commitment to this community and to its success?

## You Can Get Involved Locally and Nationally

Being an active citizen is another form of involvement. On a local level, you might take part in your community's debate over saving open space from developers. On a state level, you might contact legislators about building sound barriers along an interstate highway that runs through your town. On a national level, you might write letters to your congressional representative to urge support of an environmental, energy, or patients' rights bill. Work for political candidates who adopt the views you support, and consider running for office yourself—in your district, city, or state, or nationally.

Most important, vote in every election. Your votes and your actions can make a difference, and getting involved will bring you the power and satisfaction of being a responsible citizen. Having the right to vote places you in a privileged minority among people around the world who have no voice in how they live. In the booklet "Everything You Wanted to Know About Registering to Vote and Voting in the United States," Caty Borum writes,

For some young people, a feeling of being disconnected from government, or that "politicians don't listen to me" is the reason they say they don't vote. But elected officials must be responsive to their constituents, so your vote is actually your way of telling leaders what you care about. There may be many reasons people give for not taking advantage of the right to vote, but it's never too late to actually jump into the game, rather than sitting it out on the sidelines. There are too many issues that affect young people—such as education, jobs, health care, crime and violence—to sit it out on Election Day.

Here's the bottom line: If you don't vote, someone else is deciding your future for you. It's that simple. If you have an opinion about the cost of college tuition, jobs, the economy, or tons of other laws and issues that affect you, then you're already involved. Now take advantage of your right to determine your future. What are you waiting for?[7]

## You Can Help Preserve Your Environment

Your environment is your home. When you help to maintain a clean, safe, and healthy place to live, your actions have an impact not only on your immediate surroundings but also on others around you and on the future of the planet. Recycle and reuse: cut down on purchase of new water bottles and bags by reusing and recycling! Take responsibility for what you can control—your own habits—and develop sound practices that contribute to the health of the environment. And don't forget to do what you can to control global warming, the biggest threat to the environment and to health. Nurses are concerned and taking action. For more information on climate change and health go to the World Health Organization website: http://www.who.int/globalchange/climate/en/.

### Recycle Anything That You Can

Many communities have some kind of recycling program. If you live on campus, your college may have its own recycling program set up. What you can recycle—plastics, aluminum, glass, newspapers, magazines, other scrap paper—depends on how extensive the program is. Products that use recycled materials are often more expensive, but if they are within your price range, try to reward the company's dedication by purchasing them.

### Respect the Outdoors

Use products that reduce chemical waste. Pick up after yourself. Through volunteering, voicing your opinion, or making monetary donations, support the maintenance of parks and the preservation of natural, undeveloped land. Be creative: One young woman planned a cleanup of a local lakeside area as the main group activity for the guests at her birthday party (she joined them, of course). Everyone benefits when each person takes responsibility for maintaining the fragile earth.

### Drive Less, Take the Bus, Ride a Bike, or Walk More

Whatever you can do to reduce the use of fossil fuels like gasoline will help. Also, think about all the things you buy: Where did they come from? It takes a great deal of fuel to get that red pepper you are eating in the middle of winter from Mexico to the United States.

Remember that valuing yourself is the base for valuing all other things. Improving the earth is possible when you value yourself and think you deserve the best living environment possible. Part of valuing yourself is doing whatever you can to create the life you want to live. Activating your successful intelligence and developing your personal mission are two ways to guide yourself to that life.

## How Can You Continue to Activate Your *Successful Intelligence?*

Throughout this text you have connected analytical, creative, and practical thinking to academic and life skills. You have put them together to solve problems and make decisions. You have seen how these skills, used consistently and balanced, can help you succeed.

As you complete your work in the course, know that you are only just beginning your career as a successfully intelligent learner. You will continue to discover the best ways to use your analytical, creative, and practical thinking skills to achieve goals that are meaningful to you.

Robert Sternberg has found that successfully intelligent people, despite differences in thinking and in personal goals, have several particular characteristics in common. He calls them "self-activators"—things that get you moving and keep you going. According to Sternberg, successfully intelligent people:[8]

1. *Motivate themselves.* They make things happen, spurred on by a desire to succeed and a love of what they are doing.

2. *Learn to control their impulses.* Instead of going with their first quick response, they sit with a question or problem. They allow time for thinking and let ideas surface before making a decision.

3. *Know when to persevere.* When it makes sense, they push past frustration and stay on course, confident that success is in their sights. They also are able to see when they've hit a dead end—and, in those cases, to stop pushing.

4. *Know how to make the most of their abilities.* They understand what they do well and capitalize on it in school and in work.

5. *Translate thought into action.* Not only do they have good ideas; they are able to turn those ideas into practical actions that bring ideas to fruition.

6. *Have a product orientation.* They want results; they focus on what they are aiming for rather than on how they are getting there.

7. *Complete tasks and follow through.* With determination, they finish what they start. They also follow through to make sure all the loose ends are tied and the goal has been achieved.

8. *Are initiators.* They commit to people, projects, and ideas. They make things happen rather than sitting back and waiting for things to happen to them.

# Explore Your Personal Mission

*get practical!!*

*Work toward a concrete description of your most important life goals.*

As a way of exploring what you most want out of life, consider one or more of the following questions, which ask you to look back at the life you imagine you will have. Freewrite some answers on a separate piece of paper.

1. You are at your retirement dinner. You have had an esteemed career in whatever you ended up doing in your life. Your best friend stands up and talks about the five aspects of your character that have taken you to the top. What do you think they are?

2. You are preparing for a late-in-life job change. Updating your résumé, you need to list your contributions and achievements. What would you like them to be?

3. You have been told that you have one year to live. Talking with your family, you reminisce about the values that have been central to you in your life. Based on that discussion, how do you decide you want to spend your time in this last year? How will your choices reflect what is most important to you?

Thinking about your answers, draft a personal mission statement here, up to a few sentences long, that reflects what you want to achieve in life. Focus on the practical—on what you want to do and the effects you want to have on the world.

9. *Are not afraid to risk failure.* Because they take risks and sometimes fail, they often enjoy greater success and build their intellectual capacity. Like everyone, they make mistakes—but tend not to make the same mistake twice.

10. *Don't procrastinate.* They are aware of the negative effects of putting things off, and they avoid them. They create schedules that allow them to accomplish what's important on time.

11. *Accept fair blame.* They strike a balance between never accepting blame and taking the blame for everything. If something is their fault, they accept the responsibility and don't make excuses.

12. *Reject self-pity.* When something goes wrong, they find a way to solve the problem. They don't get caught in the energy drain of feeling sorry for themselves.

13. *Are independent.* They can work on their own and think for themselves. They take responsibility for their own schedule and tasks.

14. *Seek to surmount personal difficulties.* They keep things in perspective, looking for ways to remedy personal problems and separate them from their professional lives.

15. *Focus and concentrate to achieve their goals.* They create an environment in which they can best avoid distraction and they focus steadily on their work.

16. *Spread themselves neither too thin nor too thick.* They strike a balance between doing too many things, which results in little progress on any of them, and too few things, which can reduce the level of accomplishment.

17. *Have the ability to delay gratification.* While they enjoy the smaller rewards that require less energy, they focus the bulk of their work on the goals that take more time but promise the most gratification.

18. *Have the ability to see the forest and the trees.* They are able to see the big picture and to avoid getting bogged down in tiny details.

19. *Have a reasonable level of self-confidence and a belief in their ability to accomplish their goals.* They believe in themselves enough to get through the tough times while avoiding the kind of overconfidence that stalls learning and growth.

20. *Balance analytical, creative, and practical thinking.* They sense what to use and when to use it. When problems arise, they combine all three skills to arrive at solutions.

Make these characteristics your personal motivational tools. Return to them when you need reactivation. Use them to make sure you move ahead toward the goals that mean most to you.

## How Can You *Create and Live* Your Personal Mission?

If the trees are your goals, the forest is the big picture of what you are aiming for in life—your personal mission. To define your mission, craft a *personal mission statement*.

Dr. Stephen Covey, author of *The Seven Habits of Highly Effective People*, defines a mission statement as a philosophy outlining what you want to be (character), what you want to do (contributions and achievements), and the principles by which you live (your values). He describes the statement as "a personal constitution, the basis for making major, life-directing decisions."[9]

Here is a mission statement written by Carol Carter, one of the authors of *Keys to Success*:

My mission is to use my talents and abilities to help people of all ages, stages, backgrounds, and economic levels achieve their human potential through fully developing their minds and their talents. I aim to create opportunities for others through work, service, and family. I also aim to balance work with people in my life, understanding that my family and friends are a priority above all else.

How can you start formulating a mission statement? Try using Covey's three aspects of personal mission as a guide. Think through the following:

- **Character.** What aspects of character do you think are most valuable? When you consider the people you admire most, which of their qualities stand out?

- **Contributions and achievements.** What do you want to accomplish in your life? Where do you want to make a difference?
- **Values.** How do the values you established in your work in Chapter 2 inform your life goals? What in your mission could help you live according to what you value most highly? For example, if you value community involvement, your mission may reflect a life goal of holding elected office, which may translate into an interim goal of running for class office at college.

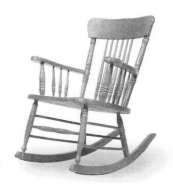

Because what you want out of life changes as you move from one phase to the next—from single person to spouse, from student to working citizen—your personal mission should remain flexible and open to revision. If you frame your mission statement carefully so it truly reflects your goals, it can be your guide in everything you do, helping you to live with integrity and to work to achieve your personal best.

## Live with Integrity

Having integrity puts your **ethics** into day-to-day action. When you act with integrity, you earn trust and respect from others. If people can trust you to be honest, to be sincere in what you say and do, and to consider the needs of others, they will be more likely to encourage you, support your goals, and reward your work.

ETHICS
A system of moral values; a sense of what is right to do.

Living with integrity helps you believe in yourself and in your ability to make good choices. A person of integrity isn't a perfect person but is one who makes the effort to live according to values and principles, continually striving to learn from mistakes and to improve. Take responsibility for making the right moves, and you will follow your mission with strength and conviction.

## Aim for Your Personal Best

Your personal best is simply the best that you can do, in any situation. It may not be the best you have ever done. It may include mistakes, for nothing significant is ever accomplished without making mistakes and taking risks. It may shift from situation to situation. As long as you aim to do your best, though, you are inviting growth and success.

And life is what we make it, always has been, always will be.

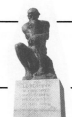

GRANDMA MOSES

Aim for your personal best in everything you do. As a lifelong learner, you will always have a new direction in which to grow and a new challenge to face. Seek constant improvement in your personal, educational, and professional life. Dream big, knowing that incredible things are possible for you if you think positively and act with successful intelligence. Enjoy the richness of life by living each day to the fullest, developing your talents and potential into the achievement of your most valued goals.

# PERSONAL TRIUMPH CASE STUDY

JOE A. MARTIN JR.

Professor of Communications, University of West Florida, Tallahassee

*Growing up around people who've been hampered by difficulties can inspire a person to make different choices. Joe Martin made the effort to achieve as a student, but that wasn't enough for him. His main focus now is his life mission to use his abilities to help and inspire others.*

I grew up in the housing projects of Miami, Florida. My mother didn't finish high school, and no one in my family even considered going to college, including me. My low GPA and SAT scores seemed to indicate I wasn't "college material."

While I was in high school, six of my friends died as a result of crime, drugs, or murder. At least 12 people I knew were in prison, five from my own family. I made a vow that if I survived the projects, I would do something constructive with my life and give something back to the community. I initially wanted to join the military, but after the recruiter told me I wasn't smart enough to go to college, I decided to prove him wrong.

I enrolled in college and, given my academic background, was shocked by my success. I ended up graduating at the top of my class, with a bachelor's degree in public relations, and was voted "Student of the Year" among 10,000 students. Competing against more than 400 other candidates, I landed a job right out of college working for the federal government. Within a year, I was able to move my mother out of the projects and afford almost anything I wanted. Life was great, but I didn't like my job and the person I was becoming.

Around that time, I heard a motivational speaker talk about the need for young professionals to give back to the community. I suddenly realized that I hadn't kept my vow. I was indulging myself, but I didn't have any passion or purpose for what I was doing with my life.

After his presentation, I asked the speaker for advice. I jotted down his suggestions on a napkin and began to implement his ideas. I discovered that I could make money doing what I do best—talking. I became a motivational speaker for students and found that my true passion was teaching. Through teaching, whether on stage or in the classroom, I discovered that I could make a difference in the lives of students who were growing up in poverty as I had.

I've given over 300 presentations and spoken to more than a quarter of a million people about student success. I've written books, recorded audio- and videotapes of my programs, and have my own television show. However, my biggest accomplishment so far has been the creation of a website called "Real World University." With the website, I'm now able to reach more than 100,000 students a month in 26 different countries.

I believe the reason many students fail is because they have no clue about their gifts and talents or about how they can use those gifts and talents to serve others. Many people are on what I call the "Treadmill Trench" of life—motivated to stay busy, but too scared to live their dreams.

My main question to students is: "If you knew you couldn't fail, what would you attempt to do professionally?" The answer to this question can help anyone find their purpose and passion in life. I also stress to students the importance of meeting a model of success—not someone you'll probably never meet, like Michael Jordan, but someone who is doing what you love to do. Then spend time with that person to find out how they did it. Once students have a clear vision of what they want to become, they're destined to succeed.

*Kaizen* is the Japanese word for "continual improvement." Striving for excellence, finding ways to improve on what already exists, and believing that you can effect change are at the heart of the industrious Japanese spirit. The drive to improve who you are and what do you provides the foundation of a successful future.

Think of this concept as you reflect on yourself, your goals, your life-long education, your career, and your personal pursuits. Create excellence and quality by continually asking yourself, "How can I improve?" Living by *kaizen* helps you to be a respected friend and family member, a productive and valued employee, and a truly contributing member of society. You can change the world.

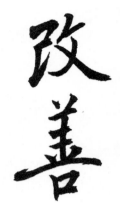

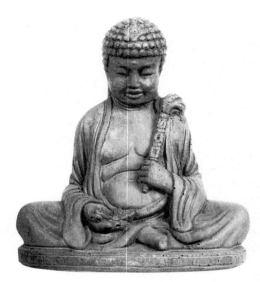

## Create Your Future

# DEVELOPING SUCCESSFUL INTELLIGENCE ——————

### *Putting It All Together*

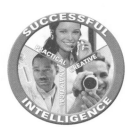

**Questions in Nursing.** Here's a way to put together what you've learned. Read the following article from *The American Nurse* (reprinted with permission from *The American Nurse*, Nov./Dec. 1999, p. 10), divide into small groups and then discuss and answer the questions that follow.

Lying for Care

A significant percentage of physicians participating in a nationwide survey indicated they'd be willing to use deception to obtain insurance coverage in certain cases, particularly when the severity of the patient's condition warrants such an approach.

In the survey, physicians were given six clinical vignettes and asked if they'd agree with a colleague's decision to deceive a third-party payer by providing inaccurate documentation to get a procedure done that otherwise would not be covered. In each scenario, the patient would be unable to pay for the treatment on her own.

In one scenario, a 55-year-old woman, homebound with occasional severe angina, wants a coronary bypass. Recently forced to switch insurance companies, she could only have the surgery for this preexisting condition if her chest pain is progressive, which it is not. About 58 percent of the 169 internists surveyed would support altering the facts of the case to her new insurance company to secure the procedure.

In another case, 47.5 percent of the respondents would approve lying to get intravenous pain medication and nutrition for a terminally ill woman who could only receive this "comfort care" if she had "recurring vomiting" and not just severe nausea after swallowing solids or liquids.

On the other hand, only 2.5 percent would sanction lying for a patient who wanted rhinoplasty because she is "sad about feeling less attractive with each passing year" by documenting that she has a deviated septum and problems breathing.

The survey results were published in the Oct. 25 *Archives of Internal Medicine* and released at a recent American Medical Association conference.

An earlier survey by the Kaiser Family Foundation also reported that many doctors—and nurses—say they have exaggerated a patient's condition to get coverage for them.

1. What ethical questions are raised?

_____

_____

_____

2. What legal questions are raised?

_____

_____

_____

3. What economic questions are raised?

_____

_____

_____

4. What is your personal reaction?

_____

_____

_____

5. As a person of science, what is your reaction? Is it different from your personal reaction and, if so, in what ways?

_____

_____

_____

# TEAM BUILDING

## *Collaborative Solutions*

As a group, read the following nursing research situation from *Reflections*. Then divide into your groups again and discuss the questions. (Reprinted with permission from *Reflections on Nursing Leadership*, Fourth Qtr. 1999, Vol. 25, No. 4, pp. 20–21, 45.)

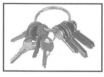

## The Pain

*by Susan Beck*

SALT LAKE CITY, August 1999—The suffering that results from cancer pain is unnecessary. In fact, according to the World Health Organization, implementation of existing knowledge of pain and symptoms can achieve critical improvements in the quality of life for cancer patients and their families (WHO, 1996). The Agency for Health Care Policy and Research (a United States government body) rigorously reviewed existing knowledge related to pain management resulting in the 1994 publication of an evidence-based *Clinical Practice Guideline on Management of Cancer Pain* (Jacox et al., 1994). The translation of this knowledge into practice is slow.

Inadequate treatment of pain is recognized as an international health problem. However, certain groups may be at higher risk. Studies in the United States indicate that minority patients and the elderly are less likely to receive adequate pain treatment. In my own research in South Africa, nonwhites had significantly higher pain levels than whites. From a health policy perspective, countries that still do not allow the manufacture or importation of opioids lack the basic tools to provide analgesia.

Studies of cancer pain prevalence indicate that approximately 30 to 50 percent of patients receiving cancer treatment experience pain. The prevalence may approach 70 to 90 percent in patients with advanced cancer.

In patients with breast cancer, two types of pain predominate (Miaskowski & Dibble, 1995). Many women suffer from a neuropathic pain syndrome following surgery for breast cancer. This type of pain is neuropathic in origin; the patient describes it as a tight, constrictive burning pain in the anterior axilla or anterior chest wall. The other common type of pain is due to metastasis to the bones. This type of pain is usually localized and is described as dull and achy. One patient aptly described it as a "tooth-ache in my bones."

This type of pain is also common in men with prostate cancer, as bone is the most common site of metastasis. Growth of prostate tumors within the pelvis can also cause pain in the back, pelvis, and lower extremities (Payne, 1993).

For persons with cancer and their family-caregivers, pain can be overwhelming as it negatively influences the quality of lives. Pain may cause or enhance the intensity of other distressing physical symptoms, such as sleep disturbances and fatigue. Pain limits an individual's ability to carry out responsibilities at home, work, and in the community. Pain causes emotional distress and has been associated with changes in mood states, including depression, anxiety and anger. Some patients may choose discontinuation of treatment, or even consider assisted suicide, because of unrelieved pain.

Individuals caring for patients in pain describe feelings of helplessness, frustration, isolation, futility and anger. As one caregiver explains, "It's just difficult . . . you're helpless. You have to watch somebody agonize, and you can't help them" (Ferrell et al., 1993).

Therapies for pain must be integrated into the overall management of the patient. If possible, the first approach to pain management is to eliminate the cause. Thus, treatments such as radiation therapy, chemotherapy, hormonal agents, biological response modifiers and surgery may be useful, depending on the type of cancer.

The mainstay of cancer pain relief is pharmacologic management. A simple method to guide pharmacological management has been developed by the World Health Organization. Three steps are summarized:

## WHO Analgesic Ladder

*Step 1.* Use non-opioid analgesics, including acetaminophen (paracetamol) and aspirin for mild pain.

*Step 2.* When pain persists or increases, add a mild opioid conventionally used orally for mild to moderate pain, including codeine.

*Step 3.* When pain is persistent, or moderate to severe at the outset, use adequate doses of a strong opioid, including morphine.

To calm fears and anxiety, additional drugs should be used. To maintain freedom from pain, drugs should be given "by the clock," that is every 3–6 hours, rather than "on demand." This three-step approach of administering the right drug in the right dose at the right time is inexpensive and 80–90% effective. Surgical intervention on appropriate nerves may provide further pain relief if drugs are not wholly effective.

*Author's note:* This section was updated February 10, 2007, from: http://www.who.int/cancer/palliative/painladder/en/.

### Dr. Susan Beck's Cancer Work in South Africa

Although health services in South Africa have been plagued by inequity and inadequate resources, new health policies have set a path to ensure universal access to health care, including palliative care for cancer. Dr. Beck's research has been distributed to governmental bodies.

Her 1998 and 1999 research validated the importance of cultural beliefs and practices for understanding cancer pain and how it is managed.

In several studies conducted to help alleviate suffering, Dr. Beck examined pain treatment to support South African efforts to improve care. Her findings showed management of pain varied by provider and setting, with major problems for access to care in the rural areas.

In African cultures, views about cancer are thought to prevent patients from seeking treatment, including for pain. Without a uniform concept of cancer as an entity, Africans have historically denied that cancer is a community problem. One resident explained, "Cancer is only for whites." In a study of 426 patients in multiple settings, nearly one-third of the cancer patients experienced pain of severe intensity. Thirty percent were not treated with adequate drugs, according to the WHO Analgesic Ladder.

## References

Beck, S. L. (1998). A systematic review of opioid availability and use in the Republic of South Africa. Journal of Pharmaceutical Care in Pain and Symptom Control 6(4), 5–22.

Beck, S. L. (1999). Health policy, health services, and cancer pain management in the new South Africa. Journal of Pain and Symptom Control 17(1), 16–26.

Beck, S. L. (In Press). Factors influencing cancer pain management in South Africa. Cancer Nursing.

Ferrell, B. R., Johnston Taylor, E., Sattler, G., Fowler, M., & Cheyney, B. L. (1993). Searching for the meaning of pain. Cancer Practice 1(3), 185–194.

Jacox, A., Carr, D. B., Payne, R., et al. (1994). Management of Cancer Pain: Clinical Practice Guideline (No. 9 AHCPR Publication No. 94-0592). Rockville, MD: Agency for Health Care Policy and Research, U. S. Department of Health and Human Services, Public Health Service.

Miaskowski, C., Dibble, S. L. (1995). The problem of pain in outpatients with breast cancer. Oncology Nursing Forum 22(5), 791–797.

Payne, R. (1993). Pain management in the patient with prostate cancer. Cancer 71(3) suppl. 1131–1137.

World Health Organization. (1996). WHO Expert Committee on Cancer Pain Relief and Active Supportive Care. Cancer Pain Relief: With a Guide to Opioid Availability (2nd edition). Geneva: WHO Technical Reports.

Using the article, answer the following questions:

1. Identify a problem. What research question could be used to direct research to help fill a "major gap in knowledge"?

_____

_____

2. What lab experiments could be conducted to answer your question? What lab equipment would you need?

_____

_____

3. What field studies could be conducted and what equipment would you need?

_____

_____

4. What is the logic behind doing research on pain?

_____

_____

_____

# WRITING ─────────────

## *Discovery Through Journaling*

*Record your thoughts on a separate piece of paper or in a journal.*

**Your Learning for Life.** Review the strategies for lifelong learning on pages 403 to 405. Which three do you feel you already do well? Which three do you think you need to develop further? For the three you want to develop, brainstorm ideas for how you will grow in those areas. Include your prediction for how this effort will benefit you.

# CAREER PORTFOLIO

## *Plan for Success*

*Complete the following in your electronic portfolio or on separate sheets of paper. When you have finished, read through your entire career portfolio. You have gathered information to turn to again and again on your path to a fulfilling, successful career.*

**A Wheel for Life.** In Figure 13.3 you see a blank Wheel of Life. Without looking at the first wheel from the beginning of the semester, evaluate

**FIGURE 13.3**   Use this new wheel to evaluate your progress

Rate yourself in each area of the wheel on a scale of 1 to 10, 1 being least developed (near the center of the wheel) and 10 being most developed (the outer edge of the wheel). In each area, at the level of the number you choose, draw a curved line and fill in the wedge below that line. Be honest—this is for your benefit only. Finally, look at what your wheel says about the balance in your life. If this were a real wheel, how well would it roll?

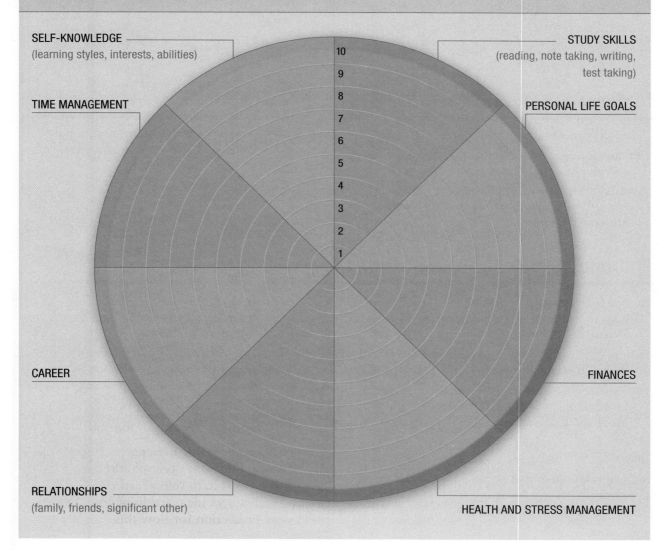

yourself as you are right now, after completing this course: Where would you rank yourself in the eight categories? After you have finished, compare this wheel with your previous wheel. Look at the changes: Where have you grown? How has your self-perception changed? Let what you learn from this new wheel inform you about what you have accomplished and what you plan for the future.

Continue to update your Wheel of Life so that it reflects your growth and development, helping to guide you through the changes that await you in the future. Add or change the categories as your college, career, and life priorities evolve.

## Suggested Readings

Blaustein, Arthur I. *Make a Difference: America's Guide to Volunteering and Community Service*. San Francisco: Jossey-Bass, 2003.

Delany, Sarah, and Elizabeth Delany with Amy Hill Hearth. *Book of Everyday Wisdom*. New York: Kodansha America, 1996.

Jones, Laurie Beth. *The Path: Creating Your Mission Statement for Work and for Life*. New York: Hyperion, 1998.

Moore, Thomas. *Care of the Soul: How to Add Depth and Meaning to Your Everyday Life*. New York: HarperCollins, 1998.

Wheatley, Margaret J., and Myron Kellner-Rogers. *A Simpler Way*. San Francisco: Berrett-Koehler, 1998.

## Internet Resources

(AmeriCorps): **www.americorps.org**

Campus Compact (site for citizenship and community service): **www.compact.org**

Hearts and Minds (clearinghouse for volunteer opportunities and civic involvement): **www. heartsandminds.org**

Queendom.com Soul Search (self-tests, personal exploration, and growth): **www.queendom.com**

## Endnotes

[1] Margaret J. Wheatley and Myron Kellner-Rogers, "A Simpler Way," *Weight Watchers Magazine* 30, no. 3 (1997): 42–44.

[2] Linton Weeks, "The No-Book Report: Skim It and Weep," *Washington Post*, May 14, 2001 p. C8.

[3] National Service Learning Clearinghouse, "Service Learning Is . . ." (2004). Retrieved May 2004, from: www.servicelearning.org/article/archive/35/.

[4] Ibid.

[5] Student essay submitted by the First Year Experience students of Patty Parma, Palo Alto College, San Antonio, Texas, January 2004.

[6] Adapted from Katherine Woodward Thomas, *Calling In the One* (New York: Three Rivers Press, 2004), pp. 298–99.

[7] Caty Borum, "Everything You Wanted to Know About Registering to Vote and Voting in the United States" (2004), Declare Yourself website. Retrieved November 2004, from: www. declareyourself.com/press/voter_guides/ voter_guide_download.pdf.

[8] List and descriptions based on Robert J. Sternberg, *Successful Intelligence* (New York: Plume, 1997), pp. 251–69.

[9] Stephen Covey, *The Seven Habits of Highly Effective People* (New York: Simon & Schuster, 1989), pp. 70–144, 309–18.

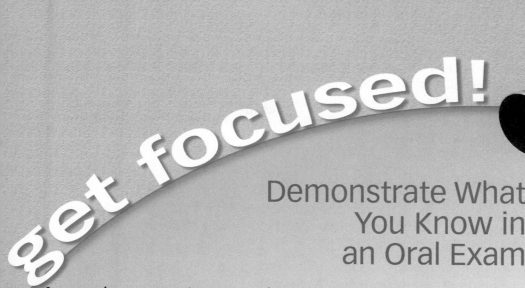

# get focused!

## Demonstrate What You Know in an Oral Exam

In an oral exam, your instructor asks you to present your responses to exam questions verbally or to discuss a preassigned topic. Exam questions may be similar to essay questions on written exams. They may be broad and general, or they may focus on a narrow topic that you are expected to explore in depth.

The material in this Study Break is designed to help you master the skills you need to perform well during an oral exam. These skills have life-long benefits. The more comfortable you are speaking in front of instructors, the more prepared you will be for any kind of public speaking situation—in school, in the community, and at work.

Keep in mind that if you have a documented learning disability that limits your ability to express yourself effectively in writing, you may need to take all your exams orally. Speak with your adviser and instructors to set up an oral exam schedule.

## Preparation Strategies

Because oral exams require that you speak logically and to the point, your instructors will often give you the exam topic in advance and may even allow you to bring your notes to the exam room. Other instructors ask you to study a specified topic and they then ask questions about the topic during the exam.

Speaking in front of others—even an audience of one, your instructor—involves developing a presentation strategy before you enter the exam room:

*Learn Your Topic.* Study for the exam until you have mastered the material. Nothing can replace subject mastery as a confidence booster.

*Plan Your Presentation.* Dive into the details. Brainstorm your topic if it is preassigned, narrow it with the prewriting strategies you learned in Chapter 8, determine your central idea or argument, and write an outline that will be the basis of your talk. If the exam uses a question-and-answer format, make a list of the most likely questions, and formulate the key points of your response.

Do, or do not. There is no "try."

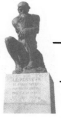

YODA (*THE EMPIRE STRIKES BACK*)

*Use Clear Thinking.* Make sure your logic is solid and your evidence supports your thesis. Work on an effective beginning and ending that focus on the exam topic.

*Draft Your Thoughts.* To get your thoughts organized for the exam, make a draft, using "trigger" words or phrases that will remind you of what you want to say.

## Practice Your Presentation

The element of performance distinguishes speaking from writing. As in any performance, practice is essential. Use the following strategies to guide your efforts:

*Know the Parameters.* How long do you have to present your topic? Where will you be speaking? Will you have access to a podium, table, chair, or whiteboard?

*Use Index Cards or Notes.* If your instructor doesn't object, bring note cards to the presentation. Keep them out of your face, however; it's tempting to hide behind them.

*Pay Attention to the Physical.* Your body positioning, voice, eye contact, and what you wear contribute to the impression you make; therefore, try to look good and sound good.

*Time Your Practice Sessions to Determine Whether You Should Add or Cut Material.* If you are given your topic in advance, make sure you can state your points in the allotted time. During the exam, make sure you don't speak too quickly.

*Try to Be Natural.* Use words you are comfortable with to express concepts you know. Be yourself as you show your knowledge and enthusiasm for the topic.

## Be Prepared for Questions

After your formal presentation, your instructor may ask you topic-related questions. Your responses and the way you handle the questions will affect your grade. Here are some strategies for answering questions effectively:

*Take the Questions Seriously.* The exam is not over until the question-and-answer period ends.

*Jot Down Keywords from the Questions.* This is especially important if the question has several parts and you intend to address one part at a time.

*Ask for Clarification.* Ask the instructor to rephrase a question you don't understand.

*Think Before You Speak.* Take a moment to organize your thoughts and to write down keywords for the points you want to cover.

*Answer Only Part of a Question If That's All You Can Do.* Emphasize what you know best and impress the instructor with your depth of knowledge. If you draw a blank, simply tell the instructor that you don't know the answer.

## Handling Your Nerves During an Exam

If you are nervous, there are things you can do to help yourself:

*Keep Your Mind on Your Presentation, Not Yourself.* Focus on what you want to say and how you want to say it.

*Take Deep Breaths Right Before You Begin, and Carry a Bottle of Water.* Deep breathing will calm you, and the water will ease a dry mouth.

*Visualize Your Own Success.* Create a powerful mental picture of yourself acing the exam. Then visualize yourself speaking with knowledge, confidence, and poise.

*Establish Eye Contact with Your Instructor and Realize That He or She Wants You to Succeed.* You'll relax when you feel that your instructor is on your side.

## Decide How Well These Techniques Work for You

Practice makes perfect, especially when it comes to public speaking. Gauge your ability to speak effectively during an oral exam with the following team exercise:

- Team up with another student to prepare for a written essay; then quiz each other as if you were taking an actual oral exam. How did your partner evaluate your presentation? What were your strengths? Your weaknesses?

- Do you think that your answers demonstrated all you know about the subject or that you could have done better in writing? If the latter, what obstacles prevented you from doing your best in your oral presentation?

- Describe three actions you will take to improve your next presentation.

    1. _____

    2. _____

    3. _____

# Index

Imbriale, William, 92
Immunizations, 343–344
Improvement, continual, 415
Income
adjusting, 382
sources of, 380–381
Information
analysis of, 141–142
clarification of, 141
evaluation of, 144–145, 277–278
gathering, 140–141
organization of, 231–232
perspectives and assumptions in, 143–144
search strategies for, 270–271
sharing of, 67
Inquiry, defined, 399–400
Instructors, 118, 261–262
Insurance coverage, 399, 415–416
Integrity, 413
Intellectual property, 283. *See also* plagiarism
Intelligence
defined, 112
emotional, 153
links to abilities, 113
and speed, 150
successful (*See* successful intelligence)
Interests, 51, 403
International Council of Nurses (ICN), 64
International nursing, 64
Internet
and academic publications, 276
defined, 275
evaluating sources on, 38, 277–278
job searches on, 376
and plagiarism, 284–285
research on, 270–271, 274, 275–278
search strategies for, 276–277
Interpretation, in listening, 212
Interview skills, 391
Introductions, of papers, 282
Involvement, local and national, 408–409

Jackson, Michael, 289
Job interviews, 377
Jobs
and school, 378–380
search plan for, 376–377
and study, 92

variety in nursing, 368
your needs from, 378–379, 392
Johnson, Crystal, 136
*Joie de vivre,* 358
Journaling
acceptance, 331
addiction, 360
choices, 167
lifelong learning, 420
memory, 238
on money, 391
observations, 73
reading challenges, 206
reflection, 39
strengths and weaknesses, 131
test anxiety, 264
time management, 105–106
writing, 294
Journals, research, 185

*Kaizen,* 415
Kanda, Lillan, 210
Katz, Janet, 86–87
Kawaide, Eiko, 4–5
*Kente,* 329
Keyword searches, 270–271, 276
Keywords, in résumés, 377
King, Martin Luther, Jr., 312
Knowledge
acquired, 84–85
application of, 119–120
building about careers, 369
cultural, 311
importance of, 262
in nursing, 55
sharing, 196
and wisdom, 129
*Kqivelv,* 163
Krauss, Kathryn, 396–397

Labeling, of groups, 308
Language barriers, 302–303, 321, 328
Leaders, effective, 197–198
Learners, lifelong, 110–111, 403–405
Learning, 70, 403–405, 406–407
Learning centers, 53–54
Learning disabilities
identification of, 125, 128
and listening, 214
management of, 128–129
and reading assignments, 181
signs of, 129

Learning styles, 110–111
in choosing a major, 121–122
in the classroom, 117–118
defined, 112
effect on careers, 373–375
and note taking, 218
and study strategies, 115
value of assessments of, 111–112
Legibility, on tests, 259
Levine, Mel, 286
Liberal arts, usefulness of, 54, 405
Librarians, help from, 273–274
Libraries
catalogues, 272
discovering your, 273
open *vs.* closed stack systems, 269
organization of, 269–270
personal, 397
search strategies for, 272
Life, Hebrew word for, 102
*Life on Earth* (Audesirk and Audesirk), 202–205
Linkages, 5
Listeners, adjusting to as a speaker, 317
Listening
active, 214–216
analysis of personal habits, 216
defined, 211–212
lapses in, 213
managing challenges to, 213–214
stages of, 212
Literacy, importance of, 206
Luck, role of, 102
Lyder, Courtney, 366–367
Lying, for care, 416–417

Mahoney, Mary Elise, 15
Main ideas, finding, 191–192
Majors
changing, 124
choosing, 118–119, 121–124
double, 123
options in, 123
Malone, Beverly L., 13
Martin, Joe A., 414
Math anxiety, 298–299
Mathematics, need for, 56, 119–120
McIntyre, Mark, 48
*Measles-mumps-rubella* (MMR) vaccine, 344
Media
defined, 195
influence of, 308

Media literacy, 195
Medical College Admission Test (MCAT), 246
Memory
  acronyms for, 234
  fragility of, 228
  long-term, 229–230
  mental walks, 233–234
  strategies for recall, 230–236
  types of, 229
  using grouping for, 232
  using songs/rhymes for, 235
  visual images for, 233
Men, in nursing, 15, 16
Meningococcal bacteria, 343
Mental health, 344–347
Mental walks, 233–234
Mentors, 5, 397
Microforms, 270
Middle, practice of, 232
Minaya, Gustavo, 328, 330
Mind maps, 224
Minority students, 313–315
*Missing Persons* (Sullivan Report), 13–14
Mission, living personal, 412–413
Mission statements, 49, 410, 412–413
Mistakes
  avoiding, 119–120
  learning from, 24, 150, 259, 261–262
  patterns in, 261
Mitchell, George, 14
Mnemonic devices, 233–235
Moidel, Steve, 182
*Mononucleosis,* 344
Montolovo, Raymond, 268
Motivation, increasing, 196, 410
Multiple intelligences
  discovering, 112–114
  and learning, 111
  in majors and careers, 125, 126–127, 373
  using, 114
Multiple Pathways to Learning, 111–113
Myers-Briggs Type Inventory (MBTI), 111, 115
*Myth of Laziness, The* (Levine), 286

National Association of Hispanic Nurses (NAHN), 19–20
National Black Nurses Association (NBNA), 18

National Center for Learning Disabilities (NCLD), 128
Native Alaska/Native American Indian Nurses Association (NANAINA), 20–21
Needs, time-related, 90
Nervousness, handling, 425
Networking, 375–376
Nightingale, Florence, 6, 37
Nonverbal cues, 319–320
Note taking
  during class discussions, 220
  Cornell system, 223–224, 225
  effective, 218–220
  hierarchy charts, 226
  and learning, 216–217
  preparation for, 217–218
  systems for, 222–226
  teams for, 237–238
  think links, 224, 226
  while reading, 188–189
Notes
  content, 280
  guided, 223
  legibility of, 228
  outline form for, 222–223
  in research, 280
  review of, 220, 245–246
  revision of, 221–222
  source, 280, 283–284
  summarizing, 221
Nurse anesthetists (CRNAs), 61, 62, 63
Nurse practitioners (NPs), 61–63
Nurse Reinvestment Act, 52
Nurses
  African American, 15, 17–18
  Asian and Pacific Islander, 18–19
  average age of, 23
  diversity in, 9, 13
  Hispanic and Latino, 19–20
  international students, 21
  Native American, 20–21
  and patient outcomes, 7
  qualifications for, 6–7
  retention of, 23–24, 52
  RNs, 6, 11, 50, 68–69
  roles of, 58, 63–64
  supply of, 49–50
Nursing
  bilingual, 302–303
  career options in, 375–377
  complexity of, 398
  defined, 26, 41
  diversity in, 4, 12–21, 304–305

future of, 398–400
in health care, 10, 22–23
importance of, 4
men in, 15, 16
minorities in, 13–14
paths in, 367–368
in public health nursing, 60
reasons for, 54–55
specialty areas in, 62
statistics on, 10–11
views of, 54–55
Nursing practitioners (NPs), 62
Nursing programs, 9–10
Nursing schools, capacity of, 49, 52
Nursing shortage
  and ethics, 398
  problem of, 3, 23–24, 49–50, 68–69
  solutions to, 52–53, 54
Nutrition, 101

Obesity, avoiding, 340–341
Observation
  in inquiry, 162–163
Observation, need for, 56–57
*Occupational Outlook Handbook,* 69
Opinion *vs.* fact, 142, 143
Opportunity, Chinese character for, 29
Options, exploration of, 122–123, 159
Oral exams, 423–425
Orders, checking, 119–120
Organizations, nursing, 306
Outlines, 281
Overview, of tests, 249

"Pain, The" (Beck), 418–419
Palliative care, 367
Paragraphs, structure of, 287
Paraphrases, 284
Parish nursing, 65, 396
Participants, effective, 197
Passivity, in communication, 322–323
Patient load, 211
Patient outcomes, 52
Patterson, Cody, 118–119
Pauk, Walter, 223
Paul, Dr. Richard, 137
PDAs (personal digital assistants), 91
Peer readers, 286, 288
Perception puzzles, 149